Dying to Please

SECOND EDITION

Dying to Please

*Anorexia, Treatment
and Recovery*

SECOND EDITION

AVIS RUMNEY

McFarland & Company, Inc., Publishers

Jefferson, North Carolina, and London

LIBRARY OF CONGRESS CATALOGUING-IN-PUBLICATION DATA

Rumney, Avis.
Dying to please : anorexia, treatment and recovery / Avis Rumney —
2d ed.
p.   cm.
Includes bibliographical references and index.

ISBN 978-0-7864-4378-9
softcover : 50# alkaline paper ∞

1. Anorexia nervosa.   2. Anorexia nervosa — Treatment.   I. Title.
RC552.A5R85   2009   362.196'85262 — dc22   2009010506

British Library cataloguing data are available

Cover photograph ©2009 Shutterstock

Manufactured in the United States of America

*McFarland & Company, Inc., Publishers
Box 611, Jefferson, North Carolina 28640
www.mcfarlandpub.com*

Acknowledgments

I am grateful to my parents, Philip and Charlotte Wadsworth, for encouraging me to seek treatment in 1978, for their support during my early years in therapy, and for the love and concern they bestowed on me to the end of their lives. I am thankful to the staff and clients at Cathexis Institute who contributed to my early recovery. I feel blessed and helped immeasurably by my twin brother, Adrian Wadsworth, and the friends, colleagues and therapists who have contributed to my journey in the 25 years since the original edition of this book was published. The richness of my life I attribute to the many unique and wonderful people with whom I have had, and continue to have, a treasured connection. I am grateful to my editor, Frances Lefkowitz, without whose help and encouragement this book would still be a sheaf of papers collecting dust on a shelf. And I give special thanks to my life partner, Larry Fritzlan, for his presence as an unfolding gift in my life.

Table of Contents

Preface to the Second Edition

Much has changed in the 25 years since I wrote the original text of *Dying to Please*— in the world, in our culture, in technology, and in our understanding of eating disorders. A revised edition seemed warranted — indeed, overdue — because of the evolution of thinking about eating disorders and the proliferation of new options and resources for treatment.

In addition, my own perspective on anorexia nervosa, both professionally and personally, has evolved. I wanted to share what I have learned from my colleagues and clients about recovery from anorexia in the past two and a half decades. I also wanted to bring current my own personal journey of healing and recovery, which has entailed deeper levels of inner work than I could possibly have envisioned at my first writing. While the text of the original volume remains valid, it is incomplete. My intention in this edition is to summarize some more recent treatment directions, provide an updated Directory of Organizations, and expand on my personal story of recovery.

Sadly, eating disorders are more prevalent in the United States than they were 25 years ago. Girls of younger and younger ages have become weight-obsessed. Fat-phobic fourth graders now diet and pre-pubescent girls are primed to critique their bodies. The incidence of anorexia, bulimia and binge eating continues to increase, with estimates suggesting that as many as 25 percent of Americans now suffer from some form of disordered eating. While diagnostic and treatment capacities have improved, deaths from anorexia have also increased (or are more accurately recorded).

Furthermore, childhood obesity (which does not indicate presence of an eating disorder but can result from an unhealthy lifestyle) has become a national health concern and statistics have risen dramatically for the occurrence of heart disease and diabetes— both conditions resulting in part from the freedom, which for some becomes an obsession, to choose non-nutritious food in excessive quantities. And this is happening in a country where 15 percent of the population has insufficient food. These facts suggest that something is sorely amiss regarding our values with respect to food, weight and lifestyle.

Meanwhile, technology has advanced exponentially. The Internet has propelled the world into a new era of communication and information dissemination. The sheer quantity of facts and resources available and the speed of data transmission are mind-boggling. However, this accessibility to profuse resources has a down side. Among the countless sites with guides for better living are some with equally explicit directions for perpetrating self-harm. Websites have sprung up which support anorexics in furthering their disease. Chat rooms abound where anorexics can share their secrets for stifling hunger or manipulating weight for medical weigh-ins and applaud each other's efforts at self-starvation.

Fortunately, treatment options for eating disorders have multiplied, and resources for information about eating disorders are also plentiful on the Web. Cognitive behavioral, psychodynamic, and family systems therapies have been refined and applied more consistently in the treatment of anorexia. Therapies have been developed for working physically with the trauma that sometimes contributes to an eating disorder. Recent research in brain physiology has revealed neurochemical abnormalities involved with eating disorders. And treatment is more affordable in some states today than it was even five years ago because in these states, including California, anorexia nervosa and bulimia are "parity disorders," meaning that insurance benefits for these disorders are on a par with benefits allowed for treatment of other medical conditions. Furthermore, with the passage of the federal Paul Wellstone and Pete Domenici Mental Health Parity and Addiction Equity Act of 2008, health insurance benefits for mental health and substance use disorders will equal those for medical and surgical benefits nationwide beginning January 1, 2010. While implementation of this law will doubtless be cumbersome, and there are restrictions on its application to some kinds of insurance plans, many more insured individuals with eating disorders throughout the country will be able to receive necessary treatment.

Back when I wrote the first edition of this book — on a typewriter! — I had graduated from one therapy program and I was a fledgling therapist. I had not yet built a career, experienced an intimate relationship without the defenses and confines of anorexia, repaired my relationships with my parents, or differentiated sufficiently to be able to engage with my parents as a mature adult. It was as if I had emerged from my few years of therapy believing I was emotionally complete, fully formed as a 34-year-old adult and developmentally on the level with my chronological peers. I discounted the fact that at that point I had spent over half my life as an anorexic who had been emotionally stunted and mentally compromised by anxiety, depression and malnutrition. I had no concept of the developmental hurdles I had not yet cleared or the life experience I had missed during my two decades of anorexia.

In my early recovery, I lacked both the personal growth and the professional experience to comprehend what internal constructs were missing, and I had no concept of the Self or lack of Self, or how my anorexia and my sense of Self were connected. Anorexia had been my identity, my motivation and the central organizing principle of my life for so many years that articulating the way it served me was like talking about building a house without ever having seen one. It was only as I continued to grow emotionally — to experience, identify and label a range of feelings and the thoughts and behaviors that accompanied them — that I began to realize what was missing. And only then did I begin to understand that through walling myself off from others and food from me, I had been trying to protect something inside me. I had not felt safe expressing my feelings, thoughts, wants or needs. Yet these comprised the only me I knew. Exposing my innermost being could make me a target for anger, criticism, and ultimately destruction. Self-preservation was my goal, even at the risk of self-annihilation. I understand now that the struggle for self-preservation is central to anorexia; the anorexic has no cohesive Self constructed through a healthy course of development, and zealously protects that kernel of Self that she has. In this version of the book, I incorporate more of my personal story as it has developed in my past twenty-five years as a recovering anorexic and as a practicing therapist treating anorexics and their families.

This book consists of two parts. The first part is devoted to an understanding of anorexia, its origins and its major attributes. I begin with what I now consider to be the heart of the book and the central feature of the disease of anorexia: the paradox of self-annihilation in service of self-preservation. Part One also includes an overview of the origins of anorexia, including some information about the role of brain chemistry in anorexia. During the past ten years, there has been considerable research regarding the biochemical basis of disease, but this is still very much a new science. Recent research in genetics has shown the existence of family patterns in the occurrence of anorexia. There are correlations of anorexia in the genetic family tree to anxiety and depression, as well as to the incidence of anorexia or other eating disorders. In addition, specific innate personality traits such as perfectionism and risk-aversion are common among anorexics.

However, genetic predisposition is not cause. Researchers have said that in the development of anorexia, genetics loads the gun and environment pulls the trigger. Aimee Liu, who has written about her two episodes with anorexia — one in adolescence and a relapse in mid-life — believes this actually should be rephrased: genetics *makes* the gun, and cultural and familial environment *load* the gun, but "it takes the experience of unbearable *emotion* to pull the trigger" (Liu, 2008, p.127). Anorexia has no single cause but rather develops through the interplay of several internal and external factors. In this book I include the contributions of the individual's physiological as well as psychological makeup, spiritual hunger, family dynamics, cultural milieu, and triggering events. I provide a brief discussion on the question of whether anorexia is an addiction. I also consider the topic of uses and misuses of the Internet.

Part One also summarizes some of the disorders that may accompany anorexia. Anxiety and depression occur commonly with anorexia, and other disorders can co-exist with anorexia as well. The remainder of Part One is devoted to a discussion of five attributes that I consider key aspects of anorexia: perfectionism, competition, unresolved grief, immature sexuality and relationships, and distorted body image.

Part Two of the book, Treatment and Recovery, is itself in two parts. In order to make sense of the approaches to treatment, discussion of recovery precedes description of treatment. The first chapter in Part Two, Understanding Recovery, explores the difficulty of defining "cure," the challenges in evaluating recovery, and the crux of recovery, which is the development of a coherent sense of Self. I also include in this section a description of my own path towards development of a cohesive Self. In 1983, I used the word "cure" in my title, knowing very little of what I have learned in subsequent years about eating disorders, addictions and recovery. Frankly, my understanding of psychological change was relatively rudimentary and I did not know how much I did not know. I was at a stable weight and had been for over two years; I had no desire to lose weight. Didn't that mean I was cured? I understand now how superficially I grasped the components and process of healing. Since the original edition, I have had the gift of many more years of personal therapy, including exposure to a variety of modalities, and have received training in several treatment approaches. As a psychotherapist, I have also had the privilege of working with many individuals and families at all stages of life.

Rather than an eating disorder being something one can "cure," I now think recovery is a journey towards wellness that eventually merges with the continuing growth that most human beings undergo throughout their lives. While I believe it is possible for an anorexic to achieve and maintain a stable weight and to develop a healthy relationship to her body, that is not where recovery stops. Recovery from anorexia nervosa is a complex process: an interwoven web of physical, psychological, emotional, social and spiritual components. There is never a point at which a person stops healing, whether from an eating disorder or from other life challenges, because human beings by nature continue to grow. Human beings possess an innate drive towards greater self-awareness and emotional health. Even physical recovery from anorexia is not an event but a process, because maintaining physical well-being and a healthy relationship with food and one's body requires daily attention, numerous choices and specific actions.

The second chapter of Part Two, Approaching Treatment, provides an overview of some modalities for treating anorexia. This chapter is informed by my personal recovery, my training and experience as a therapist specializing in eating disorders and my research regarding approaches to which I have had little or no personal exposure. My work as a psychotherapist with people with eating disorders and their families has evolved in the years since I opened a private practice as a California Licensed Marriage and Family Therapist in 1983. Much of my personal therapy and early training was cognitive and behavioral in orientation, meaning that it addressed unhealthy beliefs and behaviors. This work remains useful as a solid platform for treatment as well as providing some basic tools for change at all phases of life. In addition, fifteen years ago, I began to study and incorporate a psychodynamic approach to therapy with my own clients, entailing a focus on the person's inner world, her sense of self and of others. This new direction in my work paralleled the course of my personal psychotherapy

In discussing treatment, I list the components I believe are essential to successful treatment of anorexia and then highlight some treatment considerations. Some aspects of treatment are addressed, including treatment settings; psychotherapeutic, medical and nutritional considerations; and formats for psychotherapy. I discuss treatment options for the anorexic, and for her family. For the anorexic, I divide treatment into psychotherapeutic modalities and experiential therapies, followed by an overview of psychopharmacological treatment of anorexia. This information is meant to be a general sampling, not a complete list of possibilities. In therapy for the family, I have included both family therapy and therapy for family members, in particular for mothers of anorexic daughters. Since I have a particular interest in working with mothers of eating-disordered daughters, I have devoted a longer discussion to this topic than to some other aspects of treatment.

I include a chapter devoted to 12-Step programs and their role in aiding recovery from anorexia. While these programs may not appeal to everyone, they can be a powerful adjunct to addressing the addictive elements of anorexia, the anorexic's deficit in Self development and the spiritual void common to this disorder.

The last chapter addresses the topic of intervening when an adult anorexic either refuses treatment or refuses a different or higher level of care when treatment is not effective. As a certified interventionist as well as a licensed psychotherapist, I feel very strongly that families should seek assistance from a professional interventionist when a loved one is anorexic and is not receiving the assistance she needs. Appropriate help can prevent unnecessary suffering and loss of life.

Finally, I provide both a list of treatment centers for eating disorders and some resources for information and referral. These lists are by no means exhaustive, but include a range of treatment facilities that were available at this writing.

While this revised edition is designed to provide resources for addressing anorexia nervosa and to offer sufferers and their families hope for recovery, I also want to emphasize that continued education in the prevention of eating disorders is essential. There is more than ever a desperate need for an attitudinal shift in our culture with respect to food, weight and appearance. Currently, the diet industry grosses over 5 billion dollars a year, 98 percent of people who diet regain their lost weight, over 30 percent of Americans are obese and the vast majority of eating disorders begin with a diet gone awry.

Eating disorders result in a tragic waste of human potential, and although those in recovery and their families are rewarded by the journey, there is tremendous suffering and self-destruction that could be prevented. Girls and women need validation for their strengths as well as tools to accept and work with their shortcomings. If we promote food or weight manipulation as a salve for what ails, and if we extol weight as the measure of acceptance and worth in our society, we cloud and confuse self-acceptance and the search for a meaningful existence that every individual deserves.

Finally, a disclaimer: this book, even in its revised edition, is not intended as a comprehensive treatment manual for the complicated and capricious eating disorder anorexia nervosa. Rather, it is a compilation of information that I have encountered and found useful in my work as a psychotherapist with individuals suffering from anorexia and with their families, coupled with my personal experiences as an anorexic and in recovery. There is a vast array of information available today about anorexia, and this book offers one perspective among many.

In describing anorexia nervosa, I recognize that my own experience is just that: simply my personal experience of this illness. I grew up in *my* family, possessed *my* particular gene pool, and each member of *my* family similarly was formed by both genes and environment. Later, I was exposed to other life experiences and to certain kinds of therapy, which further molded me. Another individual, even with identical beginnings, would not necessarily act, respond, grow, balk at growing, make the choices or draw the conclusions I have. Another person with my heritage and life experience might not develop anorexia. I view my experience as a single case example, not as representative of all anorexics or even a majority of anorexics. What I have had reaffirmed countless times in working with hundreds of girls, boys, women and men suffering from anorexia is that each individual is unique, that each possesses a personal history and particular pain, resources and gifts, and that treatment must be tailored to the specific person and designed to foster that individual's path towards recovery.

Introduction

Anorexia nervosa is a morbid, life-threatening and emotionally crippling disorder which is distressing both for the anorexic, relentlessly driven by her (or his) obsession with thinness, and for her family and friends, helpless witnesses to her wasting disease. I use "she" and "her" in this text because there are many more female than male anorexics, not because the disorder is any less insidious, painful or debilitating in sufferers of either gender.

The anorexic is impelled by an unquenchable need to please others because her sense of self-worth is dependent on others' approval. At the same time, she hides the parts of herself she fears will be rejected. And so the anorexic is caught in a battle she can never win. She seeks love, but feels irrevocably unlovable, and no amount of external attention can eradicate her self-loathing. She starves herself to acquire love and approbation, but it is an endless quest. No matter how thin the anorexic becomes, she is never thin enough. She is driven by the belief that if only she were thinner — better, smarter, more talented — she would be loved. Then and only then can she acquire this elusive quality of lovability. Extreme emaciation, physical debilitation and ultimately death can result from the anorexic's pursuit.

But those suffering from anorexia can be treated, and it is my intention that this book will provide hope and direction to anorexics and their families and friends, as well as offer insight to therapists, professionals and other interested individuals. Intervention and treatment can arrest the tragic course of this disorder. Families and loved ones suffer as well, and can unwittingly enable an anorexic's illness. They, too, can be helped.

I come to this writing from the perspective of a sufferer, a patient and a therapist. I became anorexic at age 11 and suffered from the disorder for 19 years. I didn't receive effective treatment until many years after I had left home. It was not that my parents wouldn't get help for me had they known how troubled I was, but that I disguised my problems to keep my family at bay. I could not reveal my confusion and despair. I felt ashamed of my bad feelings and feared the disappointment with which I was convinced my parents would greet disclosure of my angst. In my twenties, I was depressed and pursued psychotherapy for a couple of years but abandoned it when I didn't feel helped. I discovered antidepressant medication, which kept me functioning for some time, albeit depressed and malnourished. At the age of 30, weighing 68 pounds, I embarked on two years of therapy at Cathexis Institute, a transactional analysis-oriented outpatient treatment program in Oakland, California, that closed its doors in 1990. After Cathexis — and the 1983 edition of this book — I continued in therapy as I embarked on my own career as a psychotherapist specializing in the treatment of eating disorders. This book includes a personal account of some parts of my life as an anorexic and of my path towards recovery.

PART ONE

Anorexia

1

The Paradox of Self-Annihilation in Service of Self-Preservation

In so many ways anorexia is a perplexing phenomenon. An attractive, intelligent and talented young woman deems her body despicable and her essence contemptible and resolves to lose weight. Dieting, she is certain, is the antidote to her angst. She exerts control over her body, denies her hunger and exercises away mythical body fat, believing that weight loss is the magic key to lovability. She maps her own journey, starving herself to get thinner — although she can never get thin enough — until physiology and psychology render her victim to the very quest she undertook. The pain she tried to quell is supplanted by the terror of getting fat. No longer can she *choose* not to eat; her fear *prevents* her from eating, and death can be the consequence.

What indomitable force could compel a bright and healthy person to ignore cues so salient as prolonged hunger, shivers at the slightest breeze, lightheadedness and perpetual fatigue? What threat could drive someone to choose the pain of starvation? Why would someone subject herself to the extreme asceticism and fierce deprivation of anorexia?

Only someone in grave danger would submit to such masochism. And, to the anorexic, this danger is imminent. The anorexic believes that she is at risk of losing her Self — that sacred kernel of being that she can identify as inviolately her own. She believes her very existence is in jeopardy. It is to preserve whatever shred of personhood she possesses — even a vacuous hole of next-to-nothingness which is the only Self she knows — that she will starve and suffer. It hardly matters whether intrusion by another has provoked her stance, or if she innately knows that her own exquisite psyche could not bear invasion, or whether some unchoreographed interplay of inner and outer elements has rendered this her only safe place. What is clear is that her very life — the life that she, in fact, may lose in the battle to preserve her Self — depends on maintaining a vice-like grip on her world and warding off all threats to her borders. Food, hunger, her body and her body's needs are all alien to her.

The enemy wears many guises. It can be another's words; some skill others possess that she wishes she could learn; a comfort that belies her ascetic ways; nurturing, pleasure or play in any form; or basic sustenance. Any of these elements, if allowed in, could undermine her tenacious control, mar her essence and erode the Self she so fervently holds as her own. Her defenses are constituted in her physical body, keeping her inner being sacred, untouched, untouchable. Her armor is intact. Her walls are impenetrable; her resolve endures despite her wasting body.

However, there is a point in anorexia when physiology preempts will. This is true in any addiction, and the hallmarks of addiction — loss of control, chronicity (it persists indefinitely if untreated), continuation of behavior despite adverse consequences, progressive nature of the disease — characterize anorexia with the same accuracy they do drug or alcohol dependence. For the anorexic, when starvation has depleted her neurotransmitters, distorted her brain function, and disrupted functioning of cells, hormones and organs, the choice to eat — or not eat — is no

11

longer under her control. The messages from her starving brain — self-punitive thoughts, acute anxiety and terror — override her volition. The fierce control she once exhibited is no longer hers to flaunt; her physiology and psyche now rule. Her body, both victim and vanquisher, has rendered the anorexic's will impotent. Sadly, the danger she perceived is no longer the biggest threat. Instead, the possibility of death — which she denies — is the real danger. At this point even she cannot access that vestige of Self she fought so valiantly to preserve.

Starvation is not so much a quest for thinness as an expression of a fervent desire to be invisible. Being invisible is the ultimate protection: If I can't be seen, then I can't be hurt. Of course, mental, psychological and emotional processes are not visible to begin with, although facial expressions and body language communicate volumes without intention. But being invisible seems like the solution to avoiding relationships with others, to managing the expectations of the people around her and to dispensing with her intrinsic need to comply. She has found a place to hide — from pain and emptiness, from life, from rejection.

In her quest to shrink from starvation, the typical anorexic disengages from her body and ignores physical cues. She conceives of her body as an "it" in which she is held captive; she chips away at her physical being as if scratching a hole in a prison wall. She has become so accustomed to denying her hunger and controlling her body size that she has little sense of her body as a source of pleasure or a font of feelings which express who she is. In general, not only is she out of touch with her emotions, but also she is confused about the physical and emotional sensations that she does feel. Much of her inner world is comprised not of awareness of herself as a person, but of competitive and self-critical thoughts. Instead of her body being the vehicle of her aliveness, it is the enemy she seeks to eradicate.

As the anorexic strives to disappear, her sense of herself becomes narrow and constrained. Besides being acutely sensitive to the size of her body and its every fractional part, she experiences her body as an unwieldy gaggle of appendages surrealistically strung together. Her mind is an endless stream of obsessions, disconnected from her physical being and from the real world around her. She does not have a coherent sense of who she is, an established concept of the different dimensions of her being. She has successfully walled off her body and deadened her emotions. In so doing, she has unknowingly robbed herself of the possibility of feeling whole. But she has succeeded at her goal: to cloister and preserve that secret seed of Self she can own as hers.

What *is* the Self the anorexic strives so desperately to hide? It is her real emotions, not the feelings she deems safe enough to express; her true passions, not the pursuits she has been encouraged to develop; her own thoughts, not the beliefs she's been obliged to adopt; her innate personality, not the ever-pleasant and polite shell she exhibits. She sequesters her "True Self" for fear exposure will mean invasion, usurpation and annihilation. Her salvation lies in a "False Self," a mask of placid compliance, strict defiance, rigid self-control and endless self-deprivation.

The Self of the anorexic is but a fragment of the multi-dimensional, emotionally fluent and coherent structure that comprises the Self of the developmentally mature individual. However, it is all she knows and has; she has no way to comprehend what she is missing. Her emotional growth has been curtailed, and her sense of herself is constricted and left incomplete.

The True Self, the structure the anorexic has not had the opportunity to develop, is more complex. Rosenberg, Rand and Asay, founders of Integrative Body Therapy and authors of *Body, Self and Soul: Sustaining Integration*, define this Self as "a non-verbal sense of well-being, continuity, and identity in the body, plus the verbal structure and cognitive process one learns" (Rosenberg et al., 1991, p.96). In other words, the sense of Self is the aliveness in the body, the flow of energy. It is the permanent core of being into which a healthy person can retreat for comfort and self-support. "The sense of Self provides a continuity of internal identity. When it is intact, a person knows who he truly is, independent of the rest of the world" (Rosenberg et al., 1991, p.142).

In some other therapies, the Self is conceptualized as a structure of the mind rather than of the body. But the mind is really a construct of the brain, and the brain of course is solidly housed in the body. Emotions are sensations experienced in the body, although it is the mind that gives them meaning. So even though some therapies do not speak specifically about the contribution of the body to the sense of Self, the body is the *sine qua non* for the mind, and hence for the Self, to exist.

The Self is constructed from the myriad emotional and physiological experiences of a child's growing up, especially from earliest infancy through the first several years. It is in the relationship between the infant and her primary caretaker (generally her mother) that the Self begins to develop. That initial mother-child (or caretaker-child) connection becomes a template for the child's future relationships with others, and the foundation of her inner world. The Self develops slowly, first through bonding with the mother, then through appropriate mirroring of her emotions and behavior by her mother. Gradually the crawling infant begins to experiment with first moving away and then back towards her mother and can progress towards separateness.

Nuances in the early interaction between mother and child affect the kind of attachment that the child develops. A healthy attachment requires an attunement between mother and child that results in the child feeling safe and loved. Disruptions in this attachment process portend difficulties in the child's relationships later in life. This is a matter of fact, not fault. The capacity for a healthy attachment gets passed down from one generation to the next. When the child who lacks a solid attachment becomes a parent to the next generation, she often unconsciously repeats her own parent's attachment style. Unless in the interim she has undergone some transformative growth, she can provide as a mother only what she experienced as a child.

Appropriate mirroring, which is an aspect of the attachment process, is essential for the child to develop a healthy narcissism, an internal sense of himself as an acceptable being (Rosenberg et al., 1991, pp.163–164). Mirroring is the process of reflecting another's emotions; it conveys acknowledgement and acceptance of the other person. With insufficient or inappropriate mirroring, the Self develops barricades for protection, and eventually these barricades become defensive character styles. Character styles are an overlay on the Self, and while protective in function, they impede Self-development. The ego, or personality with which one functions in the outside world, can develop despite injuries to the Self. The ego masks developmental injuries. However, the individual with the injured and unhealed Self will experience deficits in her sense of continuity and well-being.

Lack of appropriate mirroring and a thwarted attachment process can render an individual prone to developing various disorders, among them anorexia. Compulsive behaviors emerge to protect against the pain of unmet needs (Rosenberg et al., 1991, p.70). While the child is growing up, the parents may supply sufficient stability that some of these compensatory behaviors do not appear. Eventually, however, the future anorexic emerges into extra-familial relationships and a complex world with a Self that is unintegrated and shored up with corresponding character defenses. Her compliant behavior, competitiveness and striving for perfection are parts of her defense. Food restriction and weight manipulation provide more mortar for the walls that shield the parts of her she fears will be rejected. What she shows to the world is a façade that hides what she does not want to be seen or judged — this is her "False Self" that belies her real identity.

As Deborah Luepnitz points out in *Schopenhauer's Porcupines: Intimacy and Its Dilemma* (2002, p.109), the person who forges the hyper-compliant, caretaker façade of a False Self does so for good psychological reasons based on experiences in childhood. If parents are depressed or abusive, or unavailable for any number of reasons such as overwork, illness, or their own emotional stress, children learn that it is not safe to ask for attention. Survival for these children depends on tracking the adults' moods and responding accordingly. The child gives up on having a spontaneous, desiring self in order to act as the parent to his or her parents. Luepnitz cites D.W. Winnicott, a renowned British psychoanalyst and expert in parent-child relationships, who says that "in these situations the child's 'true self' goes into cold storage and a false, 'caretaker self' takes over" (Luepnitz, 2002, p.109).

Perfect parenting, impeccable attunement to a child's needs, and mothering with never a lapse in nurturance do not exist. But even with mothering sufficient to qualify as "good-enough" .in Winnicott's terminology, most of us do not emerge from childhood unscathed. However, it is not so much whether one has injuries and hence has developed compensatory character styles, but to what degree those injuries have influenced the person, how deeply entrenched are the character styles, and to what extent they impede a person's emotional and interpersonal development. In many cases, the future anorexic's genetics may have bestowed on her deficiencies in dopamine production and serotonin metabolism. The wounded future anorexic, already compensating for innate neurophysiological deficits, then constructs a rigid and impermeable barrier against the injuries of her parents' unavailability, intrusion, or unpredictability, which are the legacy of their inconsistent mirroring.

However, even with attentive parenting, there is the problem of receptivity of the infant or child. Innately, some children are more sensitive and others more stalwart; those who are constitutionally more sensitive will be more distressed by lesser infractions in attention on the part of a parent or caretaker. Generally the child who later becomes anorexic is inclined to be highly sensitive, distressed easily by change and deficient in emotional resilience.

Typically, the anorexic creates a façade which over time becomes ever more impenetrable. The common hallmarks of anorexia — perfectionism, competition, unresolved grief, undeveloped sexuality, and disturbed body image — are part of her armature. These traits (to be discussed more fully later) halt her development and create another layer of defense protecting her inner world. They are both cause and consequence of this lethal disorder.

Briefly, perfectionism provides purpose, the anorexic's unending quest for an unattainable ideal, be it in body size, academic achievement or some coveted form of excellence and superiority. Since perfection doesn't exist, her pursuit will never cease. And because perfection is an unattainable goal, striving for perfection fosters her perception of herself as a failure. It is in being a failure that her real protection resides. Being imperfect and a failure renders others' criticisms, expectations and judgments impotent — her own prejudgment is more powerful. Hence not only is she absolved of responsibility, her mask of incompetence and inadequacy ensures that others will either remain at a distance or treat her as fragile — and either way, whatever kernel of wholeness resides within her will remain hidden. Perfectionism thus is part of her shell.

Competition is the handmaiden of perfectionism. Competition aids the anorexic's façade by securing her position as the loser; although the anorexic competes incessantly with others in every imaginable arena, she does not compete to win, failing (in her mind) even with respect to weight. In being a loser, she slinks away from others and withdraws, harboring safe within her the attributes she dares not share. To excel would draw attention to her — and although in many ways she does excel, in her own eyes she does not, and hence preserves her shroud. Her self-torment and self-derision for her perceived failures keep her focused on the past, ever ruminating about her shortcomings. This stifles her development, impedes new learning and consolidation of growth, and impairs her relationships with others. Consciously, her intent is self-protection. Unknowingly, she deprives herself of mastering skills and employing resources that would offer her other avenues of safety.

Unresolved grief is another attribute of anorexia for some. Loss can be traumatic, and unexpressed feelings associated with loss can remain frozen indefinitely. The typical anorexic believes expression of most feelings—except those that are pleasant and agreeable—is dangerous and puts her at risk of judgment or ridicule. Thus, she may repress not only grief, but many emotions. Often anorexics are unable to even recognize their feelings, or to differentiate between physical and emotional signals, a condition known as alexithymia. Without access to or understanding of her feeling states, the anorexic lacks an important reservoir of self-knowledge. In her effort to preserve her Self, she loses paths to understanding dimensions of herself and nuances in her responses to the world around her that could aid her growth and integration. In this way, she remains immature, and the simplicity of her focus on her performance—whether in pleasing or competing with others, striving for perfection or becoming invisible—absolves her of facing the responsibilities of the adult world.

Among the mass of inchoate feelings that an anorexic typically represses are sexual feelings. Sexuality is an aspect of maturity and adulthood that feels too overwhelming for the anorexic to consider. To most anorexics, romantic relationships are mysterious and unappealing and sex is an intrusive and off-putting accompaniment. Her models for relationships have not been enviable and the caretakers who were unable to respond adequately to her are unlikely to have been well-attuned to each other. As malnutrition and starvation take their toll, the anorexic's body loses its womanly curves. Her breasts shrink and her hips vanish. She appears childlike, and her menstrual cycles cease. As her body is depleted of the reserves to produce female hormones, some of the raw materials of sexual thoughts and feelings disappear. And although she may not have made a conscious decision not to be a woman, this is the message her body conveys. For her, the attributes of her Self to which she clings have less to do with being female than simply with *being*. However, at some level she recognizes that as a female, her being-ness is intricately interwoven with her femaleness. Appearing feminine or womanly is too risky—it means the possibility of unwanted attention and bids from others for connection and relationship. The prospect of closeness is the very reason she has worked so diligently to erect these barriers. Her connections have been stifling, painful and injurious. If protecting herself from these threats means denying her own femaleness, it is the cost she will happily pay.

The anorexic's lack of sexual development is embedded in her body image distortion. It is her drive to be thin which transforms her body from feminine to childlike, and then to stick-thin. This is the eventual route to the anorexic's demise, because she loses the capacity to assess her body size with any objectivity. Her quest is to become thinner, smaller and truly invisible. So fervently does she maintain her pursuit, and so unable is she to see her actual size—her vision blurred in part by the fact that no amount of weight loss confers the sought after sense that she is lovable—that she is simply unaware of the reality of her increasing emaciation. In her mind, only in being invisible will she finally be free of the possibility of judgment and criticism. Only then can she be sure that the kernel of Self inside her will no longer be at risk of being usurped, defiled or rejected. Only then will there be no possibility of her being hurt. Of course, without a body, she can have no Self. However, if her sole means of preserving her Self from danger is to destroy the very body that she inhabits, then she will fight to her own demise. Thus the anorexic engages in a battle to preserve that small, sacred seed of Self, even if unwittingly in that war she risks her own death.

2

What Is Anorexia and What Causes It?

What Is Anorexia Nervosa?

Anorexia nervosa is a psychological disorder in which the individual deliberately and willfully starves, engaging in a "relentless pursuit of thinness" (Bruch, 1973, p. 3) that can be fatal. In clinical terms, the diagnosis of anorexia nervosa is applied to individuals who refuse to maintain weight above 85 percent of normal and who are intensely afraid of gaining weight. Anorexia nervosa is an illness, not a choice. This book discusses primary anorexia nervosa, which is anorexia that has not developed secondarily to another neurotic, psychotic or medical problem. Other disorders may occur along with anorexia, including depression, anxiety and obsessive-compulsive disorder.

The predominant symptoms of primary anorexia nervosa include distortion of body image, denial or non-recognition of bodily stimuli (hunger, fatigue, emotional feelings) and a "paralyzing sense of ineffectiveness" (Bruch, 1973, p.254). The anorexic goes to great lengths to please others, but continually believes she has failed to be pleasing enough. She — or he, but I use the pronoun she in this book for simplicity — struggles to assert control, and to achieve self-esteem and a sense of her own identity through starvation. Weight and size become her identity, and further development is arrested. The anorexic's attention to self-care, relationships and other life functions gradually diminishes.

The *Diagnostic and Statistical Manual of Mental Disorders, Text Revision,* compiled by the American Psychiatric Association and accepted by clinicians as the standard diagnostic tool, lists four criteria for anorexia nervosa (*DSM-IV-TR*, 2000, p.589):

1. Desire to maintain weight at or above a minimally normal weight for age and height or maintaining weight at less than 85 percent normal;
2. "Intense fear of gaining weight or becoming fat, even though underweight";
3. Disturbance in experience of body weight or shape, or "undue influence of body weight or shape on self-evaluation, or denial of the seriousness of current low body weight";
4. Amenorrhea in postmenarcheal females, defined as the absence of three consecutive menstrual cycles in girls or women who have started having periods.

The *DSM-IV-TR* identifies two subtypes of anorexia nervosa: a Restricting Type, in which the person has not regularly engaged in binging or purging behavior during this course of anorexia, and a Binge Eating/Purging Type, in which binge eating or purging (whether through self-induced vomiting or through laxative or diuretic misuse) has been present.

Anorexia generally develops during adolescence, with peak ages of onset between twelve and thirteen or between seventeen and eighteen. Anorexia is less likely to develop in the thirties or forties, except when there has been a preexisting occurrence at an earlier age. While anorexia occurs more frequently among females than males, it appears that the percent of men with the disorder is rising (Hudson et al., 2007, p.349).

How Prevalent Is Anorexia Nervosa?

Anorexia nervosa is prevalent, potentially fatal and devastating to loved ones. Statistics for occurrence and mortality from the disorder are staggering. In one of the few recent articles on anorexia for a lay audience, *Newsweek* magazine reported that 1 in 100 females in the United States develop anorexia and that 1 in 10 of those with anorexia die from the disorder or related complications (e.g. dehydration, heart failure). This means that of the approximately 1,500,000 females alive in the U.S. today, 15,000 are or will become anorexic and 1500 of these will die from this disorder or its complications (Tyre et al., 2005).

According to current statistics reported by the University of South Carolina Department of Mental Health, an estimated 3 percent of adolescent girls between the ages of ten and twenty — over half a million — suffer from anorexia. The mortality rate associated with anorexia nervosa is twelve times higher than the death rate from *all* causes of death for females from fifteen to twenty-four years old, and they also exhibit an elevated rate of suicide. *In the United States, anorexia is the mental disorder with the highest mortality rate* (University of South Carolina).

While truly reliable statistics are difficult to obtain because only the anorexics that receive medical or psychiatric treatment are formally diagnosed and counted, these numbers nonetheless suggest the enormity of the problem. Doubtless many people suffering from anorexia never seek help and still others are likely not counted because they are misdiagnosed. Furthermore, these numbers do not take into account the much smaller but still noteworthy number of males who develop anorexia. These statistics are even harder to research, because males in general are less likely to seek psychotherapy or medical help than females.

Anorexia is widespread and treatment, if sought, is successful in only a portion of cases. Psychiatrist David Herzog and co-author Kamryn Eddy estimate that fewer than 50 percent of anorexics achieve full recovery, 33 percent improve and 20 percent remain chronically ill (Herzog and Eddy, 2007, p.12). Also, 33 percent of those who recover relapse. Many anorexics who seek help leave treatment without having made significant life changes; others make some progress but not enough to consolidate their gains. Those who make only limited changes sometimes relapse later, and then die from complications of the disorder. The good news is that there are also those who find their way to treatment, usually with strong support from family and professionals, and who are able to harness the same perseverance that prolonged the disorder and instead use it to achieve and sustain health.

What Causes Anorexia Nervosa?

There is no single "cause" for anorexia; it develops from a complex interplay of physiological, psychological, familial and cultural factors. With the backdrop of these interacting factors, the onset of anorexia may be gradual, or may be more sudden, provoked by one or more triggering events. Below I have described some of the features that can contribute to the development of anorexia.

Physiological Aspects

For many years, it was assumed that anorexia was purely a psychological problem in which emotional conflicts provoked restrictive eating behaviors, which in turn led to harmful physical consequences. Among the suggested emotional causes were early trauma; major loss; family dynamics esteeming appearance over authenticity; peer competition in a culture obsessed with thinness; ostracism by peers or rejection by a boy. The individual, suffering from one or more of these emotional stressors, would resort to food restriction and weight loss to manage the pain evoked by the disturbing situation.

About fifty years ago, however, researchers demonstrated the strong interplay between physiology and psychology in anorexia. In the 1950s a group of psychologically healthy men who were conscientious objectors to the Vietnam War volunteered to participate in an experiment on starvation in lieu of conscription. After a time of reduced food intake and weight loss to 15 percent below normal, these men developed many of the same psychological and physical features common to anorexia. They became depressed, hyperirritable and afraid of weight gain. They became more withdrawn and isolated. Their sexual interest was drastically reduced. They began to obsess about food and to dream about food, to create unusual food concoctions, to hoard food, and at the same time to voluntarily restrict food intake. Their blood pressure decreased; their heart rates increased. Their bodies literally were suffering from starvation. The study was concluded and the volunteers slowly regained lost weight. However, even gradual weight gain to pre-study levels did not immediately restore normal attitudes and functions toward food; this did not happen until several months after return to healthy body weight (Garner, 1997, p.153–161). Clearly, as these non-anorexic men demonstrated, anorexia was not just a mental disorder, but had a strong physiological component driving it as well.

While anorexia begins with voluntary food restriction, once weight drops below a biologically-determined threshold, physiology takes over and induces additional psychological problems. This is the mechanism that goes into effect when a susceptible individual begins to diet and takes the diet too far. Malnourishment induces physical and psychological changes; then, as the body recognizes that sufficient food is unavailable and starvation is in progress, metabolism alters to adapt to the situation, slowing some processes and quickening others. The body diminishes its requirements for fuel in order to survive on smaller supplies, and the individual uses food rituals to prolong the time expended with the limited food that is available. Absence of metabolic raw materials triggers a slowing or even a cessation of hormonal processes and organ functions. Neurotransmitter levels decrease and brain chemistry alters, inducing anxiety, depression and fear. The ensuing shift in body perception convinces the anorexic that her need for food has decreased and that she is already too fat. This is the insidious process that can lead to serious malnutrition and eventual death.

More recently, research in neurophysiology has revealed that genetic factors may predispose someone to developing anorexia. Genetic studies of identical twins raised apart have shown that if one twin develops anorexia, the identical twin has a 50 to 60 percent probability of also developing the disorder (Liu, 2008, p.21). Family members of an anorexic are twelve times as likely to develop the disorder as people without a family history of the disorder. Familial patterns are not sufficient to confirm a genetic basis for a disorder. However, a group of researchers has now established evidence of a "susceptibility gene for anorexia nervosa on chromosome 1" (Grice et al., 2002, p.787).

Furthermore, anorexics appear to be deficient or have abnormal functioning of two neurotransmitters, dopamine and serotonin, with possible imbalances in other neurotransmitters as well. Dopamine mediates the pleasure and reward system in the midbrain. When supplies of dopamine are deficient, which can happen for genetic reasons or because of severe or prolonged trauma or stress, the individual is more prone to emotional pain, and is predisposed to repeat behaviors that provide a spike in mood. Starvation and the sense of power the anorexic achieves by restricting food intake can provide this kind of reward. In other words, the anorexic may be compensating for a dopamine deficiency by starving, which produces dopamine and improves her mood, leading her to repeat food-restricting behaviors.

Serotonin mediates calmness and a general sense of well-being. Insufficient serotonin can lead to anxiety or depression and a general sense of malaise. These symptoms are common in anorexia. Research further suggests that in anorexia there is reduced function of specific serotonin receptor sites that affect mood, anxiety level and pleasure in eating (Bailer et al., 2007, p.1090–1097). In addition, it appears that some altered serotonin function remains in anorexics after a measure of recovery has been achieved, suggesting that these serotonin abnormalities may be involved in the origin of the disorder (Kaye et al., 2005, p.17).

Hyperactivity is common to a large subset of anorexics, particularly during acute phases of the disorder. The tendency towards hyperactivity appears to be innate and can be considered as a kind of obsessive-compulsive disorder. The effect of hyperactivity in combination with food restriction can lead to an increase in serotonin metabolism. In addition, animal research has shown that hyperactivity coupled with starvation releases an opioid in the brain. This can set up an addictive cycle whereby the hyperactive anorexic finds that food restriction induces a mood-elevating opioid spike which promotes repetition of the food-restricting behavior (Kohl et al., 2004, p.492–499).

Some personality traits are also genetically determined and many anorexics exhibit a specific constellation of these traits. Individuals who develop anorexia are likely to demonstrate perfectionism, competition, risk aversion, rejection sensitivity and obsessiveness. As clinician Carolyn Costin notes, people who develop anorexia tend to be hyper-responsible and good in school, but they lack the emotional maturity to deal with their early successes (Costin, 2007a, p.197).

One additional biological factor that may in some cases contribute to the development of anorexia is the presence of food allergies or sensitivities. Individuals who are allergic to a food and develop symptoms from eating it may begin to reduce intake of *all* food because they are aware of not feeling well after eating but do not know why and do not link their discomfort to a specific food. With sufficient weight loss, the cycle of psychological and physiological factors characteristic of starvation can be set in motion, rendering the person at the mercy of her biology. Wheat, dairy, corn and eggs are the most common food allergies in the United States. Gluten intolerance, which is a reaction to gluten-containing grains such as wheat and rye, can also set up this same cycle of digestive discomfort leading to food restriction.

Psychological Aspects

Anorexia often first appears at developmental phases of separation and individuation. In the United States, these phases correspond to entering junior high or high school, around ages twelve and thirteen, and again when preparing to leave home, generally at age seventeen or eighteen. Sometimes symptoms appear earlier in childhood or manifest other times and recur periodically throughout a person's life. Depending on the extent of recovery from the earlier episodes, emotional crises later in life, such as separation, divorce, retirement of a spouse or death of a loved one, may spark a return of the disorder.

The very fact that separation can provoke the development of anorexia accounts in part for the greater prevalence of eating disorders among females than males. The process of maternal separation is gender-dependent. At birth, boys clearly differ physically from their mothers, and as infants and young children, boys are acculturated to continue to differentiate psychologically and behaviorally from females. A girl, however, physically resembles her mother, and is brought up to emulate her mother's personality and behavior. For girls to transition successfully into young women, they must differentiate themselves from their mothers. If a girl has not been encouraged to develop her unique personality and identity, this transition will be particularly challenging, and she may remain emotionally dependent on her mother. And if the girl wants to be unlike her mother, but her personal growth has lagged, she may choose a rebellious path — reacting against her mother, but still remaining emotionally dependent on her.

Psychologically — whether or not by conscious decision — the anorexic remains childlike and immature, sometimes becoming quite regressed. British psychiatrist Arthur Crisp discusses this phenomenon as a "flight from growth," in which the adolescent can avoid not only the unasked-for physical changes of puberty, but the emotional challenges as well. Anorexia nervosa can then arise in place of any attempt at normal personality development. Through vigilance and controlling her desire for food, the anorexic acquires a sense of security, achievement and competence (Crisp, 1997, pp.250–251).

Conflicts about sexuality may also contribute to the anorexic's preference for immaturity. Her concerns may stem from sexual attitudes in her family or from peer influences. Fear of replicating her parents' relationship, lack of skill in handling interpersonal relationships, and feelings of lack of control about the changes in her body may all affect her desire to avoid becoming identified as female and sexual (Crisp, 1997, p.250).

The body image disturbance central to anorexia has its psychological underpinnings both in the individual's personal development and in cultural influences. Because the body is perceived as — and is indeed part of — the self, the body reflects and shares the individual's preoccupations. The body becomes a screen on which the anorexic projects the internal states and interpersonal conflicts she is ill-equipped to handle. The more she focuses on her body, the less attention she devotes to learning skills for handling her feelings (Kearney-Cooke and Striegel-Moore, 1997, p.297). Her body thus becomes the reservoir for her negative feelings about herself. Each perceived failure augments her self-hatred, which is then expressed as body-hatred and used as justification for self-punishment. Meanwhile the media, as the envoy of culture, proclaim that appearance is all-important and beauty an essential emblem defining worth. The culture also promulgates the myth of "change your body, change your self" (Kearney-Cooke and Striegel-Moore, p.297), which means that improving one's outside appearance automatically enhances inner health and well-being. The anorexic's focus on her body and on the cultural imperative equating thinness with beauty paves the way for her to manipulate her body to feel more attractive and better about herself. Thus through starvation, the anorexic simultaneously punishes herself and her body for perceived failures and imperfections, and strives to improve her body to enhance her feelings of well-being and competence.

Spiritual Hunger

"At the center of identity is spirit," writes Courtney Martin in *Perfect Girls, Starving Daughters* (Martin, 2007, p.250). But when identity is a shell, there is no spirit. With an internal world void of significant self-structure, the anorexic experiences an acute emptiness. Food rituals and exercise regimens substitute for real meaning. She cannot fill herself with these. She has no spiritual sustenance.

Carl Jung once described an alcoholic patient who had relapsed. Jung told the man his only hope was for a spiritual or religious experience and that "his craving for alcohol was the equivalent of the spiritual thirst of our being for wholeness" (Cortright, 1997, p.216). The situation for the anorexic is similar. The anorexic craves wholeness, but lacks the internal building blocks. Instead, perfection is her god. Perfection is the antithesis of acceptance, and acceptance is a central soul principle; perfection begets endless unhappiness and the interminable quest for "more" or "better." Acceptance rests in the now, and in the experience of trust. The anorexic however, majors in mistrust — of herself and of others.

Self is a psychological and a spiritual construct. The anorexic, lacking both psychological and spiritual tools with which to build a Self, a soul, or an identity of substance and cohesion, relies instead on her quest for perfection.

Family Dynamics

Family dynamics may play a role in the development of anorexia, although certainly the once-common generalization that anorexia develops largely in families of high socioeconomic status has proven untrue. While there are some traits that seem to characterize the families of anorexics, these are not universally present. There are also many families where similar traits occur but no child develops anorexia. Some traits in families are inherited by the anorexic, such as a proclivity towards perfectionism; others, such as attachment styles, have doubtless been passed down through the family culture for generations.

In some cases, the mother of the anorexic is depressed, preoccupied or emotionally unavailable. These conditions can affect the future anorexic's sense of internal security and emotional vulnerability. If a parent is alcoholic, similar dynamics may result where the parent's erratic or unpredictable behavior affects the child's sense of security. In both of these cases, and others as well, open expression of feelings and clear communication are often to be inhibited.

Sometimes the absence of a father's attention can lead the adolescent girl to place undue emphasis on her appearance to try to win her father's acknowledgment. A girl's hunger for an emotional connection with her father can lead her to feel inadequate. Pursuit of thinness and perfection fuel her quest to feel good about herself (Maine, 2004, p.114).

There also can be situations where one or both parents may not promote self-development in their child. Without learning self-reliance and dependence on inner strengths, the child, upon reaching the appropriate age of separation, lacks the internal capacity to manage the process of separation and individuation. If she has not been encouraged to pursue her own passions, she may be better equipped to live in her parents' shadow rather than as an independent individual.

In some families, there may be undue emphasis placed on appearance, including on weight. In these situations, the family gives the message that developing inner authenticity is not as important as creating outer symbols of success. At adolescence, the child may then align with weight and body obsessions which fit both her family's and her culture's values.

In addition, sometimes features of the parental relationship can unwittingly contribute to the development of anorexia. The anorexic may flee from growth in an unconscious effort to save a strained parental relationship. In some situations the integrity of the parents' marriage depends on the stabilizing factor of a child. The child's growth and development can become a threat to this stability, and the child may unconsciously choose to remain a child in an effort to keep her parents' marriage intact (Crisp, 1997, p. 252). Without fully realizing it, the anorexic may understand that if there is parental strife, and separation or divorce is imminent, anorexia can divert the parents' attention to a common problem: saving their daughter.

Another scenario can occur when the child has been closely bonded to her father and the father has rejected the mother. When the child in adolescence begins physically and temperamentally to resemble her unloved mother, she risks loss of her father's attention and may see not growing up as her only solution (Crisp, 1997, p.252). Or if the mother and daughter are close and the father is distant, the daughter may perceive that her mother's happiness resides in the daughter's continuing to be her mother's emotional support, a support which would be threatened were the girl to grow up.

Cultural Milieu

United States culture suffers from distorted, confusing and contradictory information about food, weight, and body image. It is a wonder that anyone, particularly if female, can emerge with healthy eating habits and body satisfaction. Media images are full of retouched and Photoshopped pictures of svelte female models and actresses, and men with bulging biceps and six-pack abs. We are a visual culture when it comes to food and our bodies. But much less consideration is given to how our bodies feel when they are healthy, or the many miraculous and life-sustaining functions our bodies perform. Couple this ignorance with the constant bombardment of images and information, the increasing complexity of technology, the atmosphere of speed and immediacy, and it becomes apparent why people yearn for a means of comfort and control. Food, for many, has become that means: food offers comfort, and dieting, or food restriction, offers control. In the end, food has become separate from its primary function as a source of nutrition, sustenance and energy. With this disconnect between food and its primary purpose, it is no surprise that dieting has become a multi-billion dollar industry.

Appearance is a charged issue, especially among women, and people go to great lengths to emulate the "ideal" body. Our culture promulgates many myths that reinforce overvaluing appearance. Among them is the notion that a person's outside image reflects inner happiness. If we transform our bodies, the myth goes, we will transform our lives. Furthermore, this conversion should not require much time or effort — pills and protein drinks should suffice to create a new and better you.

The sad truth about human metabolism, however, is that diets rarely work; it is estimated that 98 percent of dieters regain their lost weight. This high rate accounts for the financial well-being of the billon-dollar diet industry. Many people lose weight only to embark on a cycle of weight lost and weight regained. In the end, it is mostly physiology that regulates size, returning each human organism to homeostasis and to the stable weight which evolution and genetics determine will protect that particular individual from famine.

The cultural emphasis on thinness is an insidious culprit in the development of anorexia. Furthermore, what was "thin" 20 years ago would not be thin enough today. Playboy centerfolds and Miss America contestants were progressively thinner from 1985 to 2005, with 2005 centerfold models 10 percent lighter in weight (with corrections made for height differences) than in 1986. If thin is desirable, when is thin too thin? The starvation-related deaths of three South American fashion models in the fall of 2006 were a tragic answer. At least the fashion industry in Milan responded by establishing a minimum weight requirement for models. Sadly, despite substantial lobbying, the U.S. fashion industry did not follow suit. And the Western cultural obsession with thinness is spreading abroad. Twenty years ago, anorexia did not exist on the Fiji Islands. But after American television and MTV found their way to this remote region, Fijian adolescent girls began to diet and to develop anorexia.

Ultimately, it is the cultural focus on appearance, the power of the ubiquitous diet industry, and the individual's desire for control of a chaotic outer *and* inner world which coalesce and set the stage for anorexia. The body is designed to maintain homeostasis, which means the anorexic has to work hard to lose weight and to fight against a strong biological imperative. However, unlike the average yo-yo dieter, the anorexic sticks to her purpose. When she does not acquire the hoped-for inner metamorphosis through weight loss, she keeps lowering her goal weight. In time, the physiology of starvation and its psychological consequences take over, operating differently in anorexia than in cyclical dieting. At this point, weight loss begets more weight loss. And therein lies the insidious nature of anorexia and the cause for the high rate of mortality from the disorder. Yes, anorexics do starve themselves to death. But more often, the actual cause of death is heart failure or severe dehydration, both horrific consequences of the disorder. And it is because the anorexic cannot stop herself from starving that she needs help to survive the disorder.

Triggering Events

Biochemical imbalances, psychological problems, family issues and cultural milieu create the backdrop for anorexia. Each is important, but there is usually a triggering event or series of events that acts as catalyst. Because it is this interplay of background elements and life events that stimulates the illness, the onset of anorexia can rarely be traced to any one particular incident. Substrate and situation collude.

To catalogue the possible triggering events would take many pages and the list would still be incomplete. Here are a few examples: separation or divorce of parents; birth of a younger sibling; moving away from a familiar neighborhood; death of a family member; development of breasts and hips; a remark made by a boyfriend about preferred weight or shape of girls; parental pressure to get good grades; the prospect of leaving high school; feelings of isolation. Just as every individual is unique, so too are the situations or events which trigger anorexia.

It is neither possible nor desirable to shield anyone from all painful life events. The human organism requires challenges to grow, and bumping up against obstacles fosters creativity, adaptability, flexibility and strength. The difficulty arises when an individual lacks sufficient internal resources or external support to handle the stressors effectively. Sometimes parents aren't equipped to provide their children with necessary guidance and support. But even with vigilant parents, anorexia can develop, as biochemical, cultural and peer influences cannot always be intercepted and neutralized. Early intervention offers the best prognosis for recovery, and the hope is that someone will notice early anorexic symptoms and suggest or provide help before the disorder progresses.

Is Anorexia an Addiction?

The main traits that characterize addiction are present in anorexia. These include continuation of behavior despite adverse consequences; lack of control; and the progressive nature of the disease. At first, an addict can generally manage the substance, behavior or drug. However, in time, the addict no longer maintains control: physiological reactions, anxiety, obsessions, distorted thinking, and impulsivity reign. So it is with anorexia. An anorexic initially chooses to restrict food intake, but she reaches a point where the choice is no longer hers; her disease takes over, and fear and anxiety drive her behavior. The addict continues self-injurious behavior despite adverse consequences—to the point of economic ruin, destruction of relationships, and sometimes death. Similarly, the anorexic continues food restriction in the face of failing health, heightened emotional distress, and physical exhaustion, eventually risking death. And just as addiction is progressive—meaning that without treatment, symptoms get progressively worse—so, too, is anorexia.

Research into the biological basis of drug and alcohol addiction has shown that an innate deficit of the neurotransmitter dopamine, or exposure to severe or prolonged distress, which depletes dopamine, lowers the individuals' capacity for pleasure and heightens sensitivity to emotional pain. Alcohol, drugs, compulsive spending, addictive sex, overeating and starvation can all produce an initial surge of dopamine and relief from emotional pain. As the addiction continues, more and more of the pleasure-or-relief-producing substance or behavior is required to attempt to replicate the initial response; this explains the progressive nature of the disease. In addiction, as in anorexia, biology overrides will. Anxiety escalates and the anorexic restricts her eating even more.

The addictive nature of anorexia means that 12-Step programs can have value in recovery. Lack of a developed Self contributes to the emptiness an anorexic typically experiences, and development of Self can entail spiritual, as well as psychological, growth. The principles, community and tools of 12-Step programs provide antidotes to spiritual and psychological emptiness.

I think of food misuse and body size manipulation as addictions. For many, body obsession is like using drugs or alcohol, acting out sexually, gambling excessively, or getting fixated on the Internet. Weight and food obsession and their associated rituals comprise another set of thoughts and behaviors that some people have latched onto to push away reality. Like any other addict, the repeated food abuser — whether he or she overeats, undereats, or binges and purges— loses control of the substance, becomes progressively more entrenched in the self-destructive behaviors, and continues use despite harmful consequences. For the anorexic, the concept of ceasing food restriction entails terror and psychological withdrawal as intense as that encountered by any addict who considers refraining from addictive behaviors.

The demise of the anorexic resembles that of any other addict. The individual who becomes anorexic likely is predisposed genetically to this illness. She probably begins to restrict her food intake voluntarily. Perhaps at first she experiences a smug sense of superiority and power, whether from the pleasure induced by the sense of control, the constriction of her world that it provides, or the physical and emotional "high" generated by sustained hunger. Then, unwittingly, the habits take on a life of their own. Where once the anorexic was in control, the disorder now controls her. She may not realize the physical or psychological toll of continuing to restrict, because her faulty brain chemistry, disturbed further by malnutrition, has undermined her capacity to think rationally and to view herself objectively. Previously she could *choose* not to eat; now an internal force has taken over. Her mind has been hijacked, an inner demon is in charge, and she couldn't *make* herself eat even if she wanted to. Starvation, once her secret ally, has become her nemesis.

3

Uses and Misuses of the Internet

The variety of resources and information available with the click of a mouse is stunning; with an Internet connection, the average adult — and even more quickly, the average child — can find out how to raise a newt or refurbish an auto engine, and research the origins of the pterodactyl or the content of the ozone layer. The Internet has connected more human beings than anything else in history, millions of times more than the radio, television and telephone combined. However, not all of the information is accurate, and not all of it is beneficial.

When it comes to anorexia, the Internet offers a wealth of resources: sites for buying helpful books; information about types of treatment; pictures and descriptions of treatment centers; and referrals to therapists who specialize in eating disorders. Many treatment facilities have Websites, and Web addresses for a number of them are listed in the back of this book.

Unfortunately, as with other subject matter accessible on the Web, not all the information about anorexia is constructive: it is not all designed to combat this deadly disorder. Sprinkled among the Websites that offer healthy advice are potentially treacherous sites that normalize and glamorize anorexia. *San Francisco Chronicle* columnist Joan Ryan termed these sites the "outlaws of the universe" (Ryan, 2003, p.D1). In the realm of anorexia, they are called "pro-ana," meaning that they promote the disease of anorexia — anorexics in the woeful world of the Web refer to themselves as "anas." Pro-anas offer pictures of waif-thin anorexics, especially models and actresses. Sometimes the photos are doctored to make the person look even thinner than she actually is. These photos are posted not as deterrents to anorexia, but as inspiration — the sites call it "thinspiration" — and as encouragement to boost the anorexic's resolve to persevere in her pursuit of starvation.

In 2001, a columnist for the online edition of *Time* magazine, Jessica Reaves, estimated that there were over 400 pro-ana sites on the Web (Reaves, 2001). While Web hosts such as Yahoo will shut down sites if notified of their existence, other sites pop up in their place — and the site names are unlikely to give away the contents, so they may not come to the immediate attention of the Web host. Reaves noted that some of the sites even offer strict warnings to anyone who is about to enter: do not open this if you are in recovery or considering recovery. But to the anorexic, this warning may pose as a dare — flaunting her competitiveness and perfectionism, the anorexic takes pride in her will to restrict, and of course she wants to be a member of the privileged club. Besides, the anorexic who enters a pro-ana chat room is further fired by competitive zeal — she may be able to share a technique that no one else has thought of.

Pro-anas offer inspiration for persevering in food restriction, tips on how to starve without feeling hungry, and even advice on how to fake weigh-ins at a doctor's office. Some sites acknowledge that anorexia is an illness and that it is dangerous. This is probably what led Vivian Meehan, former president of the National Association of Anorexia Nervosa and Associated Disorders (ANAD), to say, "Some of these sites are worded in a way that indicates the hosts do want help" (Reaves, 2001). But juxtaposed to a caveat about the life-threatening nature of anorexia is often an avowal of the pro-ana's goal: to help anorexics in their quest for the "ideal" (emaciated) body. The sites acknowledge that anorexia is hard work; but that is no news to any anorexic, who is more than willing to suffer and sacrifice to get the body she craves.

As Meehan noted, one goal of the anorexic is to convince others that her way of life is perfectly fine, and finding other anorexics who are doing exactly what she is doing reinforces her zeal (Reaves, 2001). The anorexic believes in her quest, and in fact, may cite society and its reverence for beautiful super-thin Hollywood stars as evidence for the validity of her cause (Ryan, 2003, p.D6). Of course, the anorexic cannot discern the difference between her predicament and that of most Hollywood actresses who, except for an unfortunate few, have careers that depend on their maintaining a level of vitality, and whose managers and publicists keep them in check.

Anorexia is a disease of isolation. These sites offer connection among anorexics — although, unfortunately, not for the purpose of supporting recovery. Anorexics from opposite ends of the earth can commiserate about the challenge of staving off hunger and fending off pounds. As competitive as anorexics are, the fact that their communications are not visual may help to maintain the supportive nature of their blogs. Anorexics who are together in a room compare themselves incessantly with each other. Their mission — to be the thinnest — heightens their vigilance, and the competition occurring internally is fierce. In-person encounters rarely promote personal connections among anorexics. The Internet offers visual anonymity. Unless a posting talks about weight — pounds lost, desired weight, what weight the scale registered at the doctor's office — the message content is largely about the struggles: asking for suggestions and giving advice to further the disorder.

Several clinicians have conducted covert observations of interactions in the online pro-ana community. Brotsky and Giles reported visiting a number of sites and finding that not all pro-ana sites are the same: members of some communities were hostile while those at other sites were welcoming. The authors concluded that the sites are best understood as "local cliques offering temporary relief from offline hostility" (Brotsky and Giles, 2007, p.93). Similarly other clinicians report that for pro-ana participants, anorexia represents stability and control and this kind of site offers support and guidance to those who wish to remain in the sanctuary of the disorder (Fox et al., 2005, p.944–71). One British physician noted that, although these sites glamorize unhealthy behavior, he has had some patients who entered treatment after viewing the shocking pictures and information on these sites (Head, 2007). Unfortunately, this seems to be a rare occurrence.

Even non-anorexics can be negatively affected by looking at pro-ana sites. Psychologists at the University of Missouri randomly assigned over 200 non-eating disordered female undergraduates to view either a prototypical pro-ana site, a female fashion site using average-sized models or a home-decorating site. After the Website viewing, the participants assigned to the pro-ana site showed poorer mood and lower social self-esteem; they also perceived themselves as heavier, engaged in more image comparison with other women and reported a greater likelihood of exercising and thinking about their weight in the near future. The authors of this study concluded that pro-ana Websites are a "troubling new form of thin-ideal exposure" (Bardone-Cone and Cass, 2007, pp.537–48).

Reaves has suggested that these sites could provide a window into the world of the anorexic. Certainly the blurbs posted on the pro-ana bulletin boards from anorexics in the throes of their disease recount the painful plight of starvation, the refusal to give in to hunger, the fight against the body's limitations, the tyrannical obsession with food. Perhaps this is useful to the occasional educator who really is trying to get a grip on the psyche of the anorexic. However, any practitioner who is working with anorexics doubtless is already well aware of the anorexic mind-set and needs no further immersion into the sufferer's pain. And the existence of pro-anas— which spread the illness— is a terrible price to pay for insight into the inner world of the anorexic.

There is no adequate way to police Websites. One way to get pro-ana sites removed from the Internet is for anyone invested in prevention and treatment of anorexia —clinicians, parents of adolescent girls, educators, treatment professionals— to identify sites and inform organizations such as the National Association of Anorexia Nervosa and Related Disorders (ANAD), which can then approach the Web hosts. In 2001, Vivian Meehan, then president of ANAD, spoke with a Yahoo administrator and four days later, 21 of Yahoo's 115 pro-anorexia sites had been taken down. However, Yahoo's spokesperson gave ANAD no credit, simply noting that when "content with the sole purpose of creating harm or inciting hate is brought to our attention, we evaluate it, and in extreme cases, remove it, as that is a violation of our terms of service" (Reaves, 2001). Whatever their explanation, at least the company administrators shut down some of the offensive sites.

Europeans have also been examining the issue of how to stop the proliferation of pro-ana Websites. In February 2008, British psychiatrist Ty Glover noted that while there is no way to control the existence of pro-ana sites in general, those on social networking sites such as Facebook can be pressured to remove pro-ana sites. Glover asserted that social networking sites can censor their material "and we expect them to act responsibly" (*BBC News*, February 24, 2008). In April 2008, the French health minister, Roselyne Bachelot, declared "the pro-ana movements which spread their messages of death on the Web must be the target for special attention" (Bremner and Tourres, 2008). She introduced a bill to the French legislature, aimed at the fashion industry, media and the Internet, which would levy fines of up to 30,000 euros and two years' imprisonment for offenders "who provoke a person to seek excessive thinness by encouraging prolonged restriction of nourishment" to the point of risking death or damage to health; penalties would be increased to 45,000 euros and three years' imprisonment if the person died. The bill was tabled at the time, but its proposal is a hopeful sign.

The existence of pro-ana Websites is disconcerting to those who are working to prevent and treat anorexia, as well as to anorexics and families in recovery. Raising awareness of the existence of these sites runs the risk of making them known to "wannarexics"— the pro-ana term for those who want to become anorexic — as well as to other anorexics who are already seriously ill. There probably is no way to banish the Websites altogether or to prevent new ones from being launched. However, if concerned persons continue to disseminate pro-recovery information through all media channels, to set healthier weight standards in the fashion industry, and to impose sanctions when possible against media that promote unhealthy thinness, the quantity of positive information about recovery may in time overshadow the pro-ana presence.

4

Disorders That May Accompany Anorexia

An individual may suffer from one or more psychiatric disorders at the same time that she has symptoms of anorexia. Anxiety in particular and depression as well are common among anorexics. There are several subtypes of anxiety that may be present, including obsessive-compulsive disorder, panic disorder, social phobia and post-traumatic stress disorder. An anorexic may develop bulimia, or vice-versa. Body dysmorphic disorder, which is a preoccupation with a particular defect in appearance (as opposed to the anorexic's overall dissatisfaction with body size), substance abuse or addiction, and personality disorders may also occur with anorexia. An anorexic may suffer from several disorders simultaneously. Below I briefly describe some of the disorders that can co-occur with anorexia.

Depression

Depression can accompany anorexia, sometimes co-occurring with anxiety. Depression may *precede* anorexia and contribute to its origin, or develop as a *consequence* of the malnutrition of anorexia. Sometimes depression is so intertwined with anorexia that it can be hard to differentiate the two, or to tell which came first. When any individual becomes depressed, a common symptom can be loss of appetite. Alternatively, someone who is depressed may intentionally restrict food, seeking to improve mood. When depression develops after the onset of anorexia, the depression may be caused in part by the fact that an anorexic's brain lacks sufficient nutrients to manufacture the neurotransmitters required to sustain a balanced mood.

Neurophysiological research indicates that the genes involved in alcoholism, anorexia and depression are located close together on the chromosomes, the structures which carry an individual's genetic information. These three conditions have in common a deficit in the neurotransmitter dopamine, which promotes pleasure. Genetically speaking, it is probable that some measure of depression exists in most anorexics before onset of the disorder. Some of the symptoms of major depressive disorder include feelings of worthlessness, excessive or inappropriate guilt, and fatigue or loss of energy (*Diagnostic and Statistical Manual, Text Revision [DSM-IV-TR]*, 2000, pp.369–82). These depressive symptoms could help account for the "paralyzing sense of ineffectiveness" noted by psychoanalyst Hilde Bruch as characteristic of anorexia (Bruch, 1973, p.254).

Depression may manifest as a single major occurrence, as recurrent episodes, or as a chronic condition. Clinically, there are several subtypes of depression distinguished by severity and chronicity of symptoms. Dysthymia, which is a form of depression characterized by chronic low mood or malaise, may occur with anorexia and manifest as intractable low self-esteem and hopelessness. The self-hatred and self-castigation of anorexia can aggravate depression, and depression can in turn aggravate self-hatred.

Isolation can also aggravate depression. A person who is already besieged by self-defeating thoughts is apt to ruminate when uninterrupted by the natural distractions provided by other people. Anorexics tend to withdraw and to self-isolate, in part to avoid the painful self-judgments and self-defeating comparisons that they are prone to generate in the presence of others. However, what feels self-preserving may actually aggravate pessimistic mood.

Sometimes when nutritional health is restored to an anorexic, the depression lifts. Psychotherapy can also treat depression. For some anorexics who are depressed, however, it may be critical to treat the depression pharmacologically because depression can significantly impair the individual's motivation to change and to do the work of recovery from an eating disorder. Furthermore, depression can be particularly serious in an anorexic because she is already engaged in a downward physical and emotional spiral. Severe depression coupled with anorexia can lead to suicide.

Anxiety and Anxiety Disorders

Generalized Anxiety Disorder

Anxiety is so common in anorexia that anorexia has been termed an anxiety disorder. Anxiety may co-occur with depression. With generalized anxiety disorder, the person tends to worry excessively and also to be restless, easily fatigued, have difficulty concentrating, be irritable, exhibit heightened muscle tension or suffer from a sleep disturbance (*DSM-IV-TR*, 2000, p.476).

Anxiety is regulated by neurotransmitters in the brain. Furthermore, anxiety can be genetic in origin and often runs in families. Malnutrition, which can lead to the suppressed production of neurotransmitters, can also cause anxiety. It can be difficult to determine which came first, anxiety or anorexia, and each can exacerbate the other. Starvation can intensify fears (especially of weight gain), obsessiveness, and irritability — some of the traits that characterize anxiety. When anxiety precedes anorexia, it may persist even after nutrition has been restored.

Similar to depression, anxiety can be aggravated by isolation because the individual's solitary musing can exaggerate fears. Interrupting the rumination through distraction by social contact can be helpful. However, this is a double-edged sword as the anorexic's propensity for comparison to others can escalate in social situations.

Anxiety, like depression, can be treated pharmacologically, and often the dilemma exists of whether to treat anxiety to assist resolution of anorexia, or to reverse malnutrition in order to lessen anxiety. Various forms of psychotherapy can help anorexia and anxiety together.

Obsessive-Compulsive Behavior or Obsessive-Compulsive Disorder

Obsessions are persistent, recurrent thoughts, usually of a disturbing nature. Compulsions are the repetitive behaviors devised to relieve the obsessive thoughts. Commonly, an anorexic is plagued by persistent, intrusive thoughts about food, calorie content of food, and weight. She attempts to silence her distressing thoughts through ritual behaviors. The perfectionist and competitive traits typical of anorexia aggravate the anorexic's obsessive tendencies, and her obsessions intensify her perfectionism and competition. Recurrent thoughts of "I'm too fat" or

"I'm not thin enough" can drive an anorexic to weigh herself repeatedly, exercise incessantly, limit food intake, and engage in elaborate, time-consuming rituals around acquisition and preparation of food which she may barely touch. Thoughts of "I'm bad" or "I'll never amount to anything" will also drive food- and weight-related rituals. One client described to me the hours she spent at the farmer's market every Saturday picking out a ripe cantaloupe. She picked up each melon, felt it carefully all over, smelled it several times, held it first in one hand, then the other, then both, smelled it again, put it back and repeated this performance with cantaloupe after cantaloupe. When she finally purchased one, she would feel guilty all the way home for spending money on this luxurious, perfect fruit, and she would throw it in the garbage uneaten.

If an anorexic's compulsive behaviors extend to areas beyond food and weight, and meet other criteria for frequency and persistence, she can be diagnosed as having obsessive-compulsive disorder. This is not unusual when an anorexic becomes progressively more anxious and upset with prolonged malnutrition. In these circumstances, more and more of her life begins to be preoccupied with thoughts about others, herself, her performance, how others see her, or what she is doing wrong. She develops an ever-greater repertoire of compulsive behaviors to quell the intrusive thoughts.

Panic Attack or Panic Disorder

Sometimes an individual experiences a sudden onset of acute fear or anxiety. This is termed panic attack when the fear is accompanied by such symptoms as heart palpitations or pounding, chest pains, shortness of breath, dizziness, chills, nausea, fear of losing control, or fear of dying. For the anorexic, particularly as her disease progresses, fear of loss of control is significant and panic attacks, if present, may become more frequent or severe. Panic disorder is diagnosed if a person who has experienced a panic attack worries persistently about having another one or engages in behaviors designed to avoid a recurrence. For example, a person who has a panic attack while driving on a particular road may go to great lengths to avoid driving that particular route, or even to avoid driving altogether.

Anorexics tend to be fear-driven. Fear of disapproval, and of the anticipated rejection or abandonment that might ensue, motivates much of an anorexic's perfectionism. The anorexic prizes control, or the illusion of control. She frequently seeks power in arenas where in fact she has none, such as controlling others' thoughts and feelings. However, the anorexic's fears may not necessarily culminate in panic attacks.

Social Phobia

An anorexic's fear of disapproval and rejection can predispose her to social phobia. Social phobia manifests when an individual develops an intense fear of particular social or performance situations where she will be exposed to unfamiliar people and possibly to their scrutiny. When this fear develops, the individual takes steps to avoid these situations, or is intensely distressed when in them. She may experience severe anxiety when she is exposed to one of these situations, sometimes resulting in a panic attack. Also in social phobia, the individual recognizes that her fear is excessive or unreasonable (*DSM-IV-TR*, p.456). Unfortunately, the anorexic's fear and dislike of social situations, whether or not at the level to be diagnosed as social phobia, promote her tendency towards isolation. This can set up a vicious cycle in which the more isolated the anorexic becomes, the more threatened she is by social situations and the more likely she is to avoid them.

Post-Traumatic Stress Disorder

Post-Traumatic Stress Disorder (PTSD) sometimes occurs among anorexics, particularly as trauma can be a precipitating factor in the onset of anorexia. For this diagnosis to apply, the trauma witnessed or experienced must have involved threat of death, or of serious injury or loss of personal integrity to her or to another, and she must have responded to the situation with fear, helplessness or horror. Then, when the individual is exposed to something that symbolizes or resembles the past event, she re-experiences it through intrusive recollections, distressing dreams, feelings of recurrence of the trauma, intense psychological distress, or physiological responses. The tendency in these circumstances is for the individual to prevent reminders of the event, and to avoid thoughts or activities relevant to the trauma. The individual may not recall specific details. She may feel detached or estranged from others, exhibit a restricted range of affect, or have either a diminished interest in significant activities or a sense of a foreshortened future. Persistent symptoms occur, such as sleep difficulty, irritability, difficulty concentrating, hypervigilance or exaggerated startle response (*DSM-IV-TR*, pp.467–468).

Trauma does not necessarily produce immediate symptoms of PTSD. Symptoms may be acute or chronic, and onset may be delayed. In anorexia, trauma may have occurred at an earlier time in childhood or adolescence. Sometimes a more recent event evokes thoughts or feelings relevant to the trauma. Or the trauma may be more remote and stored in the body and its effects not even evident until some time after therapy has commenced. Trauma is not necessarily a discrete event or even just a few events, but may be something that the person experienced repeatedly or consistently over a period of time.

While I am hypervigilant and experience an acute startle reflex, these symptoms occur independently of other identifying characteristics of PTSD. For me, these traits may be genetic; my mother was anxious, my father very sensitive to noise and light. Although certain events in my life, such as my grandmother's death, had significant emotional repercussions, I did not develop the constellation of symptoms typical of PTSD. In contrast, a former anorexic client of mine had been in a serious automobile accident at the age of seven. Her father was driving and she was in the passenger seat when an out-of-control motorist ran a red light and rammed into the front of their car. Although neither my client nor her father was injured, years later she experienced intrusive flashbacks, a frequent sense of physical danger when she was in a car, and an exaggerated startle reflex. She was skittish about being a passenger in a car, and when her peers were getting drivers' permits and learning how to drive, she began having nightmares, reliving the car accident by night, and feeling anxious and restricting food by day. She also avowed that she never wanted to get a drivers' license.

Body Dysmorphic Disorder

Body Dysmorphic Disorder (BDD) is diagnosed when an individual develops obsessive dissatisfaction with a specific part of her body. This can co-occur with anorexia or manifest without eating disorder features. Behaviors that are common to both disorders include preoccupation with appearance, camouflaging body shape and size, dieting, excessive exercise, and frequent comparison with others. The key difference is that anorexics wish to become thinner overall, whereas those with BDD focus on specific perceived body defects. Anorexics often direct their body-hatred toward the parts of their body associated with sexual development of a womanly figure, including size of hips and thighs or roundness of the abdomen. But their primary quest is to shrink in size and remake their bodies into stick thin figures. In BDD, sufferers seek to reconfigure particular perceived deformities rather than total body size.

Several sophisticated testing methods have been developed to increase the accuracy of diagnosis of BDD. The Body Dysmorphic Disorder Examination is a semi-structured interview that measures symptoms of negative body image as well as diagnosing specific BDD characteristics. Both anorexia and BDD produce suffering; even more serious is the plight of those in whom both disorders occur. One study in 2007 reported that 9 percent of those with BDD may also suffer from anorexia (Adams et al., 2007, p.27).

With adolescents who are plagued by distressing concerns about appearance, it can be difficult to determine whether early symptoms of *either* anorexia or BDD are present. The psychological, social and physical changes of adolescence render teens particularly prone to develop either disorder. Some new screening tools are being developed to assist diagnosis and to detect when a serious problem is present.

Bulimia Nervosa

Bulimia nervosa is a serious eating disorder that can develop in adolescence or early adulthood and often originates from causes similar to those which contribute to anorexia: biological factors, familial issues, social pressures, and trauma. In bulimia, the individual binges and purges to control her weight, but generally is of normal to slightly higher than normal weight. It is estimated that as many as 50 percent of anorexics develop bulimic symptoms (Herzog and Eddy, 2007, p.12). Bulimia differs from the bingeing-and-purging subtype of anorexia in that the bulimic individual does not possess the other symptoms characteristic of anorexia: maintenance of a low weight, intense fear of gaining weight, and amenorrhea (cessation of menstrual periods). More females than males develop bulimia.

Diagnostic criteria for bulimia nervosa include recurrent episodes of binge eating which are characterized both by consuming larger than normal amounts of food and by feeling out of control while bingeing; recurrent inappropriate compensatory behavior to prevent weight gain (e.g. excessive exercise, fasting, vomiting); and being "unduly influenced" by body shape and weight (*DSM IV-TR*, 2000, p.594). There are two subtypes of bulimia, purging and non-purging.

Some people question why a particular individual develops anorexia rather than bulimia, or vice versa. The answer is complex and probably involves more factors than those we currently understand. Briefly, genetics plays a significant role: personality traits of anorexics are not the same as those of bulimics and there are differences in biochemistry between those suffering from the two disorders. Also, the family, peer and cultural pressures and personal experiences of each individual are unique.

Alcohol or Drug Addiction

Addiction to alcohol or drugs can co-exist with anorexia. Because of the calorie content of alcohol, anorexics are less commonly addicted to alcohol than to some kind of appetite-suppressing drug. Addiction to some appetite-suppressants can induce anorexic symptoms: when an individual reduces her food intake and loses weight, she can trigger the physiological starvation response in which weight loss creates anxiety about weight gain which leads her to further restrict eating. Conversely, sometimes individuals who already exhibit anorexic symptoms will turn to use of appetite suppressants to aid weight reduction.

The most commonly used appetite-suppressants are cocaine and amphetamines, especially methamphetamine, which can be ingested orally, injected or smoked. Methamphetamine addiction causes rapid weight loss and leads to very serious physical deterioration. Meth has been called the "poor man's cocaine," because it is cheaper and more readily available than cocaine. Oxycontin, a barbiturate, also has the effect of appetite reduction and the potential for creating anorexic symptoms.

When substance addiction is present with anorexia, the substance addiction generally needs to be addressed first, and the drug use stopped, before the anorexic symptoms can be treated. If the drug use continues, it will continue to recreate the substrate for the anorexic symptoms, and treatment of these symptoms will be futile.

Personality Disorders

Personality disorders are disturbances characterized by a set of pathological personality traits, which are ingrained, habitual patterns of psychological functioning. Clinicians have discovered that a portion of clients with anorexia also suffer from a personality disorder. The presence of a personality disorder complicates treatment; both the anorexia and the personality disorder need to be addressed.

The personality disorders most commonly found to accompany the restricting type of anorexia are obsessive-compulsive personality disorder (OCD) and avoidant personality disorder (AVPD). Borderline personality disorder (BPD) and dependent personality disorders (DPD) most commonly co-occur with the binge eating/purging subtype of anorexia (Sansone and Sansone, 2007, p.84).

Briefly, OCD (also mentioned above under anxiety disorders) is characterized by perfectionism, rigidity, measurement of self-worth by productivity, and preoccupation with being perceived as self-disciplined. The individual is often controlled by perceived rules and imagined expectations of authority figures. Individuals with OCD are slow to form a relationship with a therapist because they fear having their world disrupted by chaos (Dennis and Sansone, 1997, p.445). Individuals with AVPD fear disapproval, ridicule and rejection by others, and tend to be lonely as a result. They struggle with low self-esteem, are hypervigilant to self-criticism, and experience significant self-doubt. Early therapy is particularly difficult for those with AVPD because they are very mistrusting and fear judgment. An avoidant anorexic has considerable difficulty developing supportive relationships (Dennis and Sansone, 1997, p.443).

Individuals with BPD exhibit impulsivity and a tendency toward self-destructive behaviors. Those with BPD often have difficulty with day-to-day functioning as well as with work and social interpersonal interactions. They have particularly low self-esteem and a core belief in their "badness." Also, they can have difficulty regulating feelings and may vacillate between overemotionality and being withdrawn. They generally have a chronic feeling of emptiness and an unstable identity. When an anorexic has borderline features, many anorexic symptoms, including tendency towards depression and engaging in self-harming behaviors, are aggravated (Dennis and Sansone, 1997, pp.438–439).

DPD is characterized by a pervasive sense of inferiority, submissiveness, helplessness, and self-effacing behaviors coupled by a tremendous fear of abandonment. Dependent individuals are self-sacrificing, passive participants in life. They magnify their weaknesses and belittle their abilities. They shy away from independence. Anorexia aids their avoidance of separation by reinforcing their dependence on parents or care-givers (Dennis and Sansone, 1997, pp.444–445).

5

Some Attributes of Anorexia

Perfectionism

I love flowers and gardens. The richness of color and texture, the beauty of nature, I find irresistible. Bright red geraniums, interspersed with coral and pink blossoms, lift my heart. But in the past, when the geraniums I've planted attracted budworms, I felt devastated. It's not just that I was frustrated and disappointed; I had failed. I had failed to create a garden that looked picture perfect. The evidence was clear — the colorful blooms had been decimated — and the fact that the plants I had tended, watered and fertilized now housed budworms proved that the garden was flawed and defective. And this imperfection in my garden was a direct reflection on me, the gardener. While budworms are a fact of nature, a part of the natural cycle of life and a nuisance to most geranium-growers, in my garden, infected plants were a glaring sign of my deficiency.

So it is with the trait of perfectionism: any endeavor the anorexic undertakes is another opportunity for her to excel — or fail. It hardly matters how insignificant the task is in the scheme of life. It could be composing a note for a birthday card or performing a dance recital; making her bed or graduating from school with honors; limiting her food intake or losing weight. Any outcome short of perfection she deems a failure, and a failure not only in completing the particular project, but a failure of herself as a person. Because perfection is unattainable, failure is inevitable. Thus the anorexic continually accrues more evidence to confirm that she is imperfect and never good enough.

Perfectionism — especially to such an extreme — is not consistent with a cohesive sense of Self. Someone with a solid Self does not need to shore up her identity by seeking unattainable ideals. A person with a consistent internal identity is not caught in a paradox of wanting and not wanting success; she does not ride a constant roller coaster of craving confirmation of her worth and then crashing when confirmation does not materialize. Perfectionism is part of the mask behind which the anorexic hides. In her pursuit of perfection, she has created an indelible definition of herself as the one who can't succeed. How, then, could anyone expect her to be responsible, to manage her own life, to take charge of her destiny? Perfectionism provides a cocoon of helplessness. If she can convince others of her inadequacy, they will keep their distance and erase their expectations of her.

The trait of perfectionism is central to the identity of most anorexics. In this chapter I will outline some of the clinical underpinnings of this trait, and then describe some aspects of my own personal struggle with perfectionism, both as an anorexic and in recovery.

Some of my views — as well as the views of clinicians in general — regarding the origins of perfectionism, and of anorexia, have changed in the years since I wrote the original edition of this book. Twenty-five years ago, clinicians focused on the disturbance in infancy and early childhood of the mother-child, or caretaker-child, relationship in the etiology of anorexia and of many other psychological disorders. Today, there continues to be interest and advancement in our knowledge of the attachment process in early childhood and the impact of attachment style on an individual's psychological adjustment and relationships later in life. In addition, however, there has been considerable research in neurobiology and more understanding that there is a genetic contribution to many disorders. It is now understood that perfectionism is an inborn, biologically-based personality trait that is common in those who develop anorexia.

The origins of anorexia are clearly more complex than anyone grasped two decades ago, and our knowledge about the etiology of the disorder continues to expand. What I will include here is an overview, summarizing some hypotheses about what can set the stage for perfectionism in anorexia. Other views exist, and there is still much more for all of us to learn.

Clinical Background

The anorexic is constantly driven by her quest for perfection. She must excel at whatever she does; yet no matter how well she does, she never believes her performance is good enough. The anorexic expresses her drive to be perfect in her expectation of how she should look: she is never thin enough. Any hint of a curve or suspicion of excess flesh is proof that she is too fat. No matter how much control she exerts over her eating, letting one small morsel of food pass her lips is tantamount to failure and loss of control.

The anorexic is her own worst critic, and praise from others has no impact on her. Criticism, no matter how slight, will both enrage her and reinforce her belief that she is a failure. To the anorexic, it is not her performance of one small task that is being criticized; her very self is being humiliated and scorned.

The struggle for perfection in all she does reflects the anorexic's lack of self-esteem and her belief that her worth can be measured only in terms of her accomplishments. She sets impossible goals for herself and is invariably dissatisfied with her achievements and disappointed in herself. Her performance, flawless though it may appear to others, is to her imperfect. The anorexic's continual self-deprecation precludes anyone else's criticism from being significant to her. She is in control of her own chastisement and will always criticize herself more severely than will anyone else. In this way, she exerts power over others and undermines their impact on her. She will surpass anyone's criticism with something more negative and devastating. Compliments and positive statements she shrugs off as insincere. She believes others are as critical as she is but they do not tell the truth about what they think. The anorexic doesn't trust other people and does not believe what they say.

What the anorexic really fears is rejection. By establishing a measured distance between herself and others and by maintaining control over the impact of what others say to her, the anorexic avoids the risk of rejection. If she trusts other people, allows them to be close enough to her to see her flaws and believes what they tell her, they may scorn, humiliate or reject her. Rather than make herself vulnerable to their criticism and expose herself to the possibility of humiliation, or risk the pain and loss which rejection would entail, the anorexic isolates herself from others and takes charge of her own deprecation.

In some cases, the anorexic's lack of self-esteem, her striving towards perfection and her distrust of others, begins in infancy when her mother does not respond to her with the warmth and nurturing an infant needs in order to feel loved. Her basic needs may be attended to — she may be fed and changed and bathed — but there can be a superficial and agitated quality to the caretaking if her mother is insecure and anxious. In these cases, the infant may not receive the touching, stroking and holding from her mother that gives the infant a sense of security and well-being. The infant then lacks the foundation from which to develop a sense of her own importance — she does not believe she is inherently all right, and her development of self-worth is impaired. Furthermore, in this scenario, as the infant matures and is no longer always so cute and adorable, she learns that she is taken care of not in response to her own demands but as a result of her doing something that pleases her mother. The infant begins to experience that love is conditional and that she must prove herself worthy of attention; she must perform to get the affection that she craves. Since as a baby and young child she rarely receives unconditional warmth and mothering, she learns that she does not merit love herself, but that if she is pleasing, her behavior may be rewarded with attention.

In these situations, the infant gradually learns to deny her own needs, physical and emotional, since these do not receive a response. Instead, she behaves in the ways she believes her mother wants her to, and she develops unrealistic standards for what is expected of her. No matter how well she performs, her behavior still is not rewarded with the love and caring from her mother that she seeks; whatever response she gets never addresses her deep yearning to be loved for herself. Understandably, the infant never wants again to risk experiencing the pain she feels as a result of the loss of her mother's love. By not trusting other people and keeping them at bay, she avoids exposing herself to the possibility of closeness and its seemingly inevitable consequence, the devastation of rejection.

By the age of two, the normal child asserts herself and begins to develop a sense of herself as a separate being with limits and boundaries that are fostered and reinforced by her parents. However, in many cases, the future anorexic refrains from this self-assertion. She continues to conform to her mother's expectations and to behave in the sweet and adaptable manner her mother prefers. By anticipating her mother's reactions, she robs her mother of an opportunity to set limits and control her. Instead, she in essence establishes her own internal set of standards, criticisms and punishments, which are far more severe than the judgments and boundaries that would be levied by her mother. She thereby takes charge of her own discipline so as to avoid the humiliation, anger and rejection that might ensue from not meeting her mother's standards. At the same time, she avoids establishing a sense of herself as a being independent from her mother and continues to behave in accordance with her exaggerated view of what she thinks her mother expects.

Sometimes both parents of a perfectionist child may be anxious, insecure perfectionists themselves (McNear, 1981, p.296). They respond to the child's inevitable mistakes as though they are a reflection on their abilities as parents: "If Suzie fails, it is because I am a terrible mother." The child then feels a demand to never fail, lest she hurt her parents. And with each task the child undertakes, the stakes are higher: "She thought she was a bad mother when I.... Just think how bad she will feel if I mess this one up!" As the child grows up, she becomes more anxious about the consequences of failure and more determined to succeed. But new undertakings involve greater risk — risk of failure, and hence of hurting her mother, and of causing her mother to love her less. The child learns to not take chances or expose herself to risk.

In these situations, the unresolved symbiosis of the child with her mother, as well as the thwarted boundary-setting and endless vying for control, surface in adolescence when the anorexic struggles to separate from her mother. Lacking a sense of her own identity, and both unprepared and terrified to make the break from her mother, she uses the control she exerts over her body weight to achieve a sense of autonomy. She religiously controls her food intake and exercises fanatically, constantly setting her standards higher and carrying her quest for thinness to greater extremes. Malnutrition and her own brain physiology prevail and she loses objectivity about how thin she has become. The struggle is perpetuated because no matter how emaciated she becomes, she is convinced she is never thin enough. Even in this area where she excels in her ability to perform — to starve herself — she fails. She sets ever-higher goals, and still she is too fat. No matter how thin she becomes, she does not feel loved, and she is not thin enough to satisfy her own impossible ideal of perfection. In her mind, attainment of true perfection will be signified solely by bestowal of her mother's love.

When her mother's love is not forthcoming, the daughter's only satisfaction resides in knowing that she is in charge — that it is *she*, not her mother, who controls her body, and it is she who sets her own standards. The hunger, cold and exhaustion she experiences are not as painful to her as the terrifying threat of rejection, the specter of failing to meet her mother's expectations and being denied her mother's love. Maybe she couldn't please her mother or be perfect in the other ways she has tried, but at this she can excel: she will be the thinnest.

Personal Story

When I was preparing to write about anorexia in the 1980's, I became aware that I had not come to terms with my own perfectionist principles. Given my own experience of anorexia and recovery, I thought I should to be able to write a definitive account of anorexia, its cause and treatment. Of course this expectation was unrealistic, but at the time, I was afraid I would fail to meet this imaginary ideal, and that horrific consequences would result. What if I wrote something that was insufficient or inaccurate? Would I be rejected by my peers, my teachers, or those who had supported my recovery?

As I read what various other people had written about the disorder, including a master's thesis by a former anorexic, and accounts of the etiology and treatment of anorexia by both therapists and researchers, I became scared that I couldn't match their quality and insight, or write anything new or original about the disorder. I became convinced that whatever I wrote was not going to be as good as what had already been written. Fear of ridicule and rejection immobilized me. I became depressed, and did not want to read or write anything further about anorexia.

When my adviser suggested that I have parts of my manuscript reviewed by a psychiatrist and a therapist, I balked. I was certain these experts would see only my flaws and my shortcomings. They were bound to criticize what I had written, and I would be humiliated. I wanted to run away and hide until I had read everything that had ever been written about anorexia and I had crafted the definitive book on the subject. At that point, I could announce, "It's finished. You may not like it. I hate it, I know it's awful, but it's the best I could do, even though it's not good enough." I would deflect any potential criticism with my own unforgiving judgment and no one else would be able to censure it — or me — more harshly. I could not be rejected or humiliated because I had already condemned myself.

It was only when I redefined the project and viewed it differently that I could continue. I decided that my task was to synthesize what I knew and had read about anorexia and to write my own perspective on the disorder, not to compose a comprehensive account of anorexia. Instead of wasting energy trying to be perfect or mourning the fact that I wasn't, if I stayed on track with my goal and did my best, I would accomplish what I intended.

Sometimes when I began to write a new section or read another article, my old thinking patterns reemerged and again I thought, "This will never be good enough. Why am I bothering to write it?" And once more, I would stop working on the project. Eventually, however, I realized that I would not solve my problems by avoiding them. Either I would postpone facing this predicament until I finally decided to write, or feel like a failure because I had given up. I also recognized that if I gave up, the same problems— depression, competitive thinking, fear of criticism and rejection, striving towards unrealistic goals— would surface elsewhere and interfere with other parts of my life. I was not willing to let myself be derailed and pay the price of letting these demons haunt and control me after all the time and energy I had invested in treatment, and the amount of my life I had sacrificed to anorexia. So in 1982, I abandoned my perfectionist ideals and wrote my own account of the disorder, the first edition of this book.

Twenty-five years later, in embarking on a revision of the book, I have no illusion about writing a definitive account of anorexia or of its treatment, and I am thankful that I feel no desire to try. I have established more realistic goals. My plan is simply to update the original book, to review some of what clinicians have learned about the origins and treatment of anorexia in the intervening years, and to highlight what I have discovered in this time through my own continuing process of recovery and growth as a therapist. When I remind myself of my goals, it helps me to stay focused. I don't need to consider the numerous other possibilities or think about what I'm *not* doing. I need to be competent, thorough and accurate — not perfect.

Competition

With trepidation, I entered the room where several women were already seated, chatting and sipping tea from dainty china cups. It was November 1983; my book had been published six months earlier and by some twist of fate, I had been invited to a meeting of local women authors. My stomach was in a knot, my body had turned to ice, and I knew I didn't belong here. My book wasn't famous; it wasn't an engrossing 400-page novel or a profound inquiry into the origins and evolution of Indian philosophy. In fact, it was a farce — I wasn't as "cured" as I had thought when I'd written the book, or I wouldn't be in such a state right now. My mind had gone to that familiar place of self-torment and I was comparing myself to everyone there. I looked around; I wasn't sure I recognized anyone. That didn't matter. Before anyone had even spoken, I mentally listed at least five reasons why every other woman present deserved to be there and I didn't. I desperately wanted to turn and flee: "Oh my gosh! I think I left my stove on!" or "I feel a migraine coming on!" Should I — could I — do the polite thing and sit down, smile, and somehow act like I belonged? Or was the right thing really to leave because I truly *didn't* belong?

As I berated myself for having come, fate intervened. One woman spilled her tea and ran to the kitchen for a towel. I followed her and spied a back door off the kitchen. I slipped out quickly, not caring if anyone noticed or not. It was so clear to me: I had no right to be there.

This kind of comparison continually haunts the anorexic. Years earlier, even if I had had something to write about, I would not have let myself write. And years later, I doubtless would have felt anxious, but probably could have stood my ground. But at that time, although I had managed to write the book, I lacked a center strong enough and an identity cohesive enough to connect with anything comforting inside. Similar circumstances might well make anyone feel anxious and stressed, but competing to lose, while providing a safe haven, could not help me master that situation. Nor could I learn, or grow, or interact with others with any serenity. For me, with the task of building a Self still very much in process, my means of coping was to hide.

Competition and perfectionism go hand-in-hand. Striving for perfection is fostered by competition, and losing a competition reinforces the sense of failure endemic to perfectionism. The degree to which the tendency towards either may be genetic in origin is yet to be determined. And the extent to which early attachment style and childhood circumstances are contributors is equally unclear.

Clinical Background

The anorexic typically develops a highly competitive frame of reference, or way of looking at the world. She approaches tasks, people, and every imaginable process as warranting rivalry. And in each case, she believes there will be a winner and a loser, and that inevitably she will lose. In some cases, these perpetual competitions probably originate in the infant's struggle with her mother over whose needs are going to be met: those of the infant, hungry or wet, or of the mother, perhaps preoccupied with other concerns or attempting to accomplish a variety of chores while attending to the baby. Some infants in this situation may conclude that caretaking is scarce, of limited availability, and attainable only through competition with the mother.

Developmentally, a two-year-old child vies with her parent for control. In a healthy outcome, when the parent lovingly yet firmly sets clear boundaries, the child learns to distinguish acceptable from unacceptable behaviors. However, sometimes the future anorexic never undergoes a true control struggle with her mother and over-adapts before two years of age. She remains ever pleasing, suppressing her own needs, never testing limits or engaging in the typical two-year-old's battles. Then, as the girl grows up, she continually relives the unresolved competition with her mother, both in how she sees herself and in how she views the rest of the world. She perceives situations and relationships as struggles in which opponents — or conflicting events, or tasks that need to be done, or people whose requests of her are incompatible with her own desires — are pitted against each other with only one victor possible.

This inner competition creates extreme internal conflict for the anorexic, compounding her difficulty in making decisions. She heaps on this the burden of harsh self-torment — she *should* be able to make a decision. Even the simple day-to-day activities — visiting with her friends, playing outside or puttering in her room — she views competitively, knowing that in doing any one thing, she will miss out on something else. And the thing she misses out on is the one about which she will obsess, flagellating herself for having made the wrong choice. Thus decisions about what to do become onerous and cataclysmic. There is no developed Self inside with clear preferences, no solid center from which to draw guidance, no comforting core to provide consolation. Whether the scenario includes her not choosing among options, leaving someone else to choose, or stalling until the situation develops and no choice remains, in the end she inevitably loses and misses opportunities by not defining what she wants. Her indecision becomes fodder for more harsh self-torment, as she berates herself for "failing" to make a choice.

In her relationships with peers, the anorexic generally assumes that the other person is in some way better than she is. Often she is scared to form relationships with other people lest someone notice her glaring flaws. At the same time, she can be angry and envious, although rarely overtly (and perhaps without recognizing the feelings herself) because everyone else possesses some quality that renders him or her "better" than she is. The anorexic is often particularly competitive with other women because in these relationships, the unresolved conflict with her mother reemerges, as well as her old feelings of anger and fear — she is angry at having to compete, and scared that no matter what she does, she will not feel adequate. The anorexic often views other females as having some elusive trait, "the ability to be a woman," which she lacks, and which enables them to make it in the world while she cannot. Upon casually meeting another woman, the anorexic may mentally tabulate the ways in which the other woman surpasses her. Meanwhile, she gropes frantically to retrieve her own flimsy self-definition, desperately seeking a way to come out of the encounter without hating herself more. The sole attribute the anorexic can flaunt is her thinness. But she is gripped in a deadly competition with herself about her weight, and never thinks she is sufficiently thin; thus, she dismisses any advantage she may have in this arena. There is no way for the anorexic to emerge from this situation without feeling she is the loser.

Intimate relationships with men she generally views as competitive because she believes that only one person can get what he or she wants. The anorexic who develops a relationship with a man while her issues of competition for caretaking remain unresolved is likely to undergo repeated conflicts around whose needs are going to be met. In the anorexic's frame of reference, it is the other person who always succeeds at getting what he wants; she is never the one who wins. Thus she frequently adapts to her mate's demands, and then feels angry and bitter at not getting what she wanted. For the anorexic, compromise is the same as defeat. What matters to her is not what is accomplished in arriving at an agreement, but what is lost in the settlement.

When the anorexic is involved in a love relationship, she is often jealous of her partner's friendships with other men or women, believing that her relationship with her mate is somehow inferior to his other relationships. In addition, she believes his other relationships deprive her of his attention. She is angry at her mate, as well as at his friends, for forcing her to compete with them. In the end, she believes it is inevitable that he will recognize her shortcomings and leave her for someone better.

She also may act from the belief that she does not deserve her mate's attention because he is male and powerful and has many attributes that render him superior to her. She may idealize his masculinity, athletic ability, income and intelligence. Having defined him as superior, she competes with him, continually berating herself and remarking on her own inferiority. At the same time, she can be angry about being one-down in the relationship, and may seek subtle ways to reverse the score. Her constant competitiveness ultimately undermines the relationship, either because she is hostile and bitter, or because she exasperates her mate with demands for reassurance that she is adequate and loved. Until she is willing to give up her competitive frame of reference, to acknowledge her own positive attributes as well as those of others, and to interact with people without ranking their personal qualities against her own, she will be unhappy and unsuccessful in forming relationships.

The anorexic's decision not to eat can be an expression of her competition, indirectly with others and directly with her mother, to be thinner, and hence "better" in some indefinable way. Often, the mother of an anorexic frequently frets about her own weight. The mother may in fact be a normal weight or only a few pounds heavier than her ideal, but she is dissatisfied with her weight. Furthermore, food is often a common currency in the family of an anorexic. Conversation often focuses on food and meals, and food and weight become natural arenas for expression of competition and control. The anorexic's decision to be thin — thinner than her mother — is one way in which she can compete and win. If her mother wants to be thin, the anorexic daughter determines to be thinner; by comparison her mother will be "fat." Yet she still fears rejection and must please her mother. Her mother wants her to eat, so she must give the appearance of eating; meanwhile, she rebels covertly and disguises the fact that she is not eating.

The anorexic thus experiences a continual conflict between pleasing her mother (eating) and doing what she is determined to do (not eat). She escalates the competition to an extreme either/or conflict and believes that eating and being thin are in direct opposition: she cannot both eat and be thin. Her emotional issues distort any facts about how to manage weight sensibly by eating somewhat smaller quantities or lower calorie foods. She overrides her hunger and subjects herself to starvation not because she has no appetite or doesn't want food, but because eating provokes in her such tremendous conflict.

Every facet of the decision as to when, what or how much to eat then becomes fraught with more conflict: "If I eat now, I can't go running. But if I go running before eating, I'll be too tired to run very far." Or, "If I eat two grapes, I can't eat a tomato. I want the two grapes, but they have more calories than the tomato, and no B vitamins, so I should eat the tomato." Or, "I need to eat protein to build muscle. But there's no food with protein that doesn't also have fat. So I can't eat protein." And sometimes, "I ate too much." "I'm getting so fat." And even, if she has bulimic tendencies, "I've got to get rid of what I ate so I won't get fat."

Sometimes, competition with specific categories of girls or women — models, ballerinas, gymnasts—motivates the anorexic's descent into emaciation. In an article entitled "So Thin She May Disappear," journalist Cheryl Lavin referred to an adolescent model, Tracy, who had concluded that "if thin got you attention, she would be thin. If thinner got you more attention, she would be thinner. And if she wanted the most attention, she would be the thinnest" (Lavin, 1981, p.5).

Anorexics compete most strenuously with other anorexics. If two anorexics are together in a high school class, a ballet company, or a hospital ward, the competition becomes vicious. No anorexic can tolerate anyone being thinner than herself. And always, the competition is for some imagined accolade that will be the anorexic's reward for being the thinnest—a yearned-for recognition and attention powerful enough to eclipse her deficits in self-esteem and self-worth.

Personal Story

Within my own family, competition was rife and family dynamics fostered the development of a competitive frame of reference. Statements such as "Boys are smarter than girls" and "Your father is smarter than I am" were frequent refrains from my mother when I was growing up. Certain privileges were incumbent on being a boy in my family. My grandfather taught his grandsons but not his granddaughters how to play chess, a decision my parents condoned. My brothers were permitted to skate or ride their bikes, but I was admonished not to engage in physical activities because I might hurt myself. I was born last of three children, with a brother two years older and a twin brother born eight minutes before me. My parents flaunted those eight minutes. Furthermore, from a young age, I remember my parents saying that my twin brother was the bright one, the smart one, and the one who was going to go far. He was indeed born with an exceptionally high IQ, and intelligence was highly esteemed in my family. At report card time, I did well but generally my grades weren't as good as my twin brother's. In my parents' disappointment at my performance there was always the intimation, "We know you did the best you could, you're just not as smart as your brother." At the same time, there was always the expectation that I should try harder to please my parents, to aim for perfection even though, since I was not that bright, and a girl besides, I would never succeed. I had to compete just to try to hold my own, although it was clear at the outset that I would lose. Furthermore, there was no acknowledgment of any strengths I might have possessed.

In the course of my early treatment for anorexia, I learned that not everyone viewed the world the way I did, as a battlefield rife with skirmishes between winners and losers with everyone reveling in others' faults so that he could declare himself the winner (or, in my case, the loser). I was taught that competitions had goals and were undertaken for a purpose, and that I needed to think about what I wanted from competing. If I could achieve the outcome I sought by competing, then competing was valid. However, if there was no goal that could be attained competitively, then maintaining a competitive frame of reference was counter-productive and I needed to find a different, more constructive way to pursue that end. For instance, competing with a friend over who remembered more scenes from a movie was pointless, unless there was an exam on the topic. If the purpose was to share experiences of the movie, then the point was simply for each of us to talk about what we liked.

I began to understand that by viewing my needs and wants competitively, I remained angry at the people I considered to be my competitors, as well as scared that I wouldn't get what I wanted. This tended to make me less than charming to hang out with, and ultimately my behavior made other people angry with me. Naturally, these people were even less inclined to say yes the next time I invited them to spend time with me. One person from my treatment program complained that I always seemed to be in a bad mood when things didn't go my way.

The program staff suggested that I play competitive games, and learn to play them to win, which helped me to focus competition in areas where I could use it productively. Initially, I agreed to play at least one game per day of backgammon and to win at least 42 percent of the games I played per week, which was more than I could win by chance alone. My game repertoire later was expanded to include cribbage. I agreed to play ten games per week of either cribbage or backgammon and to win a specified percentage of the games.

At first, I didn't want to play games to win. I was accustomed to playing games poorly, disliking them and losing. However, since the consequence of disappointing my therapist was more frightening than losing games, I learned to play to win, to engage in the drama and eventually even to derive pleasure from the pursuit of victory. Although I persisted in using a competitive frame of reference in many areas — as in scheduling social time when the time of events conflicted and, most painfully, comparing my achievements to those of other people — I nonetheless learned a socially acceptable way to compete by playing games.

In the intervening years, I have become acutely aware of the self-defeating and hostile nature of my internal competitions. Through exploration of my competitive tendencies in psychotherapy, I recognize now that I use competition to manage and defend against feelings of anger, fear and envy, and to ensure a predicable outcome: that I will feel bad. When I find I am comparing myself to another person, I have now learned to stop and ask myself what I am feeling and why. Generally, I become competitive when I decide that the other person has something I wish I had. It may be something material — a spectacular home or shiny new car — or it may be something intangible, such as some skill, talent, or ability. In that moment when something about their life overshadows my own, I feel angry, envious and scared that I won't ever get what they have. I bemoan the fact that life is not fair.

Fortunately, psychotherapy has helped me find an upside to acknowledging my feelings. Envy signals my desire to go after what the other person has that I don't. The other person can serve as a model. Mobilizing my anger can furnish the aggressive energy needed to pursue a goal. My fear generally dissipates when I begin to consider my options. Surprisingly, the more I think about what it is that I envy, the less I want the other person's version of it. Rarely do I actually want their house or car; I just like the idea of having a bigger house or shinier car, but without the payments or the responsibility of taking care of them. Nor do I generally want their exact talent or skill, since probably it fits their personality better than mine. What I really want is my own talent or ability, but again without the responsibility required — the investment of time or energy to hone that skill.

In the course of my recovery, the 12-Step program Overeaters Anonymous introduced me to a couple of slogans that have also helped me resist competing. One is "Compare, despair." This is so true! Comparison, if unchecked, inevitably leads me directly into suffering and feeling bad. Halting the competition before it starts can prevent me from sinking into the pit of "I'm bad" or "There's something wrong with me." Another helpful slogan is, "Don't compare your insides to someone else's outsides." This reminds me that when I am beginning to envy someone else, I don't really know what is going on inside that person — how they are feeling, what they are grappling with, how this supposed gift, ability or possession I resent is affecting them. I know I am not alone in creating stories of how someone else's life is better than mine — but seldom do these fictional versions take into account the ways the other person, too, is wrestling with feelings and problems.

The practice of writing a gratitude list has also helped me manage my competitive tendencies. This idea was suggested to me through my 12-Step affiliation, but it has other proponents as well. In competing to lose, by definition I am maligning my situation or myself and idealizing others. Writing a gratitude list forces me to refocus my attention on myself and what I am thankful for. Redirecting my thinking from negative to positive can then help relieve my feelings of anger and envy. This has been a welcome and useful tool, and an antidote to these destructive feelings.

As I have learned ways to manage my harmful competitive leanings, and to address what is underneath my need to compete, I have realized how competition has been a deterrent to the development of my Self. Focusing on other people — on what they have and I don't — is not an act of self-acceptance. And if I am not in the process of accepting myself, I am unlikely to be building a cohesive internal structure that could be a source of comfort and strength. Quite the opposite: I am actively defeating that purpose and undermining myself. And as long as I resort to feeling bad instead of exploring and understanding my own feelings, I deprive myself of self-knowledge. Feelings are a core part of one's identity. They are a person's own unique response to the environment, and they provide important information and insight for self-understanding. By learning to handle my competitive tendencies through exploring my feelings and understanding their meaning, I have created a stronger core and a more cohesive identity, both important ingredients in developing Self.

Unresolved Grief

When I was ten years old, my favorite grandmother died. My recollection of the circumstances is somewhat hazy. Early one morning while my father was away on a business trip, I was sleeping in my mother's bed. The phone rang, startling both my mother and me. It was my grandfather calling to say that his wife (my mother's mother) had just died in an operation to remove some abdominal cancer.

I remember feeling scared and lost. I didn't know what to do to help my mother, who was shaking with tears, or what to do with my own feelings. My mother needed to leave that morning to help arrange for the funeral, and my father curtailed his trip and returned early the next day. Meanwhile, friends and neighbors pitched in to cover for my parents; my brothers and I still needed to go to school and have meals. However, my mother had asked me "to help," and I interpreted that to mean she expected me to take care of the situation in any way that I could. I took charge of packing school lunches for my brothers and myself, making plans for dinner and getting laundry done. But I resented my mother's leaving. I didn't know what to do with the ache inside and I didn't really know how "to help" the rest of the family.

My grandmother was my favorite person in the world. I had loved spending Christmas holidays with her, sitting on her lap when my grandfather took us on long drives through the country, helping her bake cakes and cookies. I held the eggbeaters, thick with frosting, while she poured frosting from the bowl and he told me she didn't know how she got along without me.

I didn't go to the funeral; it was in New Jersey, a thousand miles away from our home in Illinois. I stayed home, and in about a week my mother returned. After that, I would spend a week or two each summer with my grandfather, and cook, shop and prepare meals for him just like I remembered my grandmother doing, using all her lovely flowered china, a separate salad plate — which was square and had the same pattern as the dinner plates — her cut glass stemware and the big glasses with pictures of Christmas trees on them. But I felt hollow and empty and longed for my grandmother. I couldn't talk to anyone about it, and nobody else talked about it, either. I felt so small and ineffective and incompetent because there was nothing I could do to replace my grandmother — not for my grandfather, not for my mother, not for me. My mother was so sad. I wanted to comfort her, but didn't know how.

It was a few months after my grandmother died that my problems with food began. I remember that I had learned to cook, but I was suddenly interested in feeding other people, not myself. One time I made French toast for my twin brother — not a piece or two but half a dozen pieces. I love French toast, but I didn't eat any. He finally told me to stop; he couldn't finish all the pieces that I'd cooked. Another time I asked my girlfriend, Helen, to come over to have lunch and play games. I had set up a card table and stacked all the board games my family owned in the center of the table. When Helen arrived, I told her I was going to make us sandwiches. I fixed her a huge sandwich, piled high with cheese and lettuce and mayonnaise, and I put a few pieces of lettuce on my plate. Somehow I slipped my plate behind the board games, handing her a plate bearing a five-inch high sandwich, and told her to sit down and eat. She couldn't see what I was eating (and not eating), but it was immensely satisfying to me that she was eating. Maybe I wanted to make everyone else fat so I could be the thin one.

Like me, other anorexics may have emotional issues from unresolved grief. Unmourned loss may not play a role in the etiology of anorexia for all individuals, but even those who have not experienced major loss are likely to have difficulty with expressing and managing most feelings. Most anorexics, I believe, experience an inner void, an emotional cavern in which there is no connection to inner sensations, feelings or self-understanding.

Clinical Background

Unresolved grief or loss appears to be a significant factor in some cases of anorexia. When this is an issue, sometimes it may originate from a disturbance in the mother-child attachment that occurs in late infancy. In the first few months of infancy, the mother-child dyad gives solace to the mother, and generally the mother can dependably soothe her infant. The baby relies totally on her mother, and the mother is able to respond and effectively calm her child. The mother is reasonably comforting and consistent in attending to her child, and the child senses the mother's love and caring.

However, at the age of eight or nine months, the infant becomes more demanding, less appealing, and not so easy to console. A mother whose own mothering was erratic, or who is stressed and having significant problems coping, can have difficulty with her baby's negative emotions. At this stage, she can relax when her baby smiles and acts cute, but gets uncomfortable and on edge if the baby contorts her face and cries for things. The mother may begin to respond to her infant less reliably and only when her child's behavior is pleasing. The infant may sense a shift in her mother's attentiveness and feel a withdrawal of her mother's love. At this point, the infant may experience a tragic loss: her mother is not there for her. This loss can leave the infant with a profound sense of sadness or grief. The baby's expressions of anger and grief do not elicit comfort from her mother; her mother doesn't like an angry baby. The mother may either ignore her baby's displays of anger or get angry herself. The infant then may learn to please her mother to get the attention she craves, and to stifle the expressions she intuits will upset her mother and make her mother grow more distant. Throughout infancy, childhood and adolescence, the growing girl may then continue to behave in ways that will earn her mother's smiles and elicit nurturance. In doing so, she denies and suppresses the feelings of anger and grief that cause her mother to further withdraw. She hides the pain that feels unsafe to show.

British psychiatrist John Bowlby and American psychologist Mary Ainsworth have done groundbreaking work in the field of attachment and substantiated the effect of different attachment styles on a child's development. While a few statements here can hardly do justice to the years of research conducted by these clinicians and their followers, it appears that certain attachment styles are likely to impede a child's capacity to self-soothe, express needs, and perform other developmental tasks that render the child capable of self-reliance. A "disorganized" attachment style, in which a parent is alternately present and not present, will confuse a child, who will then become overly independent or overly dependent. An "ambivalent" attachment style will produce a child with severe abandonment and rejection issues. A child who experiences an "insecure" attachment, characterized by dependence, abandonment or rejection issues, is prone to distress, loneliness and loss during life's myriad minor and major transitions. This insecurely attached infant is less equipped to self-soothe and manage these events than is the securely attached baby that receives adequate mirroring and emotional attention from the parents (Ainsworth and Bowlby, 1991, pp.336–341). Attachment style is only one of many elements impacting an individual's development, and many people experience problematic attachments without developing anorexia. However, an insecure attachment can impair a child's development of Self and can contribute to the Self deficits that are common to anorexia.

Other researchers, notably psychoanalyst Alan Sugarman and his colleagues, have attributed the sense of emptiness and loss experienced by anorexics to a serious depression, which can develop because of maternal over- or under-involvement. The infant then exhibits "a state of reduced spontaneity and expressiveness" resulting from lack of maternal responsiveness to the infant's needs. To promote healthy development, when the child reaches the exploratory phase, the mother needs both to "be there and not there," to allow and encourage freedom in order to promote the illusion of self-sufficiency, but also to be available for emotional support (Sugarman et al., 1981, p.53). When the mother is there too much, the baby submits to the mother's overprotective gestures and has no room to develop her own autonomous behaviors. She is then prone to feelings of depression and acute loss when her mother is not present. When the mother is not there enough, the baby feels lost and abandoned and ceases to explore the world around her. This experience can leave the infant with a painful sense of emptiness. The mother of an anorexic may fit Sugarman's profile of the "too much there and too much not there" parent. The quality of *either* being "there" or "not there" too much will preclude the toddler's development of self-reliance (Sugarman et al., 1981, p.46).

Research at the Topeka, Kansas, Infancy Research Project has provided a way to more directly correlate adolescent and adult behavior with infant attachment experience. In this setting, psychologist Sylvia Brody and other clinicians observed and used videotapes to monitor a number of individuals at periodic intervals from infancy to age thirty. Brody reviewed notes and taped interviews from infancy of two girls who at age eighteen reported having experienced anorexia earlier in their teens. Brody observed that infancy for both girls had been characterized by a lack of maternal nurturance and connection, and that the loneliness and absence of physical and emotional reassurance led to early and unrelieved anxieties of object loss (loss of the mother), setting the stage for these children to experience feelings of despair (Brody, 2007, p.180). From reviewing the girls' histories, Brody also concluded that their self-representations (their internal sense of themselves) were not as firm as those of infants who were held and touched (Brody, 2007, p.115). Thus, both girls in childhood were already burdened by a sense of unrelenting loss and in addition had limited internal capacity to manage these feelings. Brody also reminds us that of course it is not just early interpersonal interactions that shape the adolescent's sense of Self, including her capacity to handle painful feelings, but the continuous repetition of psychological events in various forms during infancy and their entrenchment in childhood and preadolescence (Brody, 2007, p.17).

Another factor that can contribute to the anorexic's difficulty with loss is that many anorexics innately are highly rejection-sensitive (Costin, 2007a, p.197). An anorexic is more prone both to perceive rejection and to be distressed by it than is a non-anorexic individual. Rejection, by definition, entails loss and grief. In addition, an anorexic has a limited capacity to handle her feelings, and thus she is likely to accumulate myriad ungrieved losses from infancy onwards. Thus an anorexic may be both biologically predisposed to experience loss and grief, and developmentally unequipped to manage these feelings.

With some anorexics, the problem with grief may also stem from the actual death, frequently unexpected and sometimes violent, of someone close to her. Often the anorexic in some way feels responsible for the person's death, and harbors unremitting guilt. In 1980, two British doctors, a psychiatrist and a general practitioner, studied a number of anorexic clients, some of them male, in whose families there had been at least one sudden or violent death. The anorexic in most of these cases had never properly mourned the death and had assumed some guilt, justifiable or otherwise, for the loss. After receiving therapy in which he or she was encouraged to mourn the death of the relative, the anorexic client resumed appropriate eating habits within six to fourteen months and attained normal weight again. The authors reported that fifteen of the eighteen anorexics who were allowed to have a mourning service showed improvement afterwards. The two doctors noted that the etiology of anorexia nervosa remains a mystery and that they do not know if unresolved mourning is common in all cases of anorexia, but their results suggest that "hidden guilt or lack of adequate recognition and feelings that are distinct from her mother's or mourning for a lost member of the family may be a causative factor" (McAll and McAll, 1980, p.368).

Whether stemming from attachment issues in infancy that are reinforced during childhood, an innate sensitivity to rejection, or unmourned loss from a death occurring during her life- time, an anorexic's difficulty with unresolved grief manifests in several areas of her life, includ- ing with separation-individuation in adolescence. In cases where the mother of an anorexic has been inconsistently available, and has been unable to reliably promote her daughter's strivings for autonomy, the daughter is limited in her capacity for self-reliance. The tasks of normal ado- lescence are separation of parent and child and individuation, or operating more as an individ- ual—for *both* parent and child. However, separation and individuation run counter to the anorexic's more usual stance of compliance; for the process of separation to occur, the child must be able to have her own feelings that are distinct from her mother's and be able to toler- ate the discomfort of negative feelings. But often the anorexic suppresses her feelings; she has no skills for knowing and managing her feelings, and certainly no means to handle the loss inher- ent in separation. Furthermore, the mother has come to rely on the compliance and general agreeableness of her daughter and she, too, is unprepared to master separation from her daugh- ter. Often both mother and daughter lack some foundational elements that would help them navigate this developmental hurdle.

According to Sugarman and his colleagues, the developmental demands of separation and independence in adolescence reinvoke the symbiotic wishes of the anorexic to remain bonded to her mother and make it difficult for her to survive loss. Other legacies of an insecure attach- ment and problematic early separation can include the anorexic's difficulty in knowing and voicing her own feelings and wants, her impaired ability to internalize her experiences and make them her own, and her difficulty in developing a firm boundary between herself and oth- ers. This lack of clear division further impairs the anorexic's capacity to evoke a representation, or picture, of her mother, or of anyone else, in their absence. The child is repeatedly subject to profound experiences of loss and accompanying depression whenever someone she relies on leaves or is absent. If she cannot create an internal picture of the other person, and cannot feel their love or presence when they are out of sight, she feels empty (Sugarman et al., 1981, p.47). An anorexic may then engage in eating or food-related behaviors as an attempt to fill the void and to recreate the satisfaction she felt in the presence of her mother or of another person.

Yet clearly, an anorexic is willfully dedicated to *not* eating. This apparent paradox resolves itself with the understanding that it is not food with which the anorexic attempts fill her inner emptiness, but other constructs. An anorexic develops innumerable obsessions which occupy significant mental and emotional space. The anorexic focuses her thoughts on her body, on the ounce lost or gained or on how thin she can get, and on food. She also incessantly reviews other aspects of her life — when to do what, whether she is doing the right thing, what other people are thinking about her. Her obsessions overshadow her dilemmas and temporarily dispel awareness of her inner void.

Often for an anorexic, unresolved grief contributes to her struggle with beginnings and endings. Finishing or ending anything — a meal, a project, an event — entails loss. For the anorexic, *any* loss feels overwhelming and takes her back to the inner void at her core. When undertaking a project, simply beginning is problematic, as it stirs up issues of perfectionism. Once having begun a project, the specter of completion is even more problematic: finishing means abandoning her standards of perfection. Because nothing can be perfect, nothing can truly be completed. In addition to the deflation and loss incumbent in declaring "finished" something that is imperfect, something that represents her and that she no longer has the power to mold and improve, the simple fact of ending means experiencing loss. "Finishing" in this case represents abandoning something that has become a part of her identity, as well as coping with the loss and accompanying grief inherent in ending.

With eating, the anorexic also encounters issues with beginning and ending, with loss and grief. She fears that if she begins to eat, she won't be able to stop, because she will have let slip her tenacious grip and given in to her desire for food. Once she has begun to eat, she is wracked with guilt and grief for succumbing to eating and losing control. Physically, her pattern of food restriction has made the ingestion of food uncomfortable. Almost immediately, with any sensation of fullness or food in her body, her sense of relinquishing control escalates and she is swept up in yet more feelings of grief. But then there is the problem of stopping eating, and the loss that entails. If she stops, she will be confronted by the vacuous endless void. She may deliberately put some food aside, push it to one corner of her plate, keep it there both to reassert her control — "There's food here that I'm *not* eating" — and to postpone the inevitable grief of stopping. Often, anorexics eat at an agonizingly slow pace, experiencing tremendous conflict with every morsel consumed. With each additional bite, the anorexic is scared she has lost control; simultaneously, she dare not put her fork down and surrender to the emptiness that will arise when she stops eating.

The anorexic relies on tenacious control to push away the inner void. The prospect of loss of control is frightening. Without control, she will experience the emptiness that feels threatening, cold, and deathlike. If she loses control, she will embark on a cataclysmic free-fall plunge into the void. Control — and her fear of its loss — tinges all aspects of her life. With other people, she tries to control their reactions to her. With situations, she tries to control the outcome. With her life, she tries to control how much time any task takes. With her body, she tries to control her weight. With food, she tries to control her intake. She hoards and saves food to control the presence (to her, the very existence) of food. Food becomes much more than a form of sustenance; it is something that she can hang onto that protects her from the void. An anorexic frequently carries with her a squashed cookie or a tiny chunk of ancient cheese, wrapped in a paper napkin or piece of plastic, crushed into the bottom of her purse. She may never eat the cookie or the cheese, but the presence of this morsel is critical. It is a part of her salvation, a symbol that she is in control, a comfort in the absence of internal solace, and a barrier between her and her horrific emptiness.

For anorexics, particularly when trauma or a major loss has contributed to their disorder, this sense of an inner void is intense. Emotions to most anorexics are conundrums — intolerable, unmanageable enigmas. Without tools to express and cope with feelings, anorexics bury and suppress their feelings through food manipulation and weight obsession. The anorexic does not know how to use her feelings as a window to self-understanding. Her inner world remains bereft of the central components of self-knowledge and personality. She looks outward for an identity. Her body is her anchor and controlling her weight is her rudder. She has no solid core of Self, and instead feels excruciating emptiness.

The anorexic lacks the means to understand, or to manage, the morass of grief and pain that she experiences. Her only recourse is to reinforce the walls that comprise her barricade. But a stronger outer shell prevents her from developing self-knowledge as well from developing resources that could help her cope. Her attention remains fixed on her defenses. Ironically, the more impenetrable her walls, the more frightening becomes the inner void that she is seeking to escape. Only by slowly reversing this process can she find a way out of this excruciating dilemma. And ultimately, grieving becomes a central part of her healing: to recover, the anorexic must grieve her symptom, let go of anorexia, and mourn the loss of what has become her identity.

The gift of grieving is that that the pain of loss is no longer sequestered inside, unshared with others. When these feelings are allowed to surface and are talked about or relieved in other healthy ways, the need for using self-destructive means to handle the pain diminishes. Anorexia is a self-destructive way to cope with enduring emotional pain. The more that the emotional pain and grief can be addressed, the less it will be acted out in disordered eating.

Personal Story

At the age of sixteen, I went to college fifteen hundred miles from where my parents lived. As unhappy as I was at home, I had mixed feelings about going away. I'd led a fairly sheltered life in a rural college town, and graduated from a tiny high school attended by sons and daughters of college professors. My life experience was pretty limited. And I was anorexic, obsessing about food, keeping my weight under tight control — just above the mark that would signal my family that I was in a bad place again — and struggling to feel like I was just a "normal" teenager.

At college, everything was new and different. Some of it was exciting; some was scary — new people, new freedoms, new opportunities, and new things to learn. I was overwhelmed with how much more was going on, internally and externally, than I was prepared to handle. I felt a gnawing emptiness. I ate less, exercised more and obsessed about food and weight and what people thought about me. I withdrew and isolated myself. Inside me was an enormous hole. I didn't know where it came from or how to make it go away. It felt like nothing in the world could possibly fill it. It wasn't that I actually missed my parents or my home — it felt, instead, like *I* was missing.

I had lost my grandmother several years earlier, and never fully grieved her loss. Here I was facing major change and its accompanying loss, the loss of what was familiar: my own room, the routines and structure of being at home, the people I knew. Furthermore, developmentally I was unprepared to individuate and be independent. I relied a lot on my parents for direction and decision-making; I had little clue how to handle money and very little experience taking care of myself. Chronologically, I was young; emotionally, I was even younger. There was plenty to be excited about, but I felt more scared, and sad, and empty.

I became depressed within weeks of arriving at college — or more accurately, I should say, I became more depressed; in hindsight, I think I suffered from mild to medium depression as far back as I could remember. Somehow I made it through my first year away at school, and survived the first semester of my sophomore year. But the emptiness inside me persisted. School felt irrelevant; *I* felt irrelevant.

Halfway through my sophomore year, I dropped out of college and moved to New York City, where I knew four people: my older brother, George, an aunt and uncle, and a boyfriend. I hoped that somehow in New York I would find the meaning or satisfaction that would fill me up and make me whole.

My brother George was two and a half years older than me, and I had always looked to him for protection. He possessed some "masculine" qualities which I admired and which my father lacked. George was physically strong, athletic and outgoing while my father appeared frail, hunched and somewhat withdrawn. My father started drinking heavily when I was about twelve. Although I think he continued to function adequately at his job, he was often cranky, tired and withdrawn at home. I often went to George for things I wanted but didn't think I could get from my father. When I went away to college and missed being at home, it was George, at school two hundred miles away from me, whom I would call when I was lonely and depressed. And when I left college in the middle of my sophomore year, instead of going home as my mother asked me to, I moved to New York City and lived in the loft that George had rented with a room-mate. Three months after I moved in with George, he went into the service. I didn't like it when he joined the Army, because I didn't know many people in New York. One of the few people I knew was a man my brother had introduced me to only weeks earlier, a friend and a former colleague of his. Within a few weeks after George left, I moved in with his friend. Rather than dealing effectively with the loss I experienced as a result of my brother's departure, I found a lover to fill the emptiness so I wouldn't be alone.

While in the service, my brother became very depressed. Although he received some therapy, he remained depressed even after leaving the service. Two years later, shortly after his discharge, George visited me in New York City. I introduced him to Michael, a man I had met when I had started taking classes at New York University and to whom I was engaged. George didn't much care for Michael, but he didn't seem so much opposed to the marriage as he was concerned, in a way that no one else in my family ever had been, about my being thin and not eating.

My parents and I had planned a small wedding ceremony in New York City. George said he didn't want to come to the wedding because he didn't want to see a lot of relatives. I was very disappointed but accepted his decision, and to some degree even sympathized with him as I had often found family gatherings uncomfortable. I didn't realize then how angry I was at him for missing my wedding.

Three weeks after I was married, my brother hitchhiked to California. On his way, he stopped in a little town in Arizona where he knew no one. He bought a gun, rented a hotel room, wrote a note asking that his body be donated to medical research, and shot himself. I never knew if there was any connection between my marriage and his suicide, but I thought that the timing was more than coincidental. I wondered if he viewed my getting married, especially to someone he did not particularly like, and at a time when he thought I had other problems to be concerned about, as my rejecting him and discounting both his advice and his efforts to help me. Although I didn't think that my marriage alone was his reason for killing himself, I did believe that it could have contributed significantly to his sense of helplessness and of rejection.

For a long time, I was unaware of the anger I felt toward my brother for committing suicide. In part, I was grandiose about my expression of anger and convinced that I would hurt someone or lose control if I started to get angry. Also, I was more comfortable feeling sad and morose, and experiencing a familiar malaise, than I was being mad. In time, as I talked about my brother's death in therapy, I became aware that I was indeed angry with him. I also became aware of how my unresolved feelings over his suicide had affected my relationships with other men in my life. For a long time, I believed that if I stood up for myself in a relationship, as I had with my brother in deciding to get married despite his concerns for me, my partner would feel rejected and then might hurt or even kill himself. Gradually, through a combination of several therapeutic modalities that included psychodrama, gestalt, guided imagery and bodywork, I was able to express and let go of much of the anger I felt toward my brother for taking his life.

What continued to haunt me, however, was the feeling of responsibility for my brother's death. In my professional work whenever a client became profoundly depressed or in danger of suicide, I not only felt the concern that any of my colleagues would feel in a similar situation, but I also felt responsible for making the client better. In reality, certain phases of therapy evoke depression, and that can be a part of the process of change rather than a feeling state to be eliminated immediately. However, once when I was working with an anorexic woman, I became particularly distressed. This client was not following medical orders; she was neither limiting her exercise nor maintaining her fluid intake, and several times each week she was rushed to the emergency room suffering from severe electrolyte imbalances. I knew she was in danger of killing herself if she continued to act this way. I began to feel overly responsible, as though her life was my responsibility, not hers.

On the advice of a colleague, I took a route not normally suggested in the course of therapy and went to a psychic in order to deal with my feelings of guilt and responsibility over my brother's suicide, and over the lives of others, as well. I do believe that some individuals can access information about other worlds to which most of us are not privy, and this particular psychic came highly recommended. When I met with him, he was warm and friendly, and did not seem in any way unusual. I told him I had come to learn about why my brother had committed suicide. As the psychic and I sat quietly, he went into a trance. In a voice that was different from the one in which he had spoken before, he said he was channeling a particular spirit, and he began to respond to my questions. Perhaps he just really knew what I needed to hear. In any event, he told me that my brother, George, had been in terrible emotional pain, and that his pain was unrelated to me or to anything I had done. He had chosen to kill himself because his pain was too great to bear. The psychic assured me my brother was in a better place since dying, and that George wanted me to go on and have a happy life. In some way, I think the psychic was telling me what I already knew but hadn't been able to give myself permission to believe: that I was not responsible for my brother's death.

I left the psychic that day feeling relieved. I felt like I had been given permission to shed decades of a burden that was never mine to bear. I know how common it is for family and friends of someone who commits suicide to feel unwarranted responsibility and survivor guilt, and I felt like I had been set free. There was still work I had to do: letting go of thirty years of feeling responsible for another's life doesn't happen in an instant. However, with this visit to the psychic, I began to think differently about my role in relationships, whether with family, partners or clients.

Grieving the loss of my brother, and further losses that have occurred in the intervening years, has been instrumental in my accepting other feelings, which has in turn helped me to accept still more aspects of myself. I understand now how integral my feelings are to my Self development. With my feelings cut off or frozen, it was impossible for me to have an internal sense of myself. I lacked inner cohesion and felt like I was made of jumbled, disconnected parts. Knowing what I am feeling, whether or not I express those feelings, provides rich texture to my inner experience. There are feelings I am not fond of acknowledging — anger, in particular — but it is only in owning *all* of my feelings that I can truly know who I am and can experience a solid core of Self. Resolving grief can go a long way toward helping us to accept and acknowledge feelings in general.

Immature Sexuality and Relationships

I was twelve when I asked my mother to buy me a bra. I hardly needed one — I was still flat-chested and my chest, waist and hips were pretty much the same circumference. But my gym locker mate, Carol, was older, taller and more developed than I was. The first time we changed clothes for gym class, she pulled off her sweater and I stood transfixed, my eyes level with her bosom, staring like a deer in the headlights at two full, round breasts encased in satiny white fabric. I had never seen such voluptuous breasts. My mother — who was the only other female I'd seen in a brassiere — certainly didn't look like that! I didn't want to look at Carol's chest, but I couldn't help it. She was beautiful but ... sexy. It seemed wrong to admire her, to see something so sexual as attractive. I felt myself turning red in shame and embarrassment. I turned my back and tried to hide as I inched out of my pullover, revealing my flat and naked chest beneath. I vowed to get a brassiere, not because I would ever look like Carol, but because I had to hide the fact that I was so unlike her.

Sex and sexuality were confusing to me — not only at the age of twelve, but for years afterwards. Sex wasn't mentioned in my household; at school, it seemed to be mainly a source of jokes. From what little I knew, sex seemed like a strange and not very nice phenomenon without any redeeming value. Imagining myself being sexual was as alien as imagining a visit to Mars; both were unreal, far-off, weird and mysterious. But sex was also ... bad.

For anorexics, sex is generally a confusing and conflictual topic, as it was for me. Sex is associated with growing up, which is a source of conflict to the anorexic. Sex also means being close to someone — which is anathema to an anorexic. However, without a sexual identity, the anorexic *doesn't* grow up. Sexuality has varied connotations for different people; sex can be off-putting and distasteful, or harsh and aggressive, or a means of connection and a source of vital energy. Without acceptance of her sexuality and development of healthy attitudes toward sex, however, the anorexic lacks a core part of her self-identity. She cannot have a cohesive sense of herself and omit this aspect of her being. Developing a sexual identity — a comfort with her sexual feelings, proclivities and capacities as a sexual being — is essential if the anorexic is to develop a full and coherent Self. Because sexual development is connected to becoming an adult and to the development of relationships, this section is longer than some of the others describing attributes of anorexia. As in descriptions of other aspects of anorexia, some of the conclusions drawn are based on my personal beliefs and experiences.

Clinical Background

SEX AND SEXUALITY

Anorexia nervosa is characterized by a disturbance in attitudes and a lack of information about sexuality. Generally, the anorexic is misinformed and confused about sexual matters, sex roles and sexual relationships. Physically, the anorexic generally has an immature, androgynous or asexual appearance. Since primary anorexia commonly manifests at or soon after puberty, it makes sense that there is a sexual component to the disorder. Sexual concerns— sexual trauma or fear of sex or of becoming pregnant — have at times been cited as the primary issue in anorexia, but more commonly it seems that anorexia is an expression of a general fear of growing up and of assuming adult responsibilities, and impoverished sexual development is a consequence of that.

Older theories about the connection between the origin of anorexia and pregnancy have largely been refuted. At one time, many experts believed that anorexics' dislike of feeling full derived from their confusion about the physiology of procreation: they believed they could become pregnant through eating too much food. However, psychoanalyst Hilde Bruch has observed that the rejection of eating as a defense against an unconscious fear of impregnation is rarely encountered in primary anorexia nervosa, in which anorexia theoretically develops unrelated to other neurotic or psychotic conflicts issues (Bruch, 1973, p.276).

Also once in great favor was the idea that sexual abuse is a causative agent in anorexia.

More recent research suggests this is not generally the case. British psychiatrist Arthur Crisp estimated in 1997 that approximately 30 percent of anorexics have a history of childhood sexual abuse, and noted that such an experience "can be inflamed by puberty, rendering the latter intolerable" (Crisp, 1997, p.252). Although Crisp did not provide an estimate of the number of non-anorexics with this history, he was not implicating sexual abuse as the cause of anorexia. Psychologists Patricia Fallon and Stephen Wonderlich summarized results of several studies and concluded that rates of childhood sexual abuse were no higher in eating disordered individuals than in psychiatric controls. Their opinion is that sexual abuse is a *nonspecific* risk factor in eating disorders, meaning that a history of sexual abuse may be present and may be one of many contributing features to an eating disorder (and more so in bulimia than anorexia, they found) but that no cause-effect relationship has been established (Fallon and Wonderlich, 1997, pp.398–399). Childhood sexual abuse was but one of many factors that can contribute to anorexia, according to Crisp, who affirmed, "clearly the range of maturational problems that can give rise to the condition [of anorexia] is endless" (Crisp, 1997, p.252).

However, the anorexic's active food restriction does impair physiological processes related to sexual development. These physical consequences of starvation include suppression of secondary sexual characteristics (breast development, change in hip shape and size), atrophy of ovarian tissue, and amenorrhea (lack of menstrual flow). Disturbance in eating patterns, together with restriction of food intake in general and of fat in particular, deprives the body of the raw materials for body composition. This deprivation means that elements essential to creating the ovulation-regulating hormones are in short supply, and eventually the menstrual periods stop. Commonly there is a decreased circulating level of the hormones LH and FSH, which are essential to ovulation (Mitchell et al., 1997, p.387).

In the view of psychoanalyst Helmut Thomä, amenorrhea is the physiological counterpart of the frame of mind that results in anorexia. In some cases, amenorrhea *precedes* the loss of weight and appetite characteristic of anorexia, and is itself a symptom and expression of the disorder. Probably this is a psychological phenomenon mediated through the pituitary gland, which is responsible for releasing the hormones needed for ovulation (Thomä, 1967, p.272). Thomä has also noted that amenorrhea seems to persist until the patients' attitudes have altered and their conflicts are on the way to being resolved. Hormone treatments with uncured patients, for instance, were ineffective in reestablishing menstruation (Thomä, 1967, p.273).

At puberty, an anorexic experiences confusion about body sensations and she fears and dislikes the uninvited changes in her body (Bruch, 1973, p.276). She feels helpless in the face of the physical metamorphosis happening to her; she is unprepared for it and unable to control it. The softening and rounding of her body, the widening of her hips and thighs and initial enlargening of her breasts, the onset of menstruation, and the surges of unexpected sexual feelings—all normal occurrences in puberty—are unfamiliar and unsettling to her (Bruch, 1973, p.277). Scared by the sensation that she is losing control, the anorexic become preoccupied with dieting and exercising in an attempt to take charge of her body and to force it to conform in shape and function to what is familiar to her: an undeveloped, immature form, firm, flat-chested, and curveless.

These and other aspects of sexual maturation can be confusing and frightening to an anorexic. In the years before puberty, Bruch suggests, the anorexic is typically naïve about sexual matters (Bruch, 1973, p.277). The very topic of sex may be foreign and cloaked in secrecy. Sex may not be talked about in the anorexic's household, or, if discussed, the connotation is that sex is bad and should be secret. The parents of an anorexic may lack permission themselves to be open about intimate subjects let alone to discuss sexual intimacy with their children. An anorexic may seek information from books—often furtively and covertly, because she has intuited that it is wrong for her to be curious about sex. The word "masturbation" is probably never uttered in the household. Often, neither the anorexic's mother nor her father talks with her about how to relate to boys, although they may provide a strong proscription against pregnancy in unwed women and caution abstractly against "getting too involved" with anyone of the opposite sex. The possibility that their daughter may not even be heterosexual is never entertained. If in fact the anorexic experiences sexual feelings toward a female, she is likely to be even further confused about sex. In short, an anorexic generally fears sex and dreads the signs of her own developing sexuality.

SEXUAL IDENTITY AND ADULTHOOD

Not only are the physical aspects of developing sexuality problematic for the anorexic, but so too is the matter of sexual identity. Psychologist Carol Gilligan, an authority on female development and author of *In a Different Voice: Psychological Theory and Women's Development*, notes that for girls, the "magic age" of eleven is pivotal. This is the age at which girls are expected to begin to make a psychological break from their mothers and orient themselves toward womanhood, marriage and motherhood, yet to use their mothers as their primary role model (Gilligan, 1993, p.51). Psychologist Deborah Luepnitz comments: "Given the lives of their mothers, no wonder some adolescent girls look at them and protest, verbally or otherwise" (Luepnitz, 2002, p.92). The peak ages of onset of anorexia are between eleven and thirteen, or between seventeen and eighteen, which correspond to the primary developmental phases of separation-individuation, in which the daughter is establishing herself as distinct from her mother.

Much of a little girl's sexual identification in childhood results from her relationship with her mother. In her book *The Magical Years*, Selma Fraiberg has written about the process of feminine identification, asserting that a mother is the central figure in her daughter's feminine development. Fraiberg notes that a mother who has found satisfaction herself in being a woman will communicate that to her daughter without words. Fraiberg further observes that it is through the love of the mother and identification with her that the girl achieves positive identification with her own gender. She learns to connect the symbols of femininity — nurturing herself and others, creating a home — with love and intimacy, and to achieve a positive attitude toward becoming a woman (Fraiberg, 1959, pp.230–235).

As well as fostering her daughter's femininity, a mother serves as the primary role model for her daughter. As long as the mother takes satisfaction in her roles as a woman — whether in the home or socially or at work — she will convey this to her daughter (Fraiberg, 1959, p.234). However, too often a mother is hard-working but not happy with her life or roles. She may have forfeited her own identity to take on the role of caretaker. Small wonder, then, that the anorexic girl does not want to grow up to be a woman — if that means being unhappy and unfulfilled like her mother.

Other aspects of growing up are frightening for the anorexic as well. It is during the pre-puberty years that young girls learn mastery of tasks and develop peer relationships with other girls. However, the parents of a future anorexic may have failed to encourage her to learn skills that would foster her independence and growth. Her mother has not taught her how to be a woman, and this lack of preparation for womanhood frightens the anorexic and contributes to her refusal to accept that strange and mysterious role. Out of ignorance and fear, she develops unrealistic beliefs about what it is like to be a grown-up woman. Furthermore, her ties to her mother are close and relating to others is not particularly comfortable. Rather than learning to develop and value relationships with other girls with whom she could talk about the things that overwhelm her — relating to boys and her body's changes — she tends to isolate herself and feel competitive with other girls.

Puberty for most adolescents is a time of massive confusion and inner conflict. For the future anorexic, unprepared to deal with the responsibilities of adulthood, it is overwhelming.

Writer Nancy Heischman, in a paper published in the University of California–Santa Cruz journal *Redwoods*, suggests that at puberty, the anorexic is confronted with a double bind in her gender identity. Her family encourages her to be assertive, achievement-oriented and success-minded and may even press her to pursue a traditionally male career in law or medicine. Yet women in Western society are also encouraged to be compliant, dependent and unassertive, a role the mother of an anorexic often exemplifies. Thus, anorexics are expected by their parents to behave in ways diametrically opposed to their socialization process and family modeling, and to take on traditionally male roles for which they may have no female role model (Heischman, 1981, p.18). Young women are further expected to accomplish all this "guy" and "girl" stuff naturally and effortlessly, in an over-sexualized and ultra-feminized way, the third knot in the "triple bind" oppressing modern female adolescents that Hinshaw and Kranz describe in *The Triple Bind: Saving Our Teenage Girls from Today's Pressures* (Hinshaw and Kranz, 2009, p.xiii).

According to Heischman, it is not a coincidence that anorexia became more widespread in the 1970s, along with both feminist activism and the emergence of the women's movement. She believes that the increase in anorexia during that time is in part a response to the redefinition of women's roles in society (Heischman, 1981, p.18). The fact that the anorexic has not been shown how to be assertive at home, but is expected to do so in her culture, contributes to her overwhelming sense of ineffectiveness. Unprepared to assume the role of an adult female in society, let alone to carry this out with aplomb, and eschewing the submissive, compliant role her mother likely models, the anorexic chooses, instead, to deny her own womanhood altogether: her thin and wasted form makes her appear androgynous. She transforms her ineffectiveness into a sense of power through dieting and maintaining control over her body.

In 2006, the documentary *Thin* chronicled the treatment of four young women at a Florida residential eating disorder center. *Washington Post* columnist Sandra Boodman reviewed the film, noting that all four women (aged 15 to 25) appeared immature and exhibited a childlike dependence. A 25-year-old who was admitted to the facility with a feeding tube implanted in her stomach acknowledged, "I'm really scared of being independent and being responsible and being on my own" (Boodman, 2006, p.3E). Clearly adulthood for the anorexic can be terrifying.

And dieting is the anorexic's panacea. When used appropriately, dieting is a way to take personal responsibility for improving her health and appearance. But dieting has other meanings for an anorexic; she diets to disguise her femaleness and to attain society's ideal of "thinness," a stalklike, genderless shape. And, since she manages to suppress both the curves which would give her the appearance of a woman and the ovulatory cycles which permit her to function physiologically as a woman, she removes herself both socially and biologically from the category of sexual beings: an androgynous state, in which she transcends maleness and femaleness by combining elements of both (Heischman, 1981, p.24). The anorexic regresses into an immature, safe, less complicated pre-puberty state, single-mindedly pursuing starvation. Here she can avoid the conflicts and responsibilities, sexual and otherwise, which are the province of womanhood.

RELATIONSHIP DEVELOPMENT

Difficult as adolescence and the prospect of adulthood are, in some cases the roots of an anorexic's disturbance with regard to sexuality and relationships may originate long before the disorder manifests in adolescence or later. A complex interplay of innate character traits and environmental factors influences the development of the girl who becomes anorexic. There may be a thread of developmental and relationship problems running through the peak stages of growth from infancy through the ages of two, four, early school years and pre-puberty, then becoming more acute at adolescence.

As we've seen, the parent-child relationship, and particularly the mother-child connection, from infancy onward has major impact on a child's development. Research has been conducted and conclusions drawn, with a scattering of hindsight, to explain why a young girl might develop anorexia ten or twelve or more years later. However, just as every anorexic is unique, so too is every mother-child bond, and every family's dynamics as well. What we have are some generalizations about typical family dynamics that contribute to anorexia, with a wide margin for, and an apology to, the many atypical families and atypical anorexics for whom these descriptions are not a satisfactory fit.

One issue that can contribute to the later development of anorexia is a deficit in maternal nurturance. As noted on page 45, psychologist and researcher Sylvia Brody demonstrated this in a study of infant and early childhood material from two girls who developed anorexia in adolescence. While admittedly the sample is small, nonetheless, the results of this research are telling. Working at the Infancy Research Project in Topeka, Kansas, in the 1950s and 1960s, Brody and her coworkers followed a number of individuals from birth to age seven, with follow-up studies at ages eighteen and thirty. Among the female subjects, two 18-year-olds reported they had been anorexic a few years before (Brody, 2007, pp.xi–xiv). When Brody went back to the infancy and early childhood records of the two young women and reviewed direct and filmed observations, she found that the mothers for both girls in this study exhibited little capacity to emotionally invest in their infants. The mothers rarely picked up or comforted their daughters, and demonstrated little affection for them (Brody, 2007, pp.130–135).

Anthropologist Ashley Montagu, in his book *Touching*, explored the relationship between a mother's affection for her infant and her child's later sexual development. Montagu observed that a high correlation appears to exist between maternal failure to nurture her infant and the child's preference as an adult for being held rather than for engaging in sexual activity. According to Montagu, the sexual impulse has two components. The first one that develops is related to non-sexual physical touch; the second to sexual touch. In children, before the development of sexual interests, only the first, non-sexual, tactile impulse exists. If the infant is deprived of nurturing and tactile experience, he or she fails to develop the need for sexual touch and remains fixated at the earlier, non-sexual phase of development (Montagu, 1978, p.169). In other words, the individual prefers being held to being sexual.

Montagu studied a number of depressed women who articulated a longing to be held and cuddled. Examination of their personal histories revealed that their desires reflected an unmet need from infancy and childhood. A similar failure to develop beyond a stage of wanting to "cling" and cuddle is typical in the case of some anorexics. An anorexic frequently has little interest in sex or sexual relationships, and usually fears sexual involvement, but may seek sexual partners in order to fulfill her desire for physical contact and affection. Through sexual encounters, she gets from men the nurturing that she needed and likely did not receive from her mother. However, the anorexic's desire for nurturing is complicated by her fear of being controlled, as she may have felt was the case with her mother. Furthermore, given her incomplete separation from her mother, an anorexic may fear that in a relationship she will merge with her partner and lose her already fragile autonomy. Thus the specter of a relationship is, in her mind, fraught with landmines.

An infant who later becomes anorexic may herself reject a mother's love, particularly if her mother's attention has been erratic or distracted. Whatever its components, the complex mother-infant dance generally results in the future anorexic's *feeling* unloved. Not only does she then believe that she is unlovable, she may feel incapable of giving love as well. Or she may give warily, afraid she is not doing it right and that she may be rejected. She can also develop a grandiose notion of what giving and receiving mean. For instance, she may think that her need for nurturing is too great to ever be filled, and then resent giving to others when her own resources are so limited. She may also fear that in giving love she will lose her own identity. If the anorexic possesses any of these skewed thoughts, it will be difficult for her to participate in the normal give and take characteristic of a mature relationship. In these cases, a sexual relationship can resemble a painful seesaw between rejection and smothering. The anorexic can clutch her partner tenaciously and the next moment, just as vigorously push him away.

Other developmental problems can also contribute to the anorexic's difficulties with individuation, and hence with her relationships. Sometimes, as noted on page 39, the future anorexic refrains from the control struggle in which two-year-olds naturally engage. She may be innately harm avoidant (Grilo, 2006, p.50) and shy away from risk of conflict. Compliant in demeanor, she simply withers in the face of parental dissatisfaction or potential conflict. Hence she neither tests limits nor engages in the nascent identification and separation typical of healthy two-year-olds. The complex mother-daughter dance continues and the symbiosis of infancy is prolonged. Often it is a two-way street: a mother, especially if depressed or compromised in some way, may herself shy away from limit-setting and self-defining behaviors—she may, for example, simply comply with her child's or her spouse's requests, even if it means compromising what she wants—while her young daughter intuitively follows suit. This behavior lays the groundwork for further separation difficulties in the girl's early adolescence and impacts future partnering relationships as well.

At about four years of age, a little girl normally begins to compete with her mother for her father's attention. In a healthy resolution of the oedipal struggle, the child learns from her parents' responses that she cannot displace her father. However, a future anorexic's relationship may be so enmeshed that the little girl avoids the struggle. She may employ marginally assertive behaviors, but for the most part she simply does not bother. Why engage in a battle that is already lost? This, too, has repercussions in later relationships as she tries to navigate interactions with partners. She may simply give in without ever asserting what she needs or wants.

Sometimes an anorexic develops a limited or distorted concept of how men and women relate from watching her parents interact. Her mother may be obedient and submissive, accommodating to her husband's wishes. Her father may be passive, withdrawn, and uncommunicative. Assumption and indirect communication may be the norm: family members may operate based on what they think someone else wants, rather than having a conversation about it.

By the time the future anorexic reaches adolescence, she is unprepared for adulthood. She has an unpleasant and distorted view of what it is like to be a woman. She envisions an adult woman's life as drowning in unpleasant realities: being submissive to men; bearing the burdens of a husband, children and a home; possessing a body strapped into brassieres, jammed into control-top pantyhose, trimmed sporadically by failed diets and interrupted once a month by an unwelcome discharge. In addition she fears, dislikes and doesn't understand sex. From both her parents she may receive reinforcement for behaving as a little girl and for depending on them for direction and decision-making. Typically, neither parent esteems womanhood. Her mother may appear to dislike being a woman and her father may seem to view her mother simply as the one responsible for keeping the home together. Furthermore, the anorexic despises the unwelcome and uncontrollable changes in her body. Given these circumstances, it is little surprise that the anorexic determines to halt this process. She vows to take control of her life: she starves and feels empowered. She suppresses her development, physically and emotionally, and circumvents the challenges of becoming a mature woman and a sexual being.

Personal Story

For my mother, life was an ordeal. She shouldered the burden of the family's needs with apparent distaste. Intelligent and well-educated, she'd opted for homemaking rather than a career as a librarian for which she'd trained. My mother cooked, cleaned and shopped for groceries, but all household chores were onerous. She operated according to a compendium of unspoken statutes established by my father. Anytime I asked why she maintained routines with unwavering constancy, she replied that it was what my father wanted. Dinner was served at six; the salad preceded the main course; my parents' bedroom door was always kept closed; their bedroom was unheated and ice cold; Sunday evening we had waffles for dinner and watched Ed Sullivan on TV. How she even knew what my father wanted, I couldn't fathom; when my parents talked, everything sounded vague and inconclusive. As a child, I resolved I would never be like my mother when I grew up. I didn't know then that she was depressed. To me, she was simply unhappy and dependent. But I was not going to be a housewife who lived life for a man. And I was never going to have children because I didn't want to produce miserable kids like me.

My mother was a poor model for how to find pleasure in life. Her enjoyments were few and far between — an occasional bridge club, a few minutes reading a novel or conversing with a friend. Otherwise, her life outside of family duties consisted of occasional mandatory social events related to my father's career. She owned pretty clothes that she wore on special occasions, but she complained she needed to wear them with a girdle. She put on makeup when she dressed up, but grumbled about the inconvenience. In referring to the accoutrements of womanhood, never did my mother express excitement, gratification or pleasure.

Nor was my mother able to support me in my pursuits. She taught me to make a bed with perfect corners, to vacuum meticulously and to set the table with forks and knives arranged appropriately. But she was neither creative nor artistic, and didn't encourage my creative leanings. In seventh grade home economics, I began to sew and wanted to learn to make clothes. My mother couldn't sew and discouraged my interest; fortunately a family friend, a generous, warm and nurturing woman, stepped in and patiently helped me interpret patterns and fit garments. This friend invited me to a tailoring class where I learned to sew suits and coats in the company of many mid-life ladies. Much as I liked to sew, my mother objected when I spent my allowance on fabric or my Saturday afternoons sewing. What I enjoyed doing, my mother didn't, and treated with indifference or disdain; I felt guilty for pursuing the pleasures she invalidated.

Being a homemaker appeared grim, and little else about adulthood appeared appealing. My parents seemed distant from each other, and their relationship ungratifying, although maybe it wasn't that way for them. To me it looked like my father worked all the time, though it didn't seem to make him happy. It was not until much later that I understood that my father was alcoholic, or how his alcoholism impacted my parents' relationship. Influenced by their own upbringing and culture, my parents expected me to marry a man who would earn a living, and to become a homemaker and a mother, just like my mother. Of course, they wanted me to go to college — my father had a Ph.D. and was a college professor and my mother had an M.A. and a degree in library science — but I think they expected that I'd eventually set aside my career for a family.

In my own family, the subject of sex was seldom mentioned and I never talked with my mother or father about how to relate to boys. As an adolescent, I felt embarrassed when a boy I liked looked at me, but I didn't know what to do—I certainly couldn't ask my parents for advice. My family didn't talk about feelings, and I figured embarrassment about boys was another one of those uncomfortable and unmentionable sensations that people bore in silence. I liked attention from boys because it made me feel good and gave me a whiff of self-esteem; I tried to look pretty and doubtless acted coy and seductive to attract their attention. But once I was with a boy, I got scared and didn't know what to say or do. I would get uptight and try to act cool and confident, while inside I was clueless. Consequently, I created a push-pull dynamic, and never learned how to communicate or relate to boys. I didn't understand how relationships, built on such a flimsy foundation, could ever last.

The part of growing up that related to career choice was as daunting as the specter of adult relationships. Most career options seemed unfamiliar and frightening. I was insulated — or I insulated myself — enough that I didn't look outside my immediate family for role models. Also, my mother told me when I was ten or eleven that I didn't need to decide yet what to be when I grew up. I was never really sure *when* I was supposed to figure that out, much less *how*. Maybe my parents thought if I just went to a good college it would dawn on me what I wanted to do. My brothers developed career goals even before high school, but they were boys; since I was a girl, my parents' expectations of me were different. I wonder if my parents expected me to grow up at all, given that they never encouraged me to make decisions or discover my interests. And if they didn't expect me to grow up, career choice was immaterial. Or perhaps they gave me guidance, but my emerging anorexia kept me from internalizing their advice; in any event, I remained ignorant of many life skills and clueless about career choice.

Growing up and leaving home were simply beyond my imagination. I couldn't envision a future any different from how my life had been up until then. I had visited grandparents and gone to camp, but generally felt lost and homesick when I was away. When I was ten and eleven, my parents weren't getting along that well, and I was scared that if I left home, they might split up or die. I didn't consciously decide not to grow up, but I did resolve to not eat and to get thin in reaction to an insensitive remark my mother made about my body. And once I started losing weight, I reveled in the consequences of getting thinner — I didn't look like a woman, I didn't feel like a woman, and people didn't expect me to act like a woman.

When finally I went away to college, I found there was far more to life than I'd known, and I never returned home. But the world out there was scary, I was anorexic, and I turned to men for comfort and safety. I was seldom without a relationship with a man who would nurture and take care of me. Whenever the end of a relationship was imminent, I would develop a new one to replace the old. Sex to me was something that was necessary to keep a relationship going. At age 20, I mistook sex for love, and married a man 13 years older than me because he liked having sex with me. We stayed together for over seven years, but it was an empty, unfulfilling relationship. It wasn't until much later that I actually began to enjoy sex; and it wasn't until after many years of therapy that I began to grasp the concepts of emotional intimacy and connection in a relationship.

In my early treatment at Cathexis, my therapists tutored me in healthy attitudes about sex and relationships. My primary therapist was a woman who clearly enjoyed being female. I learned to associate her warmth and love with being a woman. Also, she spoke openly with me about sex, sexuality, and comfort and pleasure in sexual relationships. My therapist enjoyed sex and sexual relationships, and knew how to relate to men without giving up her own selfhood. When my menstrual periods began again after I had stabilized at a healthy weight for about six months, she and my other therapists encouraged me to celebrate the event. And when I started to date, I talked extensively with them about the details of conversations and customs for male-female relating.

My therapists taught me to take charge of my own sexuality. They explained that being sexual did not mean being dominated or controlled by a man; it was up to me to define when and with whom I wanted to have a sexual relationship. I learned to talk with a partner about contraception, a subject I hadn't needed to consider for the previous twelve years when I wasn't having periods.

In role-playing exercises at Cathexis, clients would play themselves at a younger age, with the therapists acting as healthy parents. Role-playing a child at various ages helped clients experience and internalize healthier emotional interactions with caretakers than had occurred in their own childhood. When I played the role of an 18-month-old infant my primary male therapist played with me; I felt like I mattered, as a person and as a girl. As Fraiberg has observed, it is significant to the little girl's feminine identification that she be loved for being a girl (Fraiberg, 1959, p.232). In role-playing a two-year-old, I experienced how parents set healthy limits and establish boundaries for kids. This exercise also helped me develop more sense of myself as an individual person, separate from my caretakers. I discovered how vital it is in sustaining a relationship to have a healthy sense of myself, and how to *be* myself rather than to operate as an extension or a reflection of the other person, whether that other person is a parent, therapist, spouse or friend.

In role playing a four-year-old, I was delighted to sift through the contents of my therapist's purse and play with her makeup, to have her tell me stories and to play games with me. Also when I was acting four years old, my therapist read me the book *Where Do I Come From?* a children's book which describes in very simple, innocent language how babies are made. My therapist's openness in talking about sexuality and procreation helped dispel some of my skewed sexual attitudes.

In acting as an eleven- and twelve-year-old, I talked with peers and therapists about relating to boys. More and more I was able to understand how to relate to the opposite sex, as well as about the ways boys and men were and weren't different from girls and women. My quest for thinness was in part driven by a desire to be attractive to men, so long as at the same time I retained the prerogative to push them away. It was a revelation for me to learn that appearance and physical attractiveness were not the only qualities that guys appreciate in girls. Realizing that the capacity to laugh, listen and talk also mattered gave me a glimmer of the complexity of boy-girl relationships. I was only beginning to understand who I was beyond my long-held anorexic identity, and to discover that people were multi-dimensional in makeup, that their personalities were much deeper than their physical appearance.

In sum, my treatment at Cathexis allowed me to observe how much my therapist enjoyed being a woman and doing feminine things. Her example helped me understand how to make my life work as a woman and as an adult, and taught me how to think about problems and make choices and decisions based on what I needed and wanted. She served as a role model and her support gave me confidence in my capacity to become accomplished in feats other than starvation. Her ability to balance warmth and femininity with strength and competence were instrumental in my choice to act as an adult woman. And her open attitude in our frank discussions about sex and sexual relationships helped make those arenas safe, accessible and fun.

After leaving Cathexis, I continued in therapy. Although I had changed significantly, I soon discovered how much more growing I needed to do. My weight was stable, my periods had resumed, I felt better about myself as a woman, and I was more comfortable relating to men. However, it was not until years after I left Cathexis that I had the courage to address some deeper issues around sexuality.

I was still haunted by my family's programming, much of which dated from my parents' upbringing in an era of sexual repression, and perplexed by society's current sexual values. Certain lines seemed clear; others more arbitrary. The subject of pornography was an example. When and for whom was it legitimate? At what point did use become abuse, or cross the line to "addiction"? What about other sexual behaviors? I cringed at national rape statistics: in the U.S., a woman is raped every six minutes. Did this frequency speak to mental illness in our country, or was it a reflection of sexual repression?

Many of these questions I lacked the expertise to address. I had personal skeletons in my closet, and whether it was the culture, my family heritage, feelings about myself, lack of a safe forum to talk about my past, or a combination of things that kept me from revealing these I couldn't say. What I knew was that I felt so ashamed about two sexual experiences in my teens that I didn't divulge them for thirty years, long after leaving Cathexis. I certainly have neither the right nor the knowledge to determine "appropriate" sexual mores for our culture. However, I am clear that when someone does not talk about sexual experiences that leave a residue of anger, guilt or shame, the feelings do not vanish, but continue to fester and to color future sexual feelings, beliefs and behaviors.

It's not that finally revealing these incidents years later immediately relieved me of a burden of shame and guilt that I had been carrying for decades. But it opened the door to begin an exploration of them and a discussion that, over time, helped me to create a framework for comprehending, tolerating and learning from them. I believe that is how therapy helps: we can't erase our past, but we can become less triggered by our memories. We can develop the capacity to more quickly metabolize the feelings that reflexively emerge, and we can develop a perspective that allows us to understand our pain and to bear our memories with less angst.

Although neither of the two sexual incidents directly involved my brother George, both happened during times I visited him, and added to the weight of guilt I felt about his suicide and the remorse I carried for my comportment during his short life. The first event occurred when I was a college sophomore and was spending a weekend in New York City with George and his roommate in a large artist's loft in Soho. On Sunday morning, I woke early, put on my sweater and jacket, a miniskirt, tights and knee high boots, and went out for a walk.

I wandered through the nearby streets, meandering among many small fruit and vegetable stands run by local merchants, and noticing lots of men hanging out in the area, some alone and some in clusters, some drunk, many smoking cigarettes. Suddenly one of these men grabbed me from behind and pulled me roughly into a nearby doorway. With one leg and forearm, he pinned me to the wall. With his other hand, he pulled his penis out of his pants and began to masturbate. He pushed against me and grabbed my leg, groping under my short skirt and down through the waistband of my tights and panties to stick his fingers in my vagina. He continued to molest me, and to rub his body and his penis against me until he ejaculated. Then he ran off, leaving me slumped in the doorway, stunned and immobilized.

Eventually I crept out of the doorway and slunk back to my brother's loft. But I was too shocked and ashamed to tell him what had happened — wasn't it my fault for going out alone in a neighborhood I didn't know? Hadn't I made myself a target by wearing a short skirt and high-heeled boots? This incident remained emblazoned on my mind for years afterward, making me mistrustful of men and confused about sex, and fostering my desire to be invisible. It magnified the shame I felt about my own existence and intensified the conflict I experienced about inhabiting a female body. The residue of this experience melded into my sullied psychological and emotional imprints about sex left over from the repressed sexual attitudes I'd grown up with.

The second incident took place six months after the first. At that point, I had left college midway through my sophomore year and moved into the loft with George and his roommate. I was dating one of George's friends at the time. Several of my brother's friends stayed over at the loft one night after a late party; my boyfriend was among them. When everyone was asleep, my boyfriend woke me with a loud whisper in my ear demanding that I let him into my sleeping bag. I said "No!" in as forceful a whisper as I could muster. He persisted, tugging at my covers as I pushed him back. George was sleeping ten feet away and I didn't want to wake him with the commotion, so very reluctantly I relented. But once in my sleeping bag, my boyfriend wanted me to stroke his penis, and then to put his penis in me. I'd never been sexually intimate with anyone. I whispered "No! No! No!" and pushed his hands and his body away. But I was afraid if I were loud and aggressive I would disturb George, who would wake to witness my boyfriend in bed with me. I wasn't strong enough to push the guy away. I stopped struggling; he entered me, quickly climaxed, rolled off me, and climbed out of my sleeping bag.

I didn't know the term then, but later I recognized that this incident would be labeled date rape. It made me feel slimy, slutty, dirty, and indelibly marked, in my mind, as a filthy whore. I was also angry and disappointed — first and foremost at myself, but also at my boyfriend. I'd never imagined my first sexual experience, but had I fantasized about it, the dream would certainly not have included a partner I hadn't chosen, against my will, in a sleeping bag, ten feet away from my brother.

My shame kept me silent about these incidents for decades. Many years later, I was able to disclose the event of the man in the doorway to a therapist. The therapist responded compassionately, and helped me to distinguish my role in the situation from that of my assailant. Between my naiveté and lack of consideration for my safety and well-being, I had put myself at risk. However, my attacker's actions were uninvited, intrusive, invasive, illicit and illegal. This anonymous assailant had violated me. At no time had I agreed to this assault. My therapist also helped me differentiate one man's violence from the behavior of men in general, and to learn to take responsibility for my personal safety. Sometime later I was able to discuss with the therapist the incident of my boyfriend's forced intercourse with me. The betrayal by someone whom I had trusted and cared about, and who I thought cared about me, had made me feel physically sick, but talking about it helped relieve my pain.

It was only in speaking about these two incidents that I was able to learn from them rather than to continue to carry them as proof of my badness. Without expressing the rage, terror and shame of being held captive and violated sexually by an unknown aggressor, I couldn't own my power as a female. And without expressing the anger, disappointment, grief and betrayal I'd felt from my boyfriend's unwanted sexual intrusion, I couldn't understand about boundaries in relationships. I needed guidance from my therapist to reconfigure the confused mix of thoughts and fantasies in my head into a picture that differentiated healthy from unhealthy sexual relationships.

Time, along with therapy, allowed me to explore, grapple with, and resolve more of my conflicts about sex and relationships. More life experience with relationships, as well as conversations with friends about their ways of handling partnership concerns, helped me develop a deeper appreciation for the complexity and many dimensions of how partners relate to one another. I began to comprehend that relationships hold immense power as an avenue for growth and individuation. As psychologist and relationship expert David Schnarch affirms in his book *Constructing the Sexual Crucible: An Integration of Sexual and Marital Therapy,* two partners inevitably have differences and face conflict, but it is by standing up for oneself in a relationship that each partner becomes a stronger individual (Schnarch, 1991, p.126).

Thus, individuation is a central part of recovery from anorexia. As long as the anorexic defines herself solely through reaction or accommodation to another, she cannot develop her own core Self. Accepting herself as a female as well as a separate and capable individual is essential to her self-development. Her gender is a central part of her identity as she matures, and one that in her illness she has spurned. But sexuality is a key to her aliveness; her sexual feelings, like her other feelings, signal her response to the world and animate her experience. The process of embracing her sex and sexuality are foundational to the anorexic's development of a cohesive inner Self; sexuality also provides a potential source of pleasure in her life.

Distortion of Body Image

In the house where I grew up, a floor-to-ceiling mirror graced the entire length of the upstairs hallway. I walked by the mirror on my way from my bedroom to the stairs, or from the stairs to my room. Occasionally, I'd glance at my profile in passing, my mind absorbed by other things. When I was given a new sweater or blouse at Christmas, I'd stand in front of the mirror long enough to admire my new clothes. But then I entered junior high school, and everything about how I looked suddenly mattered. I'd put my hair in rollers and somehow manage to sleep through the night. In the morning, I'd get dressed and scrutinize myself in this giant glass. Did I look okay? How had my hair turned out? Was this style of skirt in? What would the other kids think of me?

When I was twelve years old, I was home alone for lunch one day. There were leftovers from a party the night before, and I ate three desserts at lunch. When later I announced this proudly to my mother, she looked at me with disdain. She decreed, "You're getting fat!" I was crushed. I had thought she'd be delighted that I'd enjoyed these delicious sweets. The verdict — fat — sounded worse than life imprisonment. I ran upstairs to the mirror in the hall, and peered at my reflection with disgust. It was true! I was fat and fat was me.

Had I possessed the Self of a healthy twelve-year-old, it is unlikely that my mother's aspersion would have propelled me on a journey of self-destruction that lasted almost two decades. How I really looked that day I'll never know. But the problem was not my mother's words, or her facial expression or tone of voice; it was the meaning I gave them and the fact that I could neither comprehend nor convey what was going on inside of me. There wasn't enough me to be anything but fat. My body image was distorted by my own self-loathing.

Below I discuss body image distortion in anorexia, and a few approaches to its treatment. Then I go further into my personal history, looking at how I began to distort my own body image, and how eventually I began to heal from that skewed perception.

Clinical Background

Body image distortion is a central characteristic of anorexia. The anorexic is excessively thin, yet can't actually see her own starved and emaciated appearance. This entrenched distortion renders treatment of anorexia enormously difficult: how can you help someone understand she is too thin and must gain weight if she sees herself as not thin enough? This paradox has caused many researchers to scratch their heads and wonder how this situation has developed and what can be done to address it.

The problem with a distorted body image in anorexia is much more than a simple visual one, or a disagreement around what is or is not thin. Development of body image is a complex phenomenon. Body image is a mental representation that is built in relationship to others. That is, body image is not simply a picture that an individual creates internally as if in a vacuum, but a contruct that arises and is influenced by interactions with others. The foundation of body image is developed in infancy and childhood. However, there are factors throughout life that impact body image as well. Body concept is affected by the attitudes of parents, peers and romantic partners. Cultural preferences play a role. The individual's attitude toward herself, which also grows out of interactional patterns, is key. And body image is not static. Mood, behavior and emotion can shift body image. Thus body image depends on the interplay of beliefs, perceptions, attitudes, behaviors, moods and emotions.

In early life, physical touch is of vital significance in the infant learning to sense her body. The experience of security that comes from consistent caretaking, in combination with nurturing touch and positive emotional experiences, enables the child to internalize a positive body image. Conversely, feelings of insecurity coupled with negative emotional attitudes can lead to internalization of a negative body image. In the work of many clinicians cited above, we have already seen the role nurturing touch and positive emotional interaction play in self-development, including Montagu's discussion of sexual development and the attachment work of Ainsworth and Bowlby, Sugarman, and Brody.

Also in early childhood, the infant's experience with movement influences development of body image. According to Paul Schilder, German neurologist and expert in psychosomatic medicine, how a child moves affects her capacity to define boundaries and to differentiate herself from her environment. Schilder suggests that the integration of perceptual and muscular feedback contributes to the formation of a dynamic body concept (Bruch, 1973, pp.88–89). This means, for example, when a child who reaches up to grasp a window ledge sees his arms reach and feels the pull in his arms, and also sees his short little legs straighten and feels the tautness in his legs, he begins to connect the perception of observing his arms and legs as they straighten with the internal feeling of his arms stretching and his legs supporting his body.

Sometimes in the case of a future anorexic, if overanxious parents unwittingly impose restrictions on movement and limitations to taking physical risks, they can hinder the child's conceptualization of how her body fits into space. She does not develop the capacity to be flexible and to adapt easily to changes in physical surrounding. In this situation, the child may not acquire a sense of integration or cooperative interaction of the parts of her body; if Mom rushes to pick her up each time she sets off to explore, she won't experience the variety of movements that her body is capable of or how different parts of her body work together to perform certain movements. This lack of experience could impair the child's capacity to develop a cohesive sense of her body and to feel at home in it, which can then interfere with her development of an integrated Self.

Parents' attitudes toward their own bodies and toward those of their children, whether implied or directly stated, may greatly influence children's perceptions. For example, a child may interpret derogatory remarks about her body as evidence that her body is unacceptable or even disgusting. In situations where her family has inhibitions against touching and physical closeness, the child may believe that there is something distasteful about her body, or about bodies in general. And if a parent has personal issues about body acceptance, the child can construe that as extending to her own body as well. In some cases, the mother of an anorexic derives little pleasure from being a woman and a mother, and communicates this in numerous small ways to her daughter. Thus the anorexic dislikes her body and sees it in mechanistic terms. When her body begins to morph without any permission from her, the anorexic begins to distrust her body and feel betrayed by its unasked-for changes. Reasserting control by getting thin seems like a solution to the unmanageability of the edifice that she already abhors.

A girl's relationship with her father can have direct consequences on her self-esteem, confidence, and body image. Clinician Margo Maine in her book *Father Hunger* speaks to the impact of the father-daughter relationship on the growing girl. A supportive father-daughter relationship significantly influences a woman over a long period of time, improving the likelihood for positive self-esteem and intellectual and social confidence, and positive body image (Maine, 2004, p.66). Without that relationship, when indeed a girl does feel the hunger for that connection with her father, she is more likely to resort to the dangerous "if onlys" that lead to body image and eating conflicts. A girl who yearns for her father's love may tend to feel inadequate and to turn to "if I had a perfect body." But when Dad's role has been a constructive one, a daughter will be less likely to feel drawn to these fantasies in order to feel competent and successful as a woman and comfortable with her femininity (Maine, 2004, p.28).

Child psychologist Selma Fraiberg has implicated self-attitudes as fundamental in a child's body perception. In her book *The Magic Years*, Fraiberg observed that a normal child during development learns to value her body both because it is the source of her self-feelings, her physical and substantial "I," and because it is the source of her pleasure (Fraiberg, 1959, p.230). Emotionally, the child who becomes anorexic already has a diminished sense of Self, and hence her self-feelings are equally undeveloped. The feelings she is most likely to possess toward herself even at this stage are likely to be unkind. If the anorexic as a child has internalized attitudes about bodies being unacceptable, she is unlikely to derive pleasure from her body or view her body with any compassion.

Social attitudes also influence the development of an individual's body concept. These attitudes tend to emphasize the importance of pleasing physical appearance, to define the concept of beauty, and to dictate what constitutes an attractive body type. In modern Western society, thin is beautiful, obesity (despite its prevalence) is scorned, and an unusual physical appearance may be the object of ridicule. Cultural emphasis on "the ideal" body has wreaked havoc on the concept of "acceptable body image" for most Western women, driving them to comparison, false expectations and chronic disappointment. Factors that affect self-concept also impact body-concept, and vice-versa. In her book *Body Traps*, psychologist Judith Rodin cites several studies showing that women routinely overestimate their size. The more negative their feelings about their bodies, the more oversized their self-images; and the more inaccurate their estimates, the worse they felt about themselves. Rodin concluded that "inaccurate judgments of body size and shape and feelings of low self-worth influence each other in a descending spiral of poor self-image" (Rodin, 1992, p.53). The anorexic's self-concept is blighted, at best. She harbors severe shame and self-hatred. A thousand times each day, her failure is affirmed, and each incident reinforces her body hatred.

Psychologists Ann Kearney-Cooke and Ruth Striegel-Moore suggest that negative body image may arise from a projection process. This conceptualization rests on the fact that the body simultaneously *is perceived as* and *is part of* the Self. This unique closeness of the body to the individual's identity means that the body reflects and shares the person's preoccupations and can become a screen on which she projects her most intense concerns. When an anorexic feels ill-equipped to handle internal feeling states or interpersonal struggles, she projects those experiences onto her body. At the same time, the anorexic is influenced by Western culture's "myth of transformation" and the belief that by changing her body, she can change her life (Kearney-Cooke and Striegel-Moore, 1997, pp.296–297). The anorexic projects her out-of-control feelings onto her body, believing that by shrinking her body, she can subdue her internal world. However, as she seeks mastery of her body to corral her painful feelings, she misses opportunities to learn how to manage her feelings. Nonetheless, her strategy works: the more consumed she is with her body, the less distressed she is by her insecurities.

Kearney-Cooke and Striegel-Moore speak of body image as an internalized complex, or schema, of perceptions, beliefs, feelings and behaviors. Once developed, this schema can become entrenched and form a filter through which the person views herself and the world. The fact that body image is both complicated and often deeply embedded accounts in part for the difficulty of modifying body concept. Changing negative body image requires not only decoding negative body projections, but also disentangling the complex of emotions, beliefs and behaviors elicited by the schema. An anorexic's negative perception, such as a fleeting observation that her arm looks flabby, can lead to a cascade of negative thoughts and feelings, such as thinking that she is fat or out of control or shouldn't have eaten anything that day, and feeling remorse or disgust or despair. These thoughts and feelings drive her compensatory behavior — for example, skipping her next meal. The result leads to a temporary feeling of relief or success or control, but the feeling isn't stable, because the plethora of negative thoughts and emotions lurks nearby and can easily be re-triggered. Thus negative schema need to be dismantled and alternative schema constructed in their place (Kearney-Cooke and Striegel-Moore, 1997, pp.298–300).

Children grow up believing that conformity with respect to physical appearance is a prerequisite for "fitting in." The anorexic is very conscious that being thin is the ideal, and carries that goal to an extreme. She wants to both fit in and stand out: she wants to feel accepted and loved, but she believes she has to compensate for not feeling lovable by embodying the superlative of the ideal, by being the thinnest. In order for an anorexic to develop a healthy body image, she needs to believe that her body is good enough; to identify it is as hers, not as a hated foreign object; and to accept that her appearance does not have to conform either to societal norms or to the perfectionist ideals she has adopted. She must expand her identity to include aspects of herself beyond physical appearance. The anorexic generally also needs to learn new ways of moving through her physical environment and taking up space. Her pursuit of invisibility has affected her body posture and movements, almost as if to minimize the square inches she fills and the milliliters of oxygen she breathes. While it is not uncommon for an anorexic to exercise fanatically, her movements may actually be highly repetitive, as in running or swimming. Actual freedom of movement is generally not in her repertoire.

The task of helping an anorexic to modify her body image is daunting, because so much of her identity is bound to her body shape and size. However, change in body image is a crucial part of treatment. Furthermore, gaining weight and resuming normal body size does not ensure a change in body image. Without developing a realistic body-concept, the anorexic cannot maintain lasting recovery. Many therapists have developed methods for addressing body image distortion, some of which are described later in sections devoted to specific therapies. Among these are the cognitive-behavioral approaches of Christopher Fairburn (Fairburn et al., 2003), and of David Garner, Kelly Vitousek and Kathleen Pike (Garner et al., 1997), the cognitive work of Thomas Cash (Cash, 2008), hypnosis as described by B.J. Walsh (Walsh, 2008) and guided imagery employed by Marcia Germaine Hutchinson (Hutchinson, 1994) as well as by Ann Kearney-Cooke and Ruth Striegel-Moore (Kearney-Cooke and Striegel-Moore, 1997).

Psychiatrists Edward Gottheil, Clifford Backup and Floyd Cornelison devised an intriguing approach to the body image problem by combining psychotherapy and self-image confrontation, using videotapes to combat denial and help change body concept in an anorexic client (Gottheil et al., 1969, p.238). Gottheil and his colleagues worked with a severely emaciated anorexic 17-year-old girl who had been hospitalized and was being treated by psychoanalysis. Twice a week they provided her with self-image experience sessions in a video studio. At the beginning of each session, while she was being videotaped, the client was asked some questions, such as how she felt, how she had slept, and when and what she had last eaten. At the next session a few days later, the videotape was played back and she was asked to report what she liked or disliked about herself on the film.

For the first six sessions, the girl reported that she liked what she saw on the screen. At the seventh session, however, she became angry and distressed and said she was tired of seeing how sick she looked. The girl stated then that the self-image confrontation helped her to realize how thin she really was. Furthermore, she explained that when she saw herself in the mirror, she wasn't aware of how thin she was, because she was used to her mirror image, but in a movie or film she looked different (Gottheil et al., 1969, p.244). It was not until the fifth month of videotaping that the anorexic client saw anything positive about herself in the films. Then, instead of just observing how bad she looked in the film, she began to notice both positive and negative points about her appearance. By the time she left the hospital, when she saw films of how she had looked six months earlier, she said she couldn't imagine how she could have starved herself and was shocked at her earlier indifference to her thinness (Gottheil et al., 1969, p.242). Confrontation with a distorted body concept via an accurate recording on film appears to produce cognitive dissonance, where different beliefs collide. The anorexic experiences conflict between her internal body perception and the picture of herself she sees on the screen.

Gottheil and his colleagues observed that in their work, the relative contribution of psychotherapy, self-image confrontation and other variables could not be distinguished. However, the client reported that she was not sure she would have progressed as well and as quickly without the videotape sessions. The authors observed that the changes which occurred in their client's self-image seemed to be correlated with the continued and repeated self-image confrontation sessions, and concluded that repeated self-image confrontation appeared to influence the anorexic client to develop a more realistic perception of herself (Gottheil et al., 1969, p.239–45).

Two psychologists have elaborated on why self-image confrontation appears to be effective. Harry Boyd and Vernon Sisney have used self-image confrontation to treat distortion in body concept of both neurotics and psychotics. They propose that the personality system normally tends toward integration and consistency. When an individual is presented with a conflict between the "perceived" and the "real" images, he will either deny the distorted self-image on the screen (e.g. "It's not really how I look. The camera distorts"), or change his self-image toward reality (Boyd and Sisney, 1967, p.294). In the case followed by Gottheil and his colleagues, they found that with repeated self-confrontation sessions, fortunately, their client modified her self-image and came to view thinness as ugly.

Two German psychologists suggested that distortion of body image consists of two components, one perceptual and the other cognitive. By using a number of techniques to assess the degree and the source of body image disturbance in subjects with anorexia, they found that the disturbance is not due to a perceptual deficit, but solely to a cognitive-evaluative dissatisfaction. In other words, body image distortion is not due to a skewed way the anorexic *sees* her body, but instead it is due to the anorexic's dislike of her *thoughts* about her body and the *meaning* she gives them. This distinction certainly suggests the potential benefit of cognitive techniques for treating body image disturbance in anorexia (Skrzypek et al., 2001, pp.215–221).

As our capacity to monitor brain activity has improved, information about how brains of anorexics process information offers another view of the body image distortion problem in anorexia. Recently four Australian psychologists, P. Sachdev, N. Mondraty, W. Wen and K. Gulliford, have suggested that the root of the body image distortion may lie in the way anorexics process self-images versus non-self-images (images of others). When comparing control subjects with anorexics, they found there was no difference in how both groups processed *non-self-images*, but that in viewing *self-images*, the anorexics' brains were significantly less active than the brains of the controls. The researchers found that in the anorexic subjects, the part of the brain called the attentional system or the insula is not activated in viewing self-images, and that a key to self-image correction may be this discrepancy in emotional and perceptual processing (Sachdev et al., 2008, pp.2161–2168).

Personal Story

Body-hatred consumed me during my anorexic years. There were precursors, but nothing extreme. Most of the factors were simply circumstantial: I grew faster than my twin brother but developed later than my peers; my mother was skittish, especially about girls being more fragile than boys, and discouraged me from being physically active; my family was not touch-oriented; and my mother, whose body type actually was quite different from my own, was unhappy with her body. However, each of these circumstances may have contributed to my body hatred and development of anorexia.

Before I reached three years old, I was bigger than my twin brother. He had a very slight build, and like most boys, grew slowly before adolescence. Until I became anorexic, I was taller and stockier, and heavier than him. In photographs of myself with both of my brothers when I was ten and eleven, I was midway in height between my twin, who was half a head shorter than me, and my brother two years older, who was half a head taller. People who knew there were twins in the family but hadn't seen us before would think when they met the family that the twins were my older brother and myself. I remember times when I would stand next to my smaller twin and feel as if I were the size of a house.

I don't know what made my mother scared that I might hurt myself, but she thought that girls were more delicate than boys. Perhaps she learned the same way I did, from her mother, who may have discouraged my mother's physical ventures. My mother complained that she felt clumsy, uncoordinated and poor at sports. In some ways, considering how much more solidly I was built than my twin brother, my mother's admonitions didn't really make sense. Nonetheless, she warned me: "Be careful! Don't do that! You might hurt yourself!" Prohibitions against taking physical risks made me scared to participate in activities like roller-skating and ice-skating, even though other boys *and* girls I knew liked doing those things, including both of my brothers. Any sport that could be construed as "dangerous" and a possible threat to physical safety, I was taught to avoid. And in turn, I felt awkward and clumsy in strange situations, as though I didn't quite know how to move through space.

In addition to discouraging physical activity, my family also had injunctions against touch. My parents seemed to major in above-the-shoulder "hello" and "goodbye" hugs, accompanied by a pat on the back. This confused me some, because my maternal grandmother was very affectionate, holding me in her lap when she sat in an overstuffed chair in the living room, or in the car when my grandfather was driving.

It seems that for my mother, the whole arena of having a body was problematic. Not only were movement and touch minimal, but also she didn't seem to appreciate being female. She complained of being too fat and not as pretty as her friends. She constantly battled losing the same ten pounds, while eating in a way that assured this would never happen. When she looked at herself in the mirror, she always saw all her faults, and itemized them for me: her tummy bulged, her thighs were too heavy, her waist wasn't slim. I don't believe she experienced any gratification from being female or from having a woman's body.

Not only did my mother not like her own body, she didn't particularly like mine. It was in response to an angry comment from her about my body that I began to diet, which eventually led to my becoming anorexic. That fateful day, when I had happily announced my consumption of extra desserts, and she had responded with disdain, "You're getting fat!" If she didn't like me in a fat body, I decided I would get a thin one! I would diet until there was no way she could call me fat. Dieting worked for me: I lost weight, which led to more dieting and more weight loss. I soon lost sight of how thin I was becoming.

When I was twelve and thirteen, I envied young women, usually a few years older than myself, who had matured past the amorphous prepubescent phase and developed trim, nicely shaped bodies. I wished that someday I would look like that, too. But no matter how little I ate, my body looked like a thinner version of a shapeless blob, and not at all like the mannequins and models I admired.

I entered treatment for anorexia at the age of thirty. At that point, I viewed my body as a jail which imprisoned me. No matter how long I withstood hunger or how little I ate, my body was still not thin enough and I had to run and swim and eat even less to keep the fat from engulfing me. I thought fat people were "out of control" because they did not have the willpower to diet. I envied thin bodies and was jealous of their owners. What power enabled them to stay thin without the deprivation and self-torture that I required to fend off hated pounds?

It was a problem when I entered the Cathexis program for treatment and observed instantly that all the major therapists were overweight. In fact, to me they seemed enormous. I was appalled to think that they wanted me to gain weight and be large and fat just like them. I couldn't trust these people who were so out of control of their bodies, and I resisted accepting information they gave me about good nutrition, health or weight. I began treatment because some of the staff members were caring and I believed they could help me overcome my depression. But I was adamant that I was never going to let them control how I should look or what I should weigh. It took a long time for me to trust them enough to accept either the information they gave me about food and weight or their assessment of my appearance.

Upon entering therapy at Cathexis, I agreed reluctantly to two treatment contracts: to identify and express a full range of feelings, and to gain weight at the rate of one pound per week until I reached a target weight range, and then to maintain my weight for the duration of treatment. I thought the first contract would be easy, but I had no idea how undeveloped my emotional perceptivity was. The second one terrified me, but I knew I had to do it to stay. The staff psychiatrist — who was overweight — calculated my target range based on the mathematical formula used to create actuarial tables. I didn't trust him, or the formula. But I decided that I would gain weight if that were the only way these therapists would help me with my depression, and then I would leave and lose the weight again.

As I gained weight, I felt like my body was an inflating blimp, and that control over my size had been usurped by the staff at Cathexis. Several times while in therapy, I rebelled and refused to gain weight, arguing that the target weight range was unrealistic and wrong for my body type. The staff patiently acknowledged my fear about loss of control and reminded me that if I wanted to remain in treatment, I had to maintain the contract. Each time I relented. My most acute struggle occurred when I was about five pounds away from my target range; I had adjusted to eating differently and to not being quite so thin, but I didn't want to get still *bigger*. Again I relented. By now I had become attached to the staff and students at the institute, and felt they cared about me. I belonged to a community now and was better at handling my emotions, and I was making headway at building more functional relationships. I was also less depressed than when I entered treatment. However, I knew I was not confident handling numerous situations in my life, and I would benefit from continuing therapy. I didn't want to lose the opportunity to continue healing and growing.

I continued to maintain my weight in my target range. But it was another two years before I felt much ease in my new body — this prison that I had struggled, interminably and unsuccessfully for over twenty years, to shape into the image I wanted. In part it was the gift of time that helped; I became more familiar with my changed body. Also, I looked at current photographs of myself. Although I hated seeing them, at the same time I realized that my mind still distorted and enlarged my internal picture, for the photos showed clearly that I was not oversized in the way my mind would still have me believe. In addition, I was strongly influenced by a female therapist at Cathexis who became my "contractual mother." (At Cathexis, it was a common therapeutic technique for a client and therapist to make a verbal agreement, or contract, that the therapist would act as a client's parent, and the client as the therapist's child, so the client could internalize new parent messages and undo the negative parent messages the client had received as a child.)

My contractual mother served as an excellent role model for me, given my disdain for my body and ambivalence about being female. She found joy in being a woman and in having a woman's body. She had many qualities I admired and loved. She was strong, well defined, powerful, amazingly energetic, playful, very bright and at the same time, soft, feminine, nurturing and very caring. She had been divorced for many years, but she enjoyed the company of men. She was dedicated to her work, and had a career as a school psychologist in addition to her work at Cathexis. She had two children of her own, and was the contractual mother for several clients. She loved being a woman and buying feminine clothes, putting on makeup and wearing nail polish, and she also loved being domestic, cooking for her kids and doing things with them.

Not only did I have endless opportunities to observe my contractual mother, she also invited me to participate in activities she enjoyed. Cathexis offered some degree of milieu therapy, or therapy resembling life. Staff members frequently included clients in activities outside of traditional individual and group therapy settings. I accompanied my contractual mother to her local gym and learned to get gratification from the things that she enjoyed. She relished exercising in the pool, taking saunas and steam baths, and sitting in the Jacuzzi, because they were relaxing and made her feel good. Many of these experiences were new to me, and she encouraged me to do them with her. I learned to enjoy and find pleasure in my body. Although I had exercised obsessively for many years, daily swimming a mile and a half or running several miles, I had not exercised for pleasure: I ran and swam to relieve anxiety and agitation, to push away uncomfortable feelings, to quell hunger pains or to burn calories. For a long time after entering treatment, I still thought of exercise either as a rote tool to drive away discomfort or as punishment for eating. But with the help of treatment, I began to learn that my body was more than a source of angst, and I could gradually tolerate pleasure without feeling guilty. Slowly I developed an association between exercise and feeling good.

Early in treatment, as I began to gain weight, I resolved to control the distribution of the pounds I gained. I was determined to create as perfect a body as I could, given the horrifying fact that I had to gain thirty pounds. I was disappointed that I couldn't exert the kind of control I wanted, that the curves on my thighs and hips wouldn't flatten out and assume contours like those of a wiry adolescent boy. It was not until I was able to grasp that my body was not simply a structure — an object to mold and beat into shape — but an integral part of myself, that I was able to begin to relinquish my obsession about how my body looked. One part of this process was learning to focus on other aspects of my life besides food and weight control, such as friendships, fun and work. Another was learning to take care of my body — to nurture it and treat it lovingly and "act as if" I cared about my body and not just about how it looked. I also had to learn to accept how my body looked and felt without always wanting it to be different.

Buying new clothes with my contractual mother helped me change my attitude about my appearance. I had hated shopping because I despised the way I looked in *anything* I tried on. I felt guilty spending money on clothing that wasn't "perfect." I agonized interminably before buying anything new to wear — did it make me look fat? Did my stomach or hips stick out? Was it the "right" color, and style, and fabric? Any new clothes I bought would hang in my closet for ages. I had to adjust to these garments, and accept that I could wear them and let them represent me despite their imperfections. If they hung in my closet long enough and were no longer "new," then when I wore them, I could believe it was an accident that these items had ended up in my wardrobe and I wasn't really responsible for how they looked on me.

Shopping with my contractual mother was a whole new experience. She loved to shop and made shopping fun. She was excited about different kinds of clothes and all the styles and colors that were available. She loved trying things on and bought clothes quickly and easily. Her exuberance was infectious and I picked up her excitement. Even though I didn't like the way my body looked as I gained weight, I did enjoy being able to wear nice clothes. My taste in clothing transformed. I discarded my former images: by day, an adolescent boy garbed in boys' jeans, T shirts and a denim jacket; on special occasions, a teenaged gypsy in long skirts and peasant blouses, or a dressier version of my boy-like daytime attire. First, I began to see myself as a girl, then as a young woman, and eventually as a woman with a definite style. Contemporary, feminine blouses and slacks now appealed to me. I bought a dress for the first time in years — a tailored knit, navy blue with little gold buttons down the front. In my teens and early twenties, I had loved the colors and textures of fabric and had hung out in fabric stores, wishing I had a use for the soft and silky cloth I found there. New shopping experiences with my contractual mother helped me recapture my interest in fabric varieties. On my 31st birthday, my contractual mother took me to have my ears pierced, and I was delighted with the new aura of femininity conferred by the little jewels sparkling in my earlobes. Staff members and other clients, and most important to me, my contractual mother, complimented me on my improved self-presentation. Initially, I was embarrassed by their attention and had difficulty trusting its authenticity. But over time, and with practice, I was able to take in their comments and accept the changes I had made.

I received frequent feedback on my appearance in a therapy group at Cathexis entitled Nutrition and Social Values, which was comprised of several clients who had problems with food and body image. In this group, ongoing discussion of the difference between my body perception and how others saw me helped me begin to revise my inaccurate body perceptions. I learned that a discrepancy between a "real" and a "perceived" image was a problem for other people in the group as well. Clients in the group did a drawing exercise that helped all of us to understand our body misperceptions. At one-year intervals, each member of the group drew a picture of how she thought she looked, and group members and a therapist would discuss what each drawing indicated. My self-portraits changed over time. When I entered Cathexis, I drew a stiff, rigid man with tiny hands and no feet. Besides the obvious lack of acceptance of myself as female, the small hands and lack of feet suggested I wasn't grounded or able to reach out to others. A year later, I depicted a chubby little girl. I saw myself as female, but not as a grownup. The following year, my representation had morphed into a plump and stocky woman, much heavier than I actually was. By then, I could see myself as older and as female, but I certainly didn't have a realistic picture of my size. I didn't have an opportunity to repeat the drawing again at Cathexis, but I am sure my self-image continued to change and in time would have reflected a much more accurate self-concept.

One other aspect of developing a clearer sense of myself was the process of beginning to experience and express my own emotions. Initially, I had little understanding of what it was like to feel feelings, especially anger. For years, I had denied that I had feelings of my own, and merely acted as I thought I was expected to, or, when still at home, acted out my mother's feelings. One of my therapists had me push and pull against him and at the same time yell "I'm angry! I'm angry!" in order to develop a kinesthetic sense how anger felt, in this case anger which was provoked by pushing against an immovable force. Initially, my yelling was very mechanical, but with repetition, I began both to feel angrier and to push against him more vigorously. I also recorded situations daily when I felt angry, and I was given suggestions about the level of anger that was appropriate to the circumstances, and when and how to respond to the anger I felt. Eventually, I was able to put together more of my internal sensations of anger with information about other people's reactions in similar situations. I was also able to begin to integrate the emotional sensations of anger with both thoughts and behaviors in response to it.

Developing a realistic awareness of my body also entailed learning how people normally experience hunger and fullness. I was very much aware of hunger, and of my usual means of responding to it — running, swimming, drinking water or coffee. I felt gratification from the discomfort of hunger and from testing myself to see how long I could go without giving into eating. Also, I hated to feel full. Feeling full meant I had been weak enough to allow myself to eat. My mind had learned to translate the physical sensation of feeling full into "feeling fat." I didn't realize that other people experienced hunger as unpleasant and felt a sense of satisfaction from being full. Much as I hated it, I was required to eat regular meals in treatment at Cathexis. I ate some meals with staff members who demonstrated appropriate size servings. Of course, for a long time I was certain the size serving they deemed "appropriate" was in fact guaranteed to make me fat. However, their input eventually helped me normalize my view of food portions. Neither starving nor bingeing was easy to accomplish in this setting. With my new and consistent eating habits, I began to experience getting hungry at regular intervals. And in time I was able to tolerate the sensations of having eaten or feeling full.

At Cathexis, participating in a form of bodywork also helped change my body perception. One of the therapists guided me through some exercises in wall sitting, stretching and deep breathing. These gave me a physical basis for experiencing my body in a new way. Through this work, I released some "body armor," the physical defenses I had unknowingly developed to block emotional experiences. I had a sense of being more grounded in my body, rather than the familiar experience of my body as a foreign, hated structure that held me prisoner. This was a step towards my feeling "real" and developing awareness of my body from the inside out, rather than of imposing my will and my vision on my body.

It was several years after I left Cathexis before I was able to adjust to my new weight, and still longer before I could truly accept my body. For a long time, I hovered at the lower end of the eight-pound weight range I had been given, still exerting a measure of control, although not so destructively as before. Developing an appreciation for my body and a sense of inner cohesiveness was an extended process. I had acquired the foundation at Cathexis: I was physically healthy; my weight was stable and I understood the need, physically and psychologically, for keeping it that way; I was aware of some emotions and possessed a language to label them and some tools to process them. But I still didn't feel completely at home in my body. I still didn't feel as though all the parts of me were connected. I still did not have the sense of an inner core.

In the years after Cathexis, I continued to participate in psychotherapy. This work helped me to understand and metabolize my emotional experiences, which in turn afforded me a greater measure of safety in feeling my feelings. As I felt more security in knowing and understanding my feelings, I was able to accept my body as a source of self-information rather than feeling compelled to mold my body to suppress my feelings. I pursued a few varieties of hands-on therapeutic massage — with Rosen and Hellerwork practitioners — which helped me release more physical and emotional blocks to feeling whole. I experimented with movement and dance therapy, which were opportunities to let the mood of the music inform my body's gestures and to feel more internal fluidity. Body and movement work gave me a sense of being more solidly present *in* my body, and helped diminish my attachment to how my body looked on the outside. I had the opportunity to work with a gifted practitioner of Somatic Experiencing, a form of bodywork designed to help release holding patterns resulting from life traumas. Through this work I was able to experience an inner cohesiveness I had not known before.

Prior to entering Cathexis, I had no sense of internal cohesion or of an inner core. While at Cathexis, I stopped starving and started developing an awareness of my emotions. In the years subsequent to Cathexis, I gradually developed a more solid sense of substance, wholeness and cohesiveness within my body and an acceptance and appreciation of my body, both in appearance and capacity. Today I have a sense of my body as a coherent whole and as a home for my feelings, thoughts, desires and aliveness. And I view my body as an expression of my being in the world; of being female, feminine, physically embodied and blessed with the capacity to dance and play and do and create and eat and hug and love; as having physical shape and characteristics — some that I love, some that I don't, some that I wish were different. Regardless, I experience my body now not as a hated object I stare at and disparage but as a vital and vibrant entity I inhabit, care for and enjoy.

PART TWO

Treatment and Recovery

6

Understanding Recovery

What Constitutes Cure?

In the original edition of this book, I spoke in terms of "cure" of anorexia nervosa. I had a somewhat myopic view of my own recovery at that point. Barely four years had elapsed since I had entered therapy weighing less than 70 pounds. I had achieved a healthy weight and sustained it for over three years and I had acquired many emotional and social tools. I thought this meant I was "cured."

Hindsight is always 20/20. Now I can see that what I possessed at that point was a strong foundation for recovery, but I was in no place to assess what psychological, social or spiritual work lay ahead of me. I had barely begun a career, still had many issues to work out with my family, had not been in an intimate relationship since entering treatment, and possessed a limited social circle. I had no experience with 12-Step programs nor any understanding of how anorexia might be considered an addiction, biochemically or psychologically. I had barely finished graduate school, and my work with eating-disordered clients was in its infancy.

However, whatever bias my own psychological development in 1983 might have conferred on my research findings, the truth was that the clinical understanding of anorexia nervosa also had a long way to go. Not only has the brain chemistry research of the last two decades given us a new perspective on both the origins and treatment of the disorder, it has also shown us how much more there is to learn about both.

It is debatable whether the term "cure" can be applied to any condition with psychological underpinnings. Human beings continue to grow psychologically throughout life, with or without the benefit of therapy. How can a line be drawn, with any accuracy, between the end of one cycle of growth and the beginning of another? When does an individual resolve all the issues that contributed to a particular illness such as anorexia nervosa? When does an individual become so free of inner conflict as to be deemed "well"?

The *DSM-IV-TR*, the standard used by psychiatrists and psychotherapists for diagnosing mental illness, lists several diagnostic criteria for anorexia nervosa: weight at 15 percent or more below healthy body weight, voluntary restriction of food and intense fear of gaining weight. Does this mean that no remnant of the disorder remains when an individual who has been anorexic no longer exhibits those particular symptoms? It seems more useful to acknowledge that attaining the state of no longer having symptoms is an important milestone, but not the end of the journey. Therefore, I now choose to use the word "recovery" and the phrase "in recovery" as markers of growth and progress towards wellness in healing from anorexia nervosa. As Ira Sacher and Sheila Buff note in their book *Regaining Your Self: Breaking Free from the Eating Disorder Identity*, "Recovery is not the absolute destination we would like it to be" (Sacher and Buff, 2007, p.124).

Challenges in Evaluating Recovery

Evaluating recovery in anorexia nervosa is a daunting task, although several researchers have developed methods and criteria to attempt to measure improvement. Part of the difficulty is that no two individuals begin life in exactly in the same way, nor do their illnesses follow identical trajectories. However, as therapists have sought to enhance treatment outcome, they quite understandably have wanted to determine whether an individual with anorexia has indeed improved and what may have contributed to improvement. This quest to advance therapeutic techniques and to establish the factors that promote recovery has spurred some dedicated clinicians and researchers to find ways to appraise progress in recovery from anorexia. Below, largely in historical sequence, is a summary of some of the methods for evaluating recovery, as well as the problems and limitations of these methods.

In brief, clinicians and researchers have used many criteria to evaluate recovery in anorexia nervosa. Weight restoration has proven to be an insufficient criterion. Some researchers have developed schemas that combine several parameters, such as weight restoration, eating behavior, social adjustment, vocational status and sexual adjustment. Over the years clinicians have developed a number of self-report questionnaires to assess both physical and psychological parameters of recovery. The results of these can be sorted according to specific traits, or groups of traits, and the data tabulated and statistically analyzed. For example, some questionnaires focus on body image attitudes while others evaluate quality of social relationships. Researchers sometimes combine several different questionnaires in a single study to develop a broader and a more detailed view of specific aspects of recovery. One study asked patients to identify the aspects of recovery most important to them. Recently, researchers with the capacity to measure change in brain biochemistry have evaluated very specific neurotransmitter functions and assessed levels during and after treatment for anorexia. Through all this, however, many questions still remain about which parameters to consider when assessing recovery.

Most authors have agreed that restoration of lost weight, although an important step in the process of getting well, is not itself enough to qualify as recovery, and that the older treatments designed solely to encourage weight gain are likely in the long run to meet with failure and possible relapse. Eating disorder specialist and psychoanalyst Hilde Bruch observed that weight gain may represent only a temporary remission of the disorder and may in fact be a misleading sign of progress. Bruch cites the case histories of four anorexic women who regained sufficient weight and maintained it long enough that they were considered recovered, but who later experienced relapses and died of starvation (Bruch, 1973, p.382).

In 1965, A.H. Crisp added to the criterion of weight the factors of eating behavior, sexual behavior, relationship with mother and presence of other psychiatric illnesses as criteria for evaluating treatment results. Individuals were categorized by weight as either over 12½ percent overweight, normal weight, moderately underweight (12½ to 25 percent) or grossly underweight (25 percent or more). Eating behavior was characterized as overeating, normal, undereating, vomiting or mixed. Under sexual behavior, Crisp included a category for presence or absence of menstruation and another for married or unmarried, and rated general sexual adjustment as good, moderate, poor or very poor. The current relationship with the mother was also judged as good, moderate, poor or very poor, and psychiatric illness, if present, was identified (Crisp, 1965, Table 1, p.74). The drawback in using categories such as Crisp's is that the distinction between some rankings, as between "good" and "moderate" sexual adjustment, is subjective and depends in part on who makes the assessment. However, for purposes of comparing individuals being observed by the same therapist, the categories can be useful if the clinician has a consistent method for drawing distinctions.

Two British researchers, Peter Dally and William Sargant, used a somewhat different set of criteria. They recorded average total weight gain and weight gain per week. They then evaluated each client on the basis of seven criteria: whether she was (1) menstruating regularly, (2) well-adjusted socially and of satisfactory weight, (3) very thin but working satisfactorily, (4) still requiring in-patient treatment, (5) exhibiting persistent compulsive overeating and overweight, (6) exhibiting a fear of food or of weight increase, or (7) manifesting other psychiatric disturbances (Dally and Sargant, 1960, Table VI, p.794). According to this method of assessment, one individual may belong to several categories. Without specifics as to which attributes are indicative of significant progress, or criteria for evaluating individuals with various rankings in different categories, it is difficult to extract from Dally and Sargant's results an estimation of the extent to which their clients improved.

The German psychiatrist and researcher Helmut Thomä evaluated anorexic clients after discharge from treatment. He used six social and symptomatic criteria. Social criteria included marital status as ("married in the meantime" or "unchanged") and childbearing status ("given birth in the meanwhile" or "no children"). Interpersonal relationships were rated as good, satisfactory or bad; professional adaptation as good, satisfactory or bad; eating disturbance as removed, improved, unchanged, worse or bulimic; gastroenteric symptomatology (such as nausea, diarrhea, constipation) as removed, improved, unchanged, with constipation still present or never present (Thomä, 1967, pp.53–54). Results of psychotherapy were rated as improved, not improved or improved spontaneously. The overall course of illness was judged as cured, improved, unchanged, worse or patient died (Thomä, 1967, p.51). Thomä's schema, not unlike the ideas of some of his predecessors, took into account the wide range of factors that need to be considered in assessing recovery from a disorder which manifests with a variety of symptoms.

One criterion that few of the early authors addressed specifically was that of change in body image awareness. Bruch observed that a realistic body image is essential for recovery in anorexia nervosa and that no real or lasting cure can be achieved without correction of the body image misperception (Bruch, 1973, p.90). However, it was known even then that body image disturbance is slow to resolve, and that it often takes many years beyond the restoration of body weight to develop a realistic body image. Other traits Bruch viewed as significant in evaluating success of treatment included changes in self-concept and resolution of the typical adolescent identity struggle with a resultant awareness of and control over one's function (Bruch, 1973, p.376). While it is significant in recovery for an individual to believe in her ability to take charge of her own life and to take action on her own behalf, specifying a point at which she has attained that capacity is subjective.

Alexander Lucas, Jane Duncan and Violet Piens, in 1976, put forth another perspective. They stated in the *American Journal of Psychiatry* that "the test of effectiveness of treatment rests not in the statistics of weight gain but in the patient's ability to master eating behavior as demonstrated by maintenance of both physical health and psychological integrity after treatment" (Lucas et al., 1976, p.1037). Restoration of "normal" eating behavior (itself hard to evaluate) and "psychological integrity," which can include readjustment to family and social environments (equally difficult to measure), are important aspects of recovery, but assessment of either is highly subjective. Comparison of the improvement of different individuals, particularly when judged by different therapists lacking a standardized system of assessment, has been inconsistent at best. It can be argued that one measure of recovery rests in an individual's progress from the time of diagnosis to the point of termination of treatment, but this does not allow a fair comparison of one "former" (as defined by absence of certain symptoms) to other "former" anorexics, let alone to random other individuals. The point at which someone with anorexic symptoms enters therapy, and the reasons and criteria for "termination of treatment," are as varied as the individuals seeking help. Therefore, many authors have reported treatment results based on their own set of clinical criteria for improvement applied to the particular individuals with whom they have worked.

In 1981, two American psychologists, Donald Schwartz and Michael Thompson, sought a way to standardize the evaluation process. They reviewed a number of outcome studies of anorexia nervosa treatment and made several recommendations to simplify accurate cross-study comparison. Schwartz and Thompson advised that results be broken down into anorexia-related symptoms, non–anorexic symptoms, and life (social) adjustment data, and that the results be reported separately rather than lumped together. They recommended that reports of anorexia-related symptoms should present separate data on eating behavior and weight, and eating behavior should be broken down by type, for example, dieting, bulimia, food faddism, and vomiting. For non–anorexic symptoms they advised using standardized symptom-assessment instruments, several of which existed at the time. Social adjustment scales could be broken down into separate subscales for vocational, socio-familial and sexual adjustment in order to identify subgroups of clients with different areas of social strength (Schwartz and Thompson, 1981, p.322).

Schwartz and Thompson further noted that assessment of qualitative differences among individuals and identification of subtypes would be facilitated by including variable scores for each subject in a study. They observed that reports of global recovery scales tended to obscure findings unless accompanied by detailed reporting of individual scales. While they seemed to acknowledge the significant variation among individuals recovering from anorexia, they also suggested it would be useful (but did not attempt it themselves!) to develop a standardized anorexia outcome scale (Schwartz and Thompson, 1981, p.322). Implementation of the suggestions proposed by Schwartz and Thompson may have rendered the initial collection of data in studies of anorexia more tedious. However, consistent use of their recommendations might have simplified and improved later comparison of treatment methods and results.

Over the past few decades, several instruments for assessing psychological, physical and social change in individuals with eating disorders have been developed. Most of these include a series of questions for the anorexic to respond to by selecting from a five- or six-item scale ranging from "not at all" to "all the time," or from zero to five. The results are tabulated and, based upon the meanings that have been assigned to the findings, the researchers can stipulate the severity of the individual's symptoms. These tests obviously do not take into account the unique qualities of each individual and are not a substitute for in-person interviewing and more interactive and psychologically sophisticated ways of understanding someone's recovery process. Nonetheless they do provide a system for standardizing assessment of some recovery criteria and of quantifying progress and recovery by producing data which can be subjected to more exacting statistical analysis.

Currently, two of the instruments most commonly used for assessing treatment are the Eating Attitudes Test (EAT) and the Eating Disorder Inventory (EDI). The most frequently used form of the EAT is its abbreviated version, the EAT-26, which is a 26-item self-report questionnaire that provides five levels of answers to each statement about eating or body image. The answers can be tabulated and used to assess the severity of the anorexic's eating and body image symptoms. This has been used particularly to evaluate drive for thinness, fear of weight gain and restrictive eating (Garner, 1997, pp.175–177).

The EDI, which was later refined to the EDI-2, was designed to evaluate behavioral and psychological dimensions of eating disorders. The EDI-2 includes several subscales for traits such as asceticism, impulse regulation and social insecurity. As in the EAT and EAT-26, the EDI and EDI-2 ask questions, provide a choice of answers, and produce a final tabulation that can be correlated to severity of anorexic (or bulimic) symptoms (Crowther and Sherwood, 1997, p.41).

A not quite so commonly used instrument, The Eating Behavior Rating Scale (EBRS), was designed to measure eating pathology in anorexia (Wilson et al., 1989). The individual rates herself from 0 to 5 on twelve questions such as "global assessment of eating" and "ritualistic behavior." The results quantify the severity of the anorexic's eating attitudes and behaviors.

One interesting self-report questionnaire is the Eating Disorder Recovery Self-Efficacy Questionnaire (EDRSQ), developed to help determine the readiness for recovery of anorexic patients undergoing short-term hospitalization. The test primarily evaluates self-efficacy with respect to body image and eating, meaning the extent to which the anorexic believes she can influence her own thoughts and behavior about body image and eating. This illuminates the anorexic's belief in her own capacity to influence her recovery in these areas (Pinto et al., 2007, pp.143–153).

A recent test developed specifically to screen abnormal body image attitudes and eating disorders is the Body Uneasiness Test (BUT). This is a 71-item self-report questionnaire in two parts, the first of which measures weight phobias, body image concerns and compulsive self-monitoring and the second of which looks at specific worries about body parts and functions (Cuzzolaro et al., 2006, pp.1–13).

Many other self-report tests and test subscales have been developed. Some of these specifically evaluate eating disorder behavior, such as the Eating Disorder Examination (EDE) (Crowther and Sherwood, 1997, p.39); others measure social adjustment, such as the Social Network Questionnaire (SNQ); and still others assess psychological factors, as in the Anorexia Nervosa Symptom Score (ANSS). Still other self-report instruments, originally developed to evaluate psychological symptoms in a variety of patients, have been employed to evaluate level and type of psychological disturbance in anorexics. Most anorexics experience some degree of anxiety or depression or both, and scales to measure these symptoms are frequently given to anorexics. For example, the Beck Depression Inventory, or BDI, is used to evaluate a person's level of depression. Many treatment programs and individual clinicians that use testing to evaluate symptoms and recovery in anorexia will administer a combination of several different tests when assessing an individual. This allows them to draw more detailed and comprehensive conclusions from their results.

In a study entitled "Do Anorexic Patients Return to Psychological Health?" a group of researchers in Germany combined several instruments to evaluate recovery of former anorexic patients (Deter et al., 1994, pp.155–173). The researchers used four scales, the ANSS, the EAT, the EDI and the SNQ (all described above), to assess psychological change in 103 anorexic patients, from 9 to 19 years after treatment. That the researchers were able to follow up on this many patients over an extended time period suggests their dedication to obtaining meaningful results. After subjecting their data to statistical analysis, they categorized the patients as dead (12.7 percent), desolate (29.4 percent), showing severe psychological disorders (30.4 percent) or healthy (40.1 percent). The authors concluded that a portion of patients with anorexia nervosa (their 40.1 percent) become psychologically healthy again.

Similarly, researchers at the University of Iowa in 2008 combined several tests to measure recovery in 32 anorexics receiving inpatient treatment in a one-year period. They combined results from the EAT and the EDI-2 in conjunction with the Beck Depression Inventory (BDI) and an instrument that evaluates psychopathology, the Minnesota Multiphasic Inventory (MMPI). Although this study evaluated only very early recovery, the use of a group of testing instruments enabled the authors to conclude that both disordered eating behaviors and psychological symptoms improved during the term of the study (Bowers and Ansher, 2008, pp.79–86).

Advances in analysis of brain chemistry have provided one additional approach to evaluating recovery. Rather than being based on patients' self-report, these tests rely on actual measurements of levels and function of biochemical elements. Since it appears that in anorexia there is a deficit in the production of the neurotransmitter serotonin (the neurotransmitter that mediates calmness and pleasure), researchers have wanted to assess change in serotonin function with treatment. In 2005, several researchers at the Western Psychiatric Institute and Clinic in Pittsburgh, Pennsylvania, employed positron emission tomography (PET scans) and carbonyl IIC to evaluate neuronal activity as determined by measurement of receptor binding by a specific type of brain serotonin. Explaining these methods is beyond the scope of this book, but suffice it to say that the researchers found that both anxiety symptoms and changes in functioning of the neurotransmitter serotonin persist after recovery from restricting-type anorexia nervosa (Bailer et al., 2005, pp.1032–1041). They further postulated that these alterations in brain chemistry might contribute to the origin of anorexia nervosa. While the study of brain chemistry is in its infancy, it is a field that in the future may offer us considerably more information about cause, consequence and treatment of anorexia.

In addition to evaluating overall extent of recovery from anorexia, other studies have been conducted to compare the outcomes of different psychotherapeutic approaches in treatment. Unfortunately, this has further complicated the evaluation process. Now rather than one group of therapists using somewhat systematic methods for assessing patients, treatment and results, therapists of different disciplines are pitted against each other. Asay and Lambert in 1999 said that when psychotherapies are compared, as little as 15 percent of the outcome is accounted for by factors that are unique to a specific type of therapy, because so many other issues affect the comparison. In other words, comparison of different therapeutic approaches yields very little reliable information. Eight-five percent of the results are due to either individual therapist factors (30 percent), patient and environmental factors (40 percent), or a general placebo or expectancy effect (15 percent) (Eisler et al., 2003, p.305). Understandably, psychotherapists are biased in favor of the therapeutic modality they use, and this affects their collection and evaluation of data. Eisler and his colleagues noted that in their own studies they have demonstrated that very different therapies—such as family therapy and cognitive therapy—can produce similar outcomes. They concluded that this similarity in outcomes using different approaches demonstrates that we still have limited understanding of the mechanisms of change (Eisler et al., 2003, p.306). And if our understanding of how change happens is rudimentary, then determining what factors contribute to change is mostly conjectural.

In 2007, some insightful European researchers decided to compare what patients and clinicians believed were necessary ingredients in the recovery process. Patients and therapists agreed that three important elements in treatment are improving self-esteem, improving body experience and learning problem-solving skills. (Vanderlinden et al., 2007, pp.357–365). While this study did not seek to offer comparison data, or to address methodology in achieving the desired outcome, it made clear that there is some consensus as to specific issues that effective treatment needs to address.

What is clear is that evaluation of recovery remains an inexact science with no universal set of criteria. Also, there is no real baseline, as every individual who enters treatment for anorexia nervosa is unique in her physical and psychological makeup, her stage of the disorder, the length of time she has been suffering from anorexia, other aspects of her history, the degree to which she is affected by the illness, her current social and family situations, and her motivation to change. In addition, recovery occurs at different rates for different aspects of the disorder, and physical, psychological and social attributes all have numerous subcategories of variables to evaluate, many of which are difficult to measure and to prioritize.

The use of self-report questionnaires can lend more uniformity to recovery comparison studies, and there is less room for clinician bias in computing results. While answers to the self-assessment tests are clearly subjective on the part of the patient, the results provide researchers and clinicians with some valuable data for assessing treatment and recovery. Furthermore, researchers continue to update and refine symptom assessment instruments, and to develop new ones, so that broader and more reliable information can be acquired. However, on any self-report scale, each person will have her own interpretation of criteria or questions.

It is certainly possible for any individual to analyze her own improvement using either self-report instruments or her own words, but this brings up another question: Who is the final arbiter of change in a person, especially in terms of psychological and less easily quantifiable variables? Is it the individual, the clinician, the researcher armed with test scores and norms, or the family and others with whom the client interacts? To what degree should the client's subjective sense of her own progress, and her personal feelings of happiness or fulfillment, be taken into account? Probably no one would argue that malnutrition, obsession, social fears, anxiety and depression detract from feelings of well-being, and of course no one has a crystal ball to predict what future progress any individual may attain. But it is the rare (if not delusional) human being who is free from internal conflict, insecurity or pain, and it seems that the individual's assessment of her own recovery is a key consideration. She can, at least, appraise improvement in her sense of well-being.

The Foundation of Recovery: Development of a Coherent Sense of Self

Just how does one who has been anorexic, emotionally thwarted and developmentally challenged build a coherent and cohesive Self? How does one know one has developed a Self? And how does this developed Self relate to the kernel of Self that the anorexic earlier risked her life to preserve?

Developing a Self is the work of therapy, and of life. When genetics and the experiences of infancy and early childhood have not promoted growth of a Self, individual psychotherapy and adjunctive recovery modalities (groups, family therapy, body-oriented therapies, medication where appropriate, etc.) can help the recovering anorexic to generate the missing elements. But there is never a specific moment when one can declare herself to have developed a Self. The realization is more clearly seen in hindsight, through recognition of the ways one feels more solid and connected now than before. If a former anorexic reports that she was able to stand up for herself without feeling guilty or at fault for doing so, to have sustained a belief in her own values despite dissent, to have done so not from rebellion or contrariness but because it was her truth, she has clearly demonstrated evidence of self.

Nor is there a point at which the process of self-development ceases. It is the nature of the human organism to grow, and emotional growth inevitably means growing in dimensions of the Self. Growth is seldom linear, and some areas develop faster than others.

The Self the anorexic has risked her own life to preserve remains sacred to her. It is the only reality she trusts and the only Self she knows. Initially, she cannot understand that treatment is not designed to rob her of what she has, but rather to help her expand her inner resources. She cannot know that her undeveloped Self is like a barren desert compared to the substantive, multi-faceted and cohesive Self that she can build through recovery. She has no way to comprehend that her cherished core of being is a significant but meager fragment which can be nurtured and supported through therapy to grow into a much more solid and alive core.

One factor that is crucial to the anorexic's development of a healthy Self is a therapeutic environment in which she can feel safe enough to reveal her inner world. This requires a non-judgmental, patient and empathic therapist who can above all be present and attuned to the conflicts and pain the anorexic fears unveiling. When a therapist empathically responds, mirrors, and acts as a gentle guide, the anorexic can gradually learn to trust another human being. This process demands patience — on the part of both the anorexic client and the therapist.

It is only in such a nurturing and empathic environment that a recovering anorexic can slowly add to the inner kernel of Self that she has so closely guarded. And it is only after a long time of gradually building pieces of a substitute reality that she may begin to disclose her own sacred truth. It is only then that, piece by piece, she can dare to disassemble the self-destructive defenses she has erected against humiliation, rejection and abandonment and construct in their place forms of self protection: She can put into words what she has formerly conveyed through her body. She can voice her frustration, fear and sadness. She can link her feelings to the situations that triggered them. She can ask for what she needs. She can say "no" to what she doesn't want. And she can recognize "feeling fat" as a disguise for negative thoughts or feelings.

Often, an anorexic is highly creative but has shrunk from developing or revealing this side of herself. It is a sign of growth for her to risk exposure of this tender aspect of her being. Sometimes she hides talents or passions that she fears exposing to others who might have harsh responses. For one anorexic teenager with whom I worked, it was two years into her therapy before she let me know that she wrote poetry. This was a well-guarded secret; I later discovered that her family only learned about her talent when she received an award at her high school graduation for her poetic contribution to a plaque her senior class had erected to war veterans. My client had originally contributed the poem anonymously, and did not reveal that she was the poet until the school principal ruled that the poem could be used only if its authorship were known.

Self-growth for the anorexic also entails revealing and reworking parts of her belief structure. While her former logic seems skewed and certainly clashes with new learning, it is totally reasonable in the context of the defensive structure that has ensured her safety. She is convinced that every morsel of ingested food begets excess body fat, that how she looks is the full measure of her worth, and that being a grown-up ensures a lonely and heinous life. I remember believing that women were lesser human beings than men; that it was okay for men, but not for women, to have successful careers; and that my role in life was to be constantly accommodating and pleasing, or else risk being rejected.

But developing trust, learning a language for her feelings and restructuring her beliefs comprise only part of the anorexic's journey towards developing a Self. Not only do these endeavors continue, with ever-increasing depth and breadth, but also the work of recovery has many layers and multiple dimensions. Growth is a process, and some steps must precede others. An anorexic cannot have an emotional interchange with another person until she can identify and communicate her own feelings; she cannot form a solid connection until she can tolerate another's reactions without personalizing the comments or collapsing from them; she cannot enjoy her body while mapping her own demise. Often several different forms of therapy, as well as adjunctive resources such as nutritional consultation, 12-Step support and bodywork, can be contributors along the path. And then there is the challenge of putting into practice outside the therapist's office the knowledge and skills that the former anorexic has discovered in therapy. The world thus becomes an endless laboratory for experimentation, learning and growing. Her interactions and endeavors provide infinite feedback for her to reflect on, revisit in therapy, and experiment with as she returns once again to the outside world. The development of Self is not a short-term process. For a growing child, it lasts at least from infancy to early adulthood, and it continues in some measure throughout life. For a teen or adult whose development has been derailed by anorexia, it can take several years to build a foundation, and longer still to fill in missing pieces and consolidate the parts into a felt sense of "wholeness." Self-development is a cumulative process, not an event. For the former anorexic, just as for those individuals who have not had to wrestle with this disorder, each experience in life can be a source of learning and growth that adds more cohesion, breadth and vitality to the solidifying Self.

My Journey Towards Self-Development

My personal path towards self-development may or may not resemble any other anorexic's journey towards recovery. By the time I left Cathexis, supposedly "cured," I had recognized that a consistent identity and a clear expression of needs were significant aspects of healing from anorexia. I knew that pleasing others had been a major *modus operandi* for me as it is for most anorexics, and that letting myself know and say what I wanted represented a fundamental change in perspective. I recognized that creating a life which did not revolve around body size, and dismantling perfectionism in favor of realistic goals, were important milestones, and I was grateful that I had developed a fuller life and was no longer driven to attain unreachable standards. But I had no way to comprehend the extent to which I still lacked inner cohesion or a solid identity, and no sense of either the work of recovery or potential for change that lay ahead of me. I could not understand then that the primary work of recovery from anorexia is the growth in complexity, consistency and cohesion of a central core essence, the Self.

I recognize today what I could not then: that by 1983, when I emerged from several years of therapy at Cathexis Institute, I had developed only a rudimentary framework of Self. I couldn't know then that more growth was possible or that there was more to being a whole person than what I was experiencing. It is apparent to me now that I was missing a substance and inner connectivity that characterize the healthy Self. I had progressed in many areas, but lacked a central organizing principle. Although I deemed myself "cured," and chose neither food restriction as my daily goal nor low weight as my identity, I still did not have a consistent, clear sense of "me." While I didn't feel totally whole, I also could not imagine feeling any *more* whole — I certainly felt a lot more together than I had when I entered treatment. However, instead of experiencing a safe haven inside, an inner source of comfort, I remained haunted by an undercurrent of inadequacy and feared that others would discover my rampant insecurity and chronic emptiness. I *tolerated* my body, but I could not actually *appreciate* it. My choices were still chameleon-like, influenced by my company of the moment. I had no concept of my potential for growth and no vision of how much more my life could change.

Treatment at Cathexis was founded on principles drawn from Transactional Analysis (TA), a cognitive and behavioral therapy originated by Eric Berne in the 1950s. In 1982 I attended a presentation by Dr. Steve Karpman, noted TA author and psychiatrist, who proposed one concept of recovery from anorexia that made sense to me at the time. In that presentation Karpman described what he termed "social cure" of anorexia, which he defined as the point when the individual has available in herself each of the five functional ego states, and she can elicit from another individual all five ego states. Those five functional ego states are Critical Parent, Nurturing Parent, Adult, Natural Child and Adapted Child.

According to TA, an ego state is a coherent system of thoughts and feelings manifested by a corresponding pattern of behavior. Structurally speaking, the personality of the individual is comprised of three ego states: that of the Parent, consisting of the values and injunctions adopted from one's parents; the Adult, which is the rational, reality-oriented center responsible for processing information; and the Child, comprised of feelings and desires. Functionally, the Parent ego state consists of a Nurturing Parent, which performs the supportive, caretaking duties of a parent, and a Critical Parent, which sets limits and reprimands the child. The Child ego state is exhibited as Adapted, which is to say, compliant and under the influence of the Parent; or Natural, demonstrating autonomous behavior.

The anorexic typically is highly adapted and has a severe Critical Parent that she imposes on herself as well as on others. She also exhibits contaminated Adult thinking, minimal Nurturing Parent and virtually no Natural Child behaviors. In TA, in the process of recovery, the anorexic needs to develop more Nurturing Parent and to attain a balance of the critical and nurturing aspects of her Parent ego state. She also needs to decontaminate her Adult, which is both clouded with misinformation and tainted with judgments that are really the province of her Critical Parent. And finally, she must relinquish many of the overly accommodating behaviors of her Adapted Child and free up her Natural Child.

In 1983, I might have applied Steve Karpman's definition of cure to myself something like this: In the process of treatment, I had developed a Nurturing Parent to help me soothe and take care of myself. I stopped obsessing over Critical Parent messages that urged me to try hard to be perfect and that undermined my accomplishments. I learned to differentiate fact from judgment and replaced many of my former misconceptions with accurate Adult information. I could distinguish when compliance was useful, as opposed to having it be my sole way of interacting. And I had liberated Natural Child energy that allowed me to be more spontaneous and have fun. Furthermore, I could elicit Nurturing and Critical Parent responses from others, participate in logical Adult-Adult interchanges, encourage others to adapt to my sensible Parental suggestions, and use my sense of humor to engage the Natural Child energy of others.

What seems implicit in Karpman's criteria for "social cure" of anorexia is a framework for the development of a Self. The "Self" of Rosenberg, Rand and Asay, as I described in the first chapter of this book, encompasses a continuity of internal identity, a sense of aliveness in the body, a non-verbal sense of well-being, a permanent core of being into which a person can retreat for comfort and self-support, a center which enables a person to truly know who she is without reference to the rest of the world (Rosenberg et al., 1991, p.143). In looking back, I can see that in 1983 I possessed a scaffold of a Self without a solid core. An ability to function from all five ego states indicates the presence of such a scaffold, but in addition, a person with a healthy Self possesses the capacity to move fluidly between ego states in response to internal or external cues while having an established sense of "I-ness" throughout. In other words, a person can be angry (Critical Parent) one minute, move to giving an explanation (Adult), and then a moment later be able to laugh (Natural Child), but feel like one and the same person throughout. This ability eluded me; I had barely glimpsed the substance and connectedness implied in the description by Rosenberg and his colleagues. My sense of who I was changed depending on the situation. My emotional structure was built more of Pick-up Sticks than solid beams, and my inner core was neither fully molded nor especially stable. There were inner qualities I knew I had developed and had not possessed before entering treatment, but they were fragile, apt to rapidly disappear under stress, and recapturing them was an arduous process. However, in some measure Karpman had supplied a framework — an outline that allowed limitless space to add missing details and dimensions. Seen through his description, I had a foundation on which to build and a framework in which to foster creation of the cohesive core I lacked.

In the intervening years, therapy and life experiences have helped fill in the skeletal frame of Self that I possessed back then. I still had deficits from my years of anorexia — in body acceptance, self-acceptance, emotional awareness, feelings of competence, development of personal interests, spiritual growth and pursuit of pleasure. Through many years of individual and group therapy in the intervening years, I was able to slowly progress. My growth in these areas, which I have summarized briefly below, was crucial to my developing Self.

Though I realized in 1983 the importance of attaining a healthy body image, I am not sure I understood that that meant more than not wanting to starve and be exceptionally thin. My body image awareness was still in process— although I was too much *in* the process to recognize that it *was* a process. I knew that simple restoration and maintenance of normal body weight could be carried out from an angry, adapted position without a revision of the underlying belief system that triggered the anorexic symptoms. This supported Bruch's claim that in anorexia, weight gain alone was insufficient to ensure future weight maintenance (Bruch, 1974, p.1421). Even two years into maintaining a consistent, healthy body weight, I still did not like the way my body looked. Nor did I feel that I inhabited my own body. It felt to me as though I was carrying around a superstructure that was bigger than I needed, and I was always shocked when I looked in the mirror and saw what I perceived as a thick and stocky form.

In time — and I can't say when, because it was a process that unfolded gradually — I changed from seeing myself as round and stocky to viewing myself as normal and acceptable —*without any loss of weight*. During my thinnest years, exercise helped me to control my body size and give me the sense that I could mold my body shape; early in therapy this was still my intent. But slowly I was able to accept both that I was more than my body, and that there were more dimensions to my body than simply appearance. I began to enjoy the kinesthetic feelings from running and swimming and dancing. I appreciated the experiences of physical touch and massage. And I developed more sense of continuity and identity *inside* my body, independent of how the *outside* of my body looked.

Owning my gender and my sexuality aided my sense of inhabiting my body, an important ingredient in developing Self, and eventually I learned to appreciate my femaleness and my sexuality. Sexual energy is part of being vital and alive, and owning my sexuality gave me back the gift of a life force I had suppressed.

Being able to feel and manage a range of emotions was one more step in solidifying my body appreciation and sense of feeling centered in my body. In the safety of individual and group therapy, I learned to let myself experience emotions and I sensed their presence in particular parts of my body. I felt sadness in the pit of my stomach, anger in my head, arms and shoulders, fear in my shoulders, neck and stomach. The greater the number of sensations I felt *in* my body, the less attached I became to only looking *at* my body. In addition, different kinds of breath and bodywork helped me to develop a kinesthetic appreciation and felt sense of my body. Through programs of slow stretches and small movements, I learned to enjoy the physical sensation of muscles moving rather than focusing on how my limbs looked as they moved or how many calories I was burning. Various kinds of bodywork helped me release tension in parts of my body that felt numb or blocked. I could *feel* that my hands attached to my arms at my wrists, and that my arms attached to my shoulders; that my feet attached to my legs and my legs to my torso. My body was no longer just an object to shrink and make as small and invisible as possible. Nor was it a compendium of disassociated parts. I sensed that my body was interconnected and formed a whole. No longer did my chest contain tight, impenetrable blocks that barred my breath from passage. I could breathe into areas that had been numb. And feelings were no longer inconvenient ripples that I tried to squelch. Physical sensations and their emotional meaning intrigued me. I felt alive!

As I learned to eat for nourishment, I increased my sense of body awareness and body ownership. I used to hate buffets or food-centered occasions that sported a prodigious amount of food — the challenge was to winnow food selection down to a minimal amount without feeling robbed of tasting everything. An anorexic client of mine recently exclaimed, "Thanksgiving is death!" I understood completely — I had once felt the same way. So many of our society's social activities center around food that it is both a challenge and a necessity — if one is to be social — to develop ways to manage food in social gatherings. Even for "normal" people, the setting and the companions influence food consumption. Some people tend to eat more, or less, or differently, in social situations than when alone. Developing healthy eating habits not only helped heal my body, but also allowed me to have meals with other people. This required a learning curve as eating with people was foreign. As an anorexic, I had generally eaten alone, hiding my habits — eating erratically, or only one food at a time and in minuscule amounts or painstakingly extracting the raisins from oatmeal cookies.

Achieving a sense of competence and effectiveness was crucial to my developing an internal source of identity, a criterion which Rosenberg, Rand and Asay deem as a critical aspect of self-development (Rosenberg et al., 1991, p.142). Power, effectiveness and self-esteem for the anorexic depend on her capacity to control her weight, and controlling her weight is her identity. By 1983, I had grown in competence both in taking care of myself and in getting along better in the world. I had developed better interpersonal abilities and honed skills as an administrative assistant in several part-time jobs, first in real estate and then for a contruction company. I had worked effectively as the intake coordinator for the treatment center where I had formerly been in therapy. What I lacked most was a belief in my competence. And my identity was hinged to my feelings of inadequacy.

Since then, with the patient help of my therapist, augmented by intentional, if erratic, reframing on my part, I am better able to own my competence and less likely to dismiss my abilities as trivial. Significant restructuring of my beliefs coupled with psychodynamic work to dislodge attachment to my prior self-view have helped offset my attitude of "learned helplessness," which programmed me to see myself as incompetent no matter what my accomplishments demonstrated. Furthermore, through learning how to manage areas in which my skills are challenged while accepting my shortcomings, I have adopted a more realistic and consistent sense of myself. I know that I possess a continuum of capacities, some better developed than others. Formerly my "all or nothing" perspective had demanded that I be competent in anything I tried, or not undertake it at all. Without the sense of chronic failure that my former perfectionism conferred, I can accept having a range of abilities. I also know that who I am does not depend solely on what I have accomplished. What is consistent for me is the knowledge that I am capable, that I have areas of competence and a track record of some achievements, and that I can learn new skills.

The sense of aliveness so integral to the experience of Self is also embodied in a capacity for pleasure and joy, and this was vital to my self-development. Laughter and joy are fonts of positive energy. Anorexics approach life with a seriousness appropriate to the life-and-death struggle in which they are engaged. An anhedonic attitude, grounded in the absence of pleasure, may even be endemic to the family of an anorexic. Life with a deficit of joy—which characterizes my anorexic years—is, in the famous words of Thomas Hobbes, "solitary, poor, nasty, brutish and short." He was describing the natural state of mankind without government, but he could just as easily have been talking about the anorexic without treatment. Anorexics are prone to depression and anxiety, and I had my share of both.

Fortunately, there are various ways to increase dopamine, the pleasure neurotransmitter that seems to be in short supply in anorexics. One thing that helped me to experience more joy was to deliberately increase the number and quality of pleasurable activities I pursued, both through revisiting endeavors from earlier in my life and through introducing new ventures. I had loved riding my bicycle as an eight- and nine-year-old, but hadn't been on a bicycle since I was a teenager. I was hesitant to borrow a bike, but delighted when I did, at age 37, to find that not only did I still know how to ride, but also that I could recreate the sensation of freedom and power I had experienced years earlier from breezing downhill at high speed!

Often growth in capacity for pleasure requires "acting as if" the activity is pleasurable until it actually becomes so. Pleasure and fun, and anything new, were initially tinged with fear for me. I was petrified to learn to water-ski, but had friends who enjoyed the sport. Fortunately, they were patient and skillful teachers, and I was up and flying over the surface of the water in no time.

Being with fun-loving people also helped increase the pleasure in my life. Earlier in my life, when I was depressed, I attracted men who also were depressed. What a joyless couple we made! As I have developed friendships with more people for whom joy is a necessary part of life, I have come to value and seek it myself. I have also learned to reframe situations or events that feel heavy and negative in order to discover something positive. Barring that, at least at those times I think about what I'm grateful for in my life. I do my best to find out what I can learn from negative experiences instead of wallowing in my gloom.

Allowing my love of color and visual beauty to surface was another source of pleasure and an asset in growing my identity. I had repressed my artistic inclinations for many years, or expressed them in a constricted fashion invisible to the eyes of potential critics. In the midst of my anorexic years, I learned to make cloisonné jewelry, but relinquished that and other artistic pursuits as my disease progressed. Only after a significant period of treatment did I feel psychologically able to pursue artistic ventures. I resumed making cloisonné jewelry for a time, working with a private instructor, and later learned to work in silver and to set rings and pendants. There was a correlation between my increasing strength to tolerate others' reactions — and even more, my own — and my willingness to share my creations. Attending watercolor classes was a courageous move because, in a room with other students representing all levels of ability, I had to keep my competitive voice in check and deflect self-criticism. I love color — in nature, in flowers, in paintings, in interior design and apparel. During my anorexic years, my asceticism largely curtailed my indulging this love of color.

As I progressed in recovery, and felt more entitled to pleasure and to pursuit of my interests, my psychotherapist encouraged me to resume some of my earlier creative hobbies. At one time, I had enjoyed the color and texture of fabrics and had created cloth collages from textile scraps used for upholstery and drapery. I began perusing fabric stores, and eventually constructed a collage. I talked about the piece I had made for a long time before actually letting my therapist see it; when I did finally show it to her, I was relieved that she was empathic about my fear of her reaction, appreciative of the work the collage had required and complimentary about the fabric choices and design. I also began to spend time combining clothing and accessories, savoring the color and style of the arrangements. Originally, my creations never left the confines of my own bedroom. In time, I took another step towards exposure and felt brave enough to wear ensembles with a select friend or two, and then gradually I was able to wear them in social and work settings. Eventually friends were asking me for help with their wardrobes! Without psychotherapy, I wonder if I would have progressed past making tiny cloisonné pieces that I hid in a drawer. Today, I consider my love of color, and of visual beauty, to be an integral part of my identity. In the words of Ira Sacher and Shelia Buff, "When people with eating disorders discover their passions, they discover their own true selves" (Sacher and Buff, 2007, p.87).

The capacity to self-soothe is one more factor that contributed to my developing the sense of a solid inner core and reliable identity. Food manipulation and weight obsession had been my major sources of comfort, as they are for most anorexics. According to Rosenberg, the healthy Self possesses an internal retreat for comfort and self-support (Rosenberg et al., p.142). For many years after entering treatment I longed for a way to fill the void inside. Communicating my needs, developing friendships and pursuing my passions all helped strengthen my identity and provide more substance, but these didn't satisfy my longing to feel whole. I envied those of my friends who seemed to find contentment through a spiritual practice. I searched for many years to find a spiritual home — it wasn't religion or the Episcopal learning of my childhood that I sought, but a sense of inner peace that eluded me. I tried attending a number of churches, and enjoyed the music, but the prayers and rituals did not speak to me.

It was finally through the support and teachings of the 12-Step program Overeaters Anonymous that I was able to find some solace. Overeaters Anonymous (OA) is a program that welcomes anyone who wishes to stop eating compulsively, and despite my anorexic history, I also could go to the opposite extreme, not by bingeing per se, but by becoming very enamored of a specific food and structuring the next several days around my quest for that particular food. Meditation and prayer are integral parts of 12-Step recovery, as is the concept of a higher power. I had practiced meditation several times previously, but never in the context of a belief system.

In OA, I struggled for some time with the concept of "surrender" because control had been so fundamental to my functioning. Nonetheless, I began to develop a sense of faith in something greater than myself. When, surprising myself, I was eventually able to embrace the concept of surrender, I felt relieved. It was reassuring to accept that my job is to do what I can, and to do my best, but that I am not in charge of the outcome.

While my journey may not mirror those of other anorexics in recovery, I believe that many of the elements that were instrumental in my healing and development of Self can echo aspects of their recovery. And my journey continues; I don't want to stop growing. How different this is from my attitude before I entered treatment! Back then I was stuck in an endless cycle of despair, self-hatred and weight obsession. I thought this was my future and my fate. I knew no way to escape. Fortunately, the people I turned to over the years had maps and methods. They were able to lead me out of my quagmire, to guide and support me in growing and changing. Still others emerged to pilot me beyond what at first appeared to be the farthest point where treatment would take me. They encouraged and helped me — and continue to do so — so that I can expand and solidify, create more inner connections, develop a deeper sense of well-being, and build and strengthen the spirit and substance that today I call "me" — my Self. This is why I believe in therapy: it can save a life. It can foster immense, enduring change. It can transform a person. It transformed me; I've seen it transform others.

7

Approaching Treatment

Essential Components in the Treatment of Anorexia Nervosa

Anorexia Nervosa is a bio-psycho-social-spiritual disorder, and effective treatment generally includes the following components:

1. Medical monitoring of individual's physical condition and guidelines to restore and maintain baseline standards of physical health, including weight, heart rate, blood pressure, and electrolyte balance.

2. Nutritional assistance as needed to restore nutritional balance and to work towards optimal health and well-being.

3. Recognition of the disease, the "voice" of the eating disorder, and learning to disempower that voice.

4. Developing an awareness of feelings and needs physically, emotionally and cognitively, including the feelings that manifest as negative body thoughts.

5. Developing non–food-related ways to identify, modulate and manage emotions and conflicts.

6. Developing of a healthy relationship with food.

7. Increasing acknowledgment and tolerance of discomfort and expanding acceptance of self, others and reality.

8. Learning to distinguish those areas one can control from those one cannot, and learning to let go of those which one cannot control.

9. Development of both body awareness and body understanding that are not dependent on visual or appearance-oriented criteria.

10. Developing a Self: acknowledging, valuing and expanding one's inner world of thoughts, beliefs, values, emotions, preferences, boundaries and fantasies, and increasing one's capacity for interpersonal relationships and intimacy.

11. Developing acceptance of being female and a capacity for healthy sexuality.

12. Restructuring beliefs about self-worth, personal competence, and the capacity and responsibility to manage one's own life, including acknowledgment of both strengths and weaknesses.

13. Participation in family therapy to facilitate open, non-critical expression of feelings and communication that enhances emotional connection among family members. Family therapy should assist each family member in identifying and expressing feelings, needs and wants, establishing personal boundaries and differentiating from other family members.

14. Redirecting creativity and passion towards healthy, self-chosen pursuits.

15. Incorporating pleasure and joy in life to help replenish neurotransmitter deficits and aid in motivation for healing, expand self-development and spark energy and zeal for life.

Considerations in Treatment

Management of both the medical and psychological aspects of anorexia nervosa are crucial in addressing this life-threatening disorder. Medical assessment is essential to ensure an anorexic's safety. Adequate nourishment is required for physical stability, and physical stability is necessary to undertake the psychological work of recovery. Inpatient treatment provides specialized staff to address each aspect of this disorder; outpatient treatment requires a comprehensive, integrated team approach. Treatment requires a warm, personal, compassionate attitude. Empathy and understanding on the part of all treatment providers are prerequisites for the anorexic to feel safe. Early recovery for an anorexic entails a delicate balance of building trust with treatment providers and improving nutrition. Ongoing therapy requires a two-track approach which addresses both the eating problems and the psychological issues which have led the anorexic to use self-destructive behaviors to cope.

Recovery from anorexia is a developmental process which addresses the emotional deficits and physical, familial, cultural and spiritual concerns that have rendered the anorexic dependent on starvation to manage life's demands. Often, the issues of adolescence and moving towards becoming a separate person have been a trigger, but frequently emotional setbacks from younger ages also are a problem. Recovery must address internal and relational difficulties from all phases of life, and prepare the anorexic to grow towards adolescence and then adulthood.

Much of psychological recovery from anorexia can be subsumed under the heading "developing a Self." However, this is a complex and multidimensional evolution which requires foremost that the anorexic develop sufficient trust and safety in another person to reveal her inner world and to explore and experiment with new and frightening behaviors and ways of thinking. In treatment, the anorexic must learn to use the mirroring, empathy and guidance she receives to restructure her inner world, to test her new knowledge in the world at large, and then ultimately to separate from her guides. Since an anorexic protects herself by building walls against intrusion, it is a major challenge for her to take in the help that formerly she has spurned; overcoming this barrier, however, is an important step towards self-development which can enable her to absorb the wisdom, skills and guidance of others that she can reconfigure as her own.

Also deeply embedded in the anorexic's psyche is her need for validation and approval, the consequence of her terror of rejection and abandonment. While learning to accept herself as an individual with her own identity, the anorexic must reformat her life objectives in terms of responding to her own needs and setting her own goals rather than pleasing others. This is no small task.

Self-development integrates expansion of emotional awareness and expression, adoption of self-care behaviors, relating to others in new ways, and gradually building a healthier self-view, including the right to exist and to have a place in the world. For the anorexic, recovery entails creating a self-identity and a sense of competence and agency in her own life that is not based on controlling her body shape and size. Creating a more accurate picture of herself in the world also requires developing a reality-based body image. Healing is a complex, multi-layered, energy-demanding and time-intensive process of change and growth. Solid recovery prepares the former anorexic for the ultimate test of self-development: becoming an emotionally healthy, responsible and functional adult.

Given the complexities of developing a Self, it is no wonder that treatment of anorexia is multidimensional. This chapter and the ones that follow are an introduction to the aspects, settings, types and modalities of treatment. It is my hope that this information can both provide a context for understanding the treatment of anorexia and serve as a guide to the variety of treatment possibilities.

Aspects of Treatment

There are many different aspects to treatment of anorexia nervosa, and several variables to consider when deciding on a treatment strategy. The first consideration is the level of care required, and hence the appropriate setting. Can treatment be conducted safely and effectively on an outpatient basis or is a partial hospitalization or inpatient setting required? If outpatient treatment is the choice, what professionals should the family or individual look to for assistance? Which approach to therapy is best? Is the involvement of a physician needed for outpatient treatment? Should a nutritionist be included? What about family therapy: when is that helpful and when is it not? Should other family members aside from the anorexic be seeking support? Is group therapy useful, and if so when?

Every anorexic is unique, and so is each anorexic's family; therefore, for many of these questions there are no universal answers. In addition, both the availability and quality of resources can vary, depending on the geographical location. Finances and insurance coverage may also be considerations. Treatment of anorexia is rarely short term, although the duration of treatment and the prognosis for recovery does generally improve with earlier intervention.

When anorexia may be an emerging issue but has not developed into a serious illness, finding a psychotherapist who is an eating disorder specialist is the best way to begin. It is important to find someone who feels like a good fit: a psychotherapist to whom one can speak openly, who listens well, and is empathic and responsive to one's concerns, and who speaks to both the behavioral and psychological aspects of the problem. It is also important to remember that for an anorexic, discussions about emotional issues, weight, and body image are likely to be uncomfortable with *any* therapist (although it may also be a relief for her to no longer hold these worries inside). Also, the patient or patient's family may not like *any* therapist's treatment recommendations because it can be difficult to acknowledge the existence or extent of the problem.

In this chapter and those that follow, I provide information to help with some of the questions about treatment, and to guide the reader to possible appropriate avenues for recovery. (At the end of this book, a list of some eating disorder facilities and an appendix with other sources for information and referral provide more resources for finding treatment.) In the remainder of this chapter I will first summarize some types of *treatment settings*—inpatient hospitalization, partial hospitalization, residential treatment center, intensive outpatient program and therapist-managed outpatient care — and list reasons why one setting might be more appropriate than another for an individual's needs. Generally the decision as to what level of care is needed is made either by a physician who has evaluated the client's condition or by a therapist in conjunction with a physician, in collaboration with the anorexic and her family. All inpatient and intensive outpatient programs also provide assessment to determine appropriate level of care. In this section, I also include a summary of *psychotherapeutic, medical and nutritional considerations* in outpatient treatment, since the coordination of these three aspects of care is essential to treatment of anorexia.

In Chapter 8, I discuss individual therapy for an anorexic, beginning with a number of different *psychotherapeutic modalities* used in the treatment of eating disorders. Many outpatient eating disorder specialists incorporate aspects of several approaches in their work, as clients' needs evolve during the course of treatment. All of the approaches are valid and have been used effectively in working with anorexics. Some clinicians just prefer specific approaches to others, and some clients simply respond better to certain approaches. Also, at different points in treatment, one modality may be more appropriate than another. Several *experiential modalities* also can be valuable adjuncts in the treatment of anorexia, and I discuss several of these. Given that anorexia is a body-centered and body-harming disorder, an anorexic can benefit greatly from new and pleasurable ways to experience her physical self through the experiential and body-based therapies.

Many anorexic clients do several courses of treatment in different settings or with different therapists in the process of recovery. Residential treatment centers generally incorporate more than one psychotherapeutic modality and several experiential therapies. With outpatient treatment, an anorexic may use both psychotherapy and experiential therapy at the same time, for instance, combining individual psychotherapy with therapeutic bodywork.

In addition to psychotherapeutic and experiential therapy, sometimes treatment involves medication. I close Chapter 8 with remarks on the use of *psychopharmacology* in anorexia.

Chapter 9 addresses therapy for families as a whole and for individual family members. I devote a special section to therapy for mothers of anorexic daughters because this is an area of particular interest for me. I believe that mothers have received far too little support in handling the painful and difficult situation of raising a daughter who develops the life-threatening disorder of anorexia.

Chapter 10 is a brief discussion of *12-Step programs* as an adjunct to treatment of anorexia. Anorexics tend to self-isolate; 12-Step programs provide a supportive community. Anorexics commonly experience a profound sense of despair, hopelessness and meaninglessness; a 12-Step philosophy can offer solace.

Chapter 11 addresses *intervention*. Sadly, it is characteristic of anorexia to believe that one is in control and doesn't need help, or that help in fact will make things worse; this is the very nature of the disease. With anorexics who are minors, it is the responsibility of their parents or caretakers to ensure that they receive treatment. However, when the anorexic is an adult and is not seeking treatment, friends and family members can feel overwhelmed, confused and helpless. In these situations, family members can meet with a professional interventionist to help them cope with their feelings and to approach their loved one in a caring, supportive way. The family, guided by the interventionist, can share their concerns, help the anorexic understand the severity of her condition, and express their wish that she get help. Family therapy is an integral part of the intervention process.

Clinicians working with an adult anorexic who either is making no progress in treatment or is refusing a higher level of care are faced with legal and ethical considerations. Sometimes clinicians can benefit from reassessing the anorexic's treatment history and implementing a new approach to therapy.

Treatment Settings

Possible settings in the treatment of anorexia nervosa include inpatient hospitalization, partial hospitalization program, residential treatment program, intensive outpatient treatment program and outpatient therapy.

Inpatient Hospitalization

Hospitalization is necessary when someone with anorexia is in danger, medically or emotionally. Possible dangerous medical conditions include very low blood pressure, very low heart rate, electrolyte disturbance or dehydration. Malnutrition and dehydration can cause electrolyte disturbance, which can, in turn, cause heart failure. Severe starvation can cause all of these conditions, any of which can be life threatening. Mortality rates for anorexia nervosa are high, often estimated at over 20 percent of individuals diagnosed with the disorder, so hospitalization is an appropriate and essential course of action in some cases.

Psychiatric hospitalization is required when an anorexic is actively suicidal or is so seriously depressed as to not be able to function on her own. Anorexia is a slow, almost passive, form of suicide and severe depression can precede or accompany anorexia. Furthermore, depression in an anorexic is generally aggravated, if not caused, by poor nutrition.

Hospitalization is generally a short-term intervention designed to help the anorexic stabilize medically and psychiatrically.

PARTIAL HOSPITALIZATION PROGRAM/DAY HOSPITAL PROGRAM

There are very few partial hospitalization programs for the treatment of anorexia. However, where they exist, these programs offer intensive treatment, consistent medical care and nutritional rehabilitation at a lower cost than inpatient treatment. This kind of program can work when outpatient therapy is insufficient or has not worked, but where there is not an acute medical or psychological crisis requiring round-the-clock medical care. Partial hospitalization is less expensive than residential treatment, which sometimes is a factor in choosing treatment. One advantage of this kind of treatment is that the anorexic may find it less confining and regimented, than inpatient or residential settings allowing her a little more freedom and autonomy. This freedom, however, can also be a disadvantage, as it does not offer the same sense of containment as an inpatient program. Some clients, therefore, can de-stabilize at the initial stage of their treatment, particularly when they are first experiencing major stress around changing their eating patterns (Kaplan and Olmsted, 1997, pp.354–7).

RESIDENTIAL TREATMENT PROGRAM

Residential treatment can be a valuable phase in the treatment of anorexia. Residential treatment can last from 30 days to six months or longer. Unfortunately, length of stay can be limited to 30 days when insurance coverage dictates the extent of treatment based on "medical necessity." Most case managers for insurance and managed care companies are not well-versed in the breadth and severity of psychological problems that can accompany anorexia. The concept of "medical necessity" does not take into account the fact that physical recovery and psychological growth sufficient to benefit and to protect from relapse are rarely accomplished in one month of residential treatment. Unfortunately, residential treatment is costly, although some programs offer scholarship plans. It is expensive to provide the quality and breadth of care present in well-run residential eating disorder treatment centers. However, longer-term stays are valuable when financially possible.

Residential treatment offers the advantage of providing many kinds of support not available on an outpatient basis. One advantage is the provision of substantial balanced meals prepared with the guidance of a dietitian or nutritionist to ensure that the recovering anorexic will be given appropriate nutrition. In addition, staff members are available to provide support at mealtime to help the anorexic manage the physical and psychological discomfort that eating can provoke. Not having to make food choices can be a relief to the anorexic in the early part of treatment. Many residential centers then gradually increase the individual's participation in food choices, food preparation and food shopping, and even arrange outings to experience meals in restaurants. This prepares the anorexic to manage food and eating when she returns home after treatment.

Residential treatment also offers a vast array of therapy groups, including groups that focus on body image, creative expression, emotional management, relaxation, meditation, stress management and cognitive skills. This abundance of psycho-educational opportunities helps the anorexic to address the complex assortment of issues she faces in recovery. Her previous unswerving focus on food and weight control has narrowed her range of coping abilities and stunted her development of many life skills. To a large degree, the anorexic's emotional development has been arrested at the stage when she began using food restriction to manage her life. Group therapy offers opportunities for the anorexic to develop emotional, social and life skills.

Family therapy is often a part of the treatment protocol at residential programs. Whether family therapy takes place during a weekend or extends for a full week, it provides a forum for the anorexic and her family members, guided by a therapist, to express feelings, discuss family issues and concerns, and begin to plan for the anorexic's transition home, if that is her destination after treatment. Family therapy is invaluable, whether in residential or outpatient therapy, because an anorexic does not develop her disorder in a vacuum. Even if the anorexic is no longer living with her family, her psychological development occurred in the family environment, and addressing her current psychological issues is greatly assisted by involving the individuals who were a part of the arena in which her belief system and emotional development originated.

Often a psychiatric evaluation is conducted during residential treatment. Given that many anorexics suffer from depression, anxiety, obsessive thinking, compulsive behaviors or other psychiatric conditions, expert evaluation and prescription of appropriate psychotropic medication can sometimes assist an anorexic's overall functioning, and thereby enhance her capacity to benefit from treatment. In early recovery, medication can also assist the anorexic's nutritional restitution, since mood influences appetite and digestion. The question that ultimately needs to be answered is what portion of the anorexic's psychological issues result from malnutrition and will self-correct when nutritional health is restored. However, the answer to this question may remain unclear for some time into recovery.

Intensive Outpatient Treatment

Residential treatment is not always possible, nor is it always necessary in the treatment of anorexia. Some residential centers offer an onsite, extended-care program, which resembles an intensive outpatient program (IOP). Other IOPs will take patients either after or instead of residential treatment. An IOP generally provides many of the same treatment opportunities and care as a residential center, but allows the anorexic to be in a less regulated environment outside of the program hours. This atmosphere can be a good transition between a highly structured residential program and the minimally structured environment of returning home. It can also be a good option that provides a structured treatment setting which is less intense and less expensive than a residential center.

Outpatient Treatment

Effective outpatient therapy requires a comprehensive, collaborative approach in which the primary psychotherapist, who should be an eating disorder specialist, acts as a case manager and coordinates treatment with a physician and other practitioners involved in a client's care. The primary therapist needs to be aware of the medical and nutritional status of the client, as these affect her emotional condition. Therefore, the primary therapist maintains communication with the physician, nutritionist, family therapist, group therapist, psychiatrist or any other adjunctive practitioners involved in the client's treatment.

Psychotherapeutic, Medical and Nutritional Considerations

In outpatient treatment of anorexia, the therapeutic, medical and nutritional aspects should be addressed in concert. Focusing on any one without the other two will not provide the anorexic with a solid foundation for recovery. The physician, nutritionist and psychotherapist all need to be experienced in working with anorexics; treatment of anorexia requires specialized knowledge and specific experience. In general, it is the therapist who coordinates treatment, but a close collaboration among all three practitioners is essential, especially when the anorexic is in early recovery.

PSYCHOTHERAPEUTIC CONSIDERATIONS

Psychotherapeutic treatment of anorexia requires a two-track approach with attention both to issues related to weight control and dieting, and to psychological issues of emotional expression, self-concept, perfectionism, and interpersonal relationships. The psychotherapist works with both of these aspects, often moving back and forth between the two, focusing more on weight and dieting concerns early in therapy (Garner et al., 1997, p.108). In this work, the therapist relies on the physician and nutritionist to cover the medical and nutritional fronts, so as to establish a foundation of physical recovery, while the therapist addresses the related emotional issues.

Individual, family and group therapy are all of potential value in recovery from anorexia. Each has its particular strength and function in the recovery process. Individual psychotherapy is generally the central part of treatment. Sometimes the individual therapist will also act as a family therapist or lead a therapy group that the anorexic attends. In other cases, the individual therapist may recommend that the anorexic see another therapist for family or group therapy. With written authorization from the client, the therapist will consult with any other practitioners involved in the client's care.

A group that offers education in building specific skills, such as cognitive behavioral therapy or dialectical behavioral therapy, can be a useful adjunct to individual therapy. A general eating disorder support group may be useful, as isolation is common to anorexia. In a group setting, the therapist generally establishes a format or structure that creates a feeling of safety and routine. A group can be a supportive environment where people with similar issues can share their struggles and successes, particularly around implementing specific skills taught in the group. While it can be daunting initially to open up to a group of strangers, in time the client can experience caring and support from this group.

Family therapy can be important in the recovery process because anorexia has an impact on family members, who in turn have an impact on the anorexic. Family members can experience a lot of pain and confusion about their role in the anorexic's recovery. Furthermore, they often worry that they may have "caused" the anorexic's disorder, and the guilt they feel about this possibility sometimes leads them to feel responsible for "fixing" the anorexic. One focus of family therapy is helping family members understand that multiple factors contribute to the origin of the disorder. Another focus is identifying and addressing issues in the family that may unwittingly contribute to prolonging the anorexia.

Chapter 8 offers an overview of some approaches to individual therapy. Chapter 9 gives further information about therapy for families and family members.

MEDICAL CONSIDERATIONS

Medical monitoring is essential because of the risks, particularly of cardiac problems, resulting from starvation. Only by measuring vital signs and monitoring electrolyte balance with blood tests can a person's physical condition can be assessed with any accuracy. An anorexic may report that she is "feeling fine." In fact, she may not remember what "feeling fine" feels like, and she may have become accustomed to feeling exhausted, cold and light-headed. Furthermore, if an anorexic is at a low weight, it is the physician who should establish the weight limit and other medical parameters which would make hospitalization necessary. Some of the acute medical concerns in anorexia include cardiac arrhythmias, very low blood pressure or heart rate, and inability to maintain core body temperature.

In my practice, I find a complete medical evaluation at the outset of treatment essential to establish a baseline for the client's physical status. It is generally the physician who establishes the frequency of subsequent medical visits, which will be determined by the client's physical condition. Initial evaluation includes weight measurement; temperature; evaluation of heart rate and blood pressure, and particularly of shift in blood pressure from lying down to standing up; blood tests to assess red blood cell count and sedimentation (indicators for anemia, which is not uncommon in anorexia) as well as white blood count, and levels of minerals such as magnesium (an indicator of heart function) and phosphorus (which affects breathing). Thyroid function may be disturbed in anorexia; other hormones may be imbalanced, and specific blood tests can indicate these levels. An EKG is valuable to establish heart rhythms. Anorexics may suffer a loss in bone-mineral density, and establishing baseline bone density at the outset of treatment is helpful, but not as critical as the various metabolic measurements. Some physical parameters improve as nutrition improves; others may need specific medical treatment.

NUTRITIONAL CONSIDERATIONS

The nutritional component of outpatient care is essential to help the anorexic eat and regain weight. Sometimes the therapist handles the nutritional issues along with the therapy. However, it is more frequently the case that a nutritionist manages the program for restoring healthy nutrition while the therapist addresses the psychological components of treatment. Anorexics are terrified of eating, but nutritional restoration is essential for healing. Early in recovery, addressing the anorexic's fears about eating and weight gain is central to the work both of therapy and of nutritional consultation.

Nutritional treatment, like psychotherapy, needs to be individualized for the client. It is essential to dispel a client's misconceptions about food and weight gain, and anorexics need explanations and clarification of the reasons behind specific nutritional suggestions. Anorexics also need considerable encouragement to make any small change in their eating behavior. Educating an anorexic in detail about any aspect of her current medical condition and any potential medical complications of anorexia is important, even if both her physician and her therapist are also providing similar information. Each practitioner is likely to provide a slightly different slant, and the client may only be able to process a portion of what she is told at any one time.

It is also essential that the anorexic understand in detail what changes to expect as her body takes in added nutrients. Fear or dislike of her body's development at puberty — and what that represented — may have been a trigger in the onset of her anorexia. After a course of controlling her food intake and her weight, she is likely to be even more fearful of the ways her body will begin to alter. Furthermore, results of starvation studies have shown that weight gain after starvation does not follow the same path initially as weight gain in the course of normal development. With a 25 percent loss of weight, there is a 70 percent loss of fat and a 40 percent loss of muscle; with refeeding, a greater proportion of the "new weight" is fat (i.e., over 70 percent of lost fat returns), and that weight initially tends to settle in the mid-section. In other words, initially an anorexic may gain weight in proportions and areas that she would prefer not to, making her feel even *more* out of control. However, after about nine months, body weight and body fat tend to return to pre-starvation ratios (Garner, 1997, pp.159–160). In addition, the physical discomfort the anorexic may experience from changing eating habits can be significant. Finally, increasing the quantity the anorexic eats must be done slowly to minimize discomfort from "refeeding syndrome." When a starved individual eats too much too soon, the resulting dramatic changes in blood mineral levels can be dangerous, possibly causing cardio-respiratory irregularities (Costin, 2007a, p.241).

Often a nutritionist will suggest that an anorexic keep journals in which she records levels of hunger and fullness, as well as amounts and types of food eaten. The client may benefit from sharing her journal with her psychotherapist as well. While it can be hard for anyone with eating issues to see on paper the reality of what she is consuming, a written record can also offer the anorexic an objective perspective on her food intake, and an opportunity to notice correlations between incidents of under- or over-eating and specific emotionally triggering events.

An anorexic in recovery should work with a registered dietitian (RD) who is a specialist in eating disorders. The educational and certification requirements for an RD are far more rigorous than those for a nutritional consultant (NC). Unlike NCs, RDs are required to update their knowledge and certification through obtaining continuing education credits. RDs are certified by the credentialing agency of the American Dietetic Association (ADA) (www.eat right.org).

8

Therapy for an Anorexic

Psychotherapeutic Modalities

There is no single psychotherapeutic protocol which has been shown to be universally effective in treating anorexia nervosa. Each client is unique; a specific approach may be better suited to working with a particular client, or with that client at a particular phase of treatment. Various experiential therapies and body-oriented approaches can be valuable adjuncts as well. It is helpful when a psychotherapist who is working in an outpatient setting with an anorexic can be flexible and draw from different disciplines depending on the particular needs of a client at any given time. As Kaplan and Noble have pointed out, "Adherence to one single theoretical framework is insufficient to effectively treat these patients.... A working knowledge of psychotherapeutic paradigms that embrace self psychological, cognitive, behavioral, interpersonal, motivational and psychodynamically informed principles is necessary to provide optimum outpatient management for patients with anorexia nervosa" (Kaplan and Noble, 2007, p.132). In addition, when the anorexic is an adolescent, family therapy is an essential component of treatment.

Psychotherapy with anorexia generally requires a two-pronged approach: attention needs to be directed both at the eating behaviors themselves, and at the psychological meaning and beliefs which the food behaviors represent. However, the starving patient is not able to benefit from cognitive or psychodynamic psychotherapy. Doing effective psychotherapy with a starving patient "is analogous to trying to address underlying issues with an alcoholic patient who is intoxicated" (Garner et al., 1997, p.103). Therefore, for the seriously underweight anorexic, some level of nutritional restitution must precede any significant psychological work.

In the pages that follow, I describe a few of the primary psychotherapeutic approaches used in the treatment of anorexia. Where I have had experience with a particular approach, I include a personal note.

Behavior Modification

Behavior modification is designed to reinforce some behaviors and reduce others through a system of rewards and punishments. It is based on fundamental axioms of human behavior: we seek pleasure over pain and we tend to repeat a behavior or action that is rewarded and to discontinue a behavior or action that is punished. Behavior modification is a technique which has proven effective, but it has drawbacks that are important to consider.

In the treatment of anorexia, behavior modification has been used to work with behaviors related to food restriction. One disadvantage of this approach is that unless behavioral treatment is conducted in a hospital or residential setting, it can be difficult to monitor. Furthermore, if it is used for weight restoration, there is the danger that this weight gain will cause the anorexic additional psychological distress because she feels less in control of her body. Also, neither change in eating behaviors nor change in weight gain addresses the psychological under-pinnings of anorexia nervosa. Nonetheless, there is a delicate balance in the treatment of a severely underweight anorexic: without re-nourishment, she cannot effectively process cogni-tive and psychological issues; and without addressing psychological problems, she is unlikely to maintain the weight gained or to continue implementing newer eating behaviors. Therefore, early treatment in anorexia generally requires a slow and skillful integration of both behavioral and psychological work.

Since the 1960s, behavior modification has been used effectively with some anorexics to change their eating behavior (Touyz and Beaumont, 1997, p.362). The technique has been of particular value because it can directly address the life-threatening aspect of the disorder: star-vation. Because "not eating" is learned behavior, healthier food-related responses can be selec-tively strengthened and eating habits can be changed. The way this works is that a stimulus is presented, which occasions a response. The consequences of the response will then determine whether that response will recur. When a "reward," or positively reinforcing event, is associ-ated with a response elicited by a particular stimulus, this will promote repetition of that par-ticular response so that the stimulus, in turn, will evoke new, more positive associations. Then repetition of the new response or new behavior pattern serves to reinforce it, while with dis-use, the old behavior fades from the individual's behavior repertoire. In treatment of anorexia, the goal is to reward, increase and reinforce food-consuming behaviors while diminishing food-restricting and food-avoidance activities.

In anorexics, the stimuli of hunger and of food or meal-related events generally elicit behav-iors either to postpone eating (perhaps rearranging the silverware in the drawer) or to allay hunger (such as excessive activity or increased fluid intake). The anorexic has associated these behaviors with the image of thinness, which for her is a very positive motivator. In a hospital or residential setting where reinforcing events can be controlled, the goal is to change the anorexic's behavior by rewarding *eating* in contrast to her old behavior in which she rewarded herself for *not eating*. So, if the anorexic attends regular meals and eats specified amounts of food, she is rewarded with visits with friends, walks outdoors, or other pleasurable pastimes. Her new eating behavior is reinforced by the positive events that follow it. Furthermore, if meals are made more enjoyable and associated with attractive table settings and agreeable social inter-actions, then hunger and mealtimes will evoke positive connections in her mind, thus reinforc-ing new eating behavior.

Several studies have shown that behavioral modification techniques have successfully changed eating behavior in anorexic clients. In one rather stark example, clinicians Arthur Bachrach, William Erwin and Jay Mohr treated a chronically anorexic 37-year-old woman with a 20-year history of anorexic symptoms who had been hospitalized for malnutrition. The cli-nicians placed the woman in a barren hospital room furnished with only a chair, a bed and a sink. They then established a reinforcement system in which the client's access to radio, books, records and visitors was contingent upon her eating a certain amount of food. If she ate the specified amount of food, she was allowed an hour of listening to music, for instance. Gradu-ally, the amount she had to consume in order to receive a reward was increased. She gained 14 pounds after 6 weeks in the hospital and was then released. With this particular patient, the family was able to continue the behavior modification program when the patient went home. Three years after admission to the hospital the client was maintaining her weight (although at a slightly lower than normal amount), working and going to business school (Bachrach et al., 1965, pp.156–162).

In another study, weight gain was monitored and reinforced in five hospitalized adoles-cent girls who had lost from 34 to 42 percent of their weight. They were rewarded with overnight or weekend passes, or physical activity such as a twenty-minute walk, contingent upon increased weight. At the outset, both the goals and the accruing privileges were clearly defined for each patient, and each adolescent was made to feel responsible for her own weight. During the six- to twelve-week course of treatment, the five girls regained to between 87 and 95 percent of their pre-anorexic weight. Previously, four of the five young women had been treated unsuccessfully with tube feeding, insulin and drug therapy, but behavior modification was effective in achieving weight restoration and promoting new eating habits in all five girls. The researchers concluded that behavior modification is useful in treating weight loss in anorexics, but also that it constitutes only one part of a total therapeutic program (Garfinkel et al., 1973, pp.431–432).

In behavior modification programs for anorexia, some controversy has existed over whether *eating behavior* or *weight gain* ought to be rewarded. Researchers James Brady and William Rieger concluded that direct reinforcement of eating behavior was less desirable than rewarding weight gain, and that the patient should be allowed to choose what or how she eats. The patient then is permitted maximum choice and freedom with respect to food, which facilitates her autonomy and independence in a more appropriate arena than that of choosing to eat or not eat (Brady and Rieger, 1978, p.60). These same clinicians noted in another study that applying behavior modification techniques to the treatment of anorexia both promotes a rapid restoration of lost weight and lays the groundwork for subsequent treatment of the psychological problems accompanying the disorder.

Some researchers have demonstrated the effectiveness of a combination of negative reinforcement, using tube feeding, and positive reinforcement, in the form of receiving mail, phone calls and visitors. Tube feeding entails either surgically implanting a port for a tube into the small intestine, or inserting a naso-gastric tube through the patient's nose and into the esophagus. Through this tube, liquid sustenance is introduced directly into the digestive system. Not only is tubal insertion invasive and uncomfortable, but this procedure puts medical staff fully in control of the patient's intake. In a study of a group of eight hospitalized anorexics, rewards were contingent on a *weight gain* of half a kilogram (a little over a pound) over a five-day period, while loss of weight was negatively reinforced by tube feeding, which continued until the lost weight was regained. The anorexic patients remained in the hospital an average of a little more than six weeks, and in that time each gained an average of over 19 pounds. The cooperation of their families was enlisted to maintain the patients on a behavior modification program after hospital discharge. Any loss of weight was followed by threat of readmission to the hospital and tube feeding. Seven months after hospital discharge, all eight patients were maintaining appropriate weights and none had required re-hospitalization. The researchers concluded that this strategy for promoting weight restoration in anorexics was effective. How these patients fared after their first seven months is unknown, however, as the study included no long-term follow-up results (Halmi et al., 1975, p.96).

The simplicity of behavior modification techniques and the rapidity with which the treatment can produce an increase in weight are two advantages of this approach. However, this form of treatment is not without its drawbacks. The need for careful monitoring of each patient limits use of this technique to settings such as inpatient facilities where the environment can be strictly controlled. While in some cases family members can administer the program, this can be dicey because of potential difficulties with family dynamics. Also, rapid weight gain can cause physiological complications, including water and electrolyte imbalance. However, if the rate of weight gain is regulated, physiological complications can be avoided. Also, physiological parameters can be monitored closely to guard against development of significant imbalances (Halmi et al., 1975, p.95).

Eating disorder specialist Hilde Bruch raised another objection to the use of behavior modification for changing eating patterns or encouraging weight gain: the very quality for which the technique is admired — the rapidity of weight gain achieved — provokes serious psychological damage. As Bruch states, "Its very efficiency increases the inner turmoil of the patients who feel tricked into relinquishing control over their bodies and their lives" (Bruch, 1974, p.1421). As discussed earlier, control is a central issue in anorexia, and lack of control over body changes at puberty can be a factor in triggering the disorder. Fear of becoming fat is a primary concern for any anorexic. As clinician Kelly Bemis noted regarding weight gain in anorexia, "more is not necessarily better" (Bemis, 1987, p.459). Rapid weight gain can easily be misconstrued by the anorexic as what she most fears: loss of control over her body, which now she sees as horrifically and irrevocably fat.

Another criticism levied against behaviorists, especially by psychodynamically-oriented theorists, is that modification of the symptom does not eradicate the underlying pathology. While this is true, eliminating the problematic behavior can be a significant step in treating anorexic pathology, as it is precisely this aspect of the disorder which is responsible for the physical and psychological deterioration of the client. The starving patient is not amenable to psychotherapy; she simply is neither physically nor psychologically capable of benefiting from psychotherapy until her weight and health stabilize. It is doubtful that behavior modification unaccompanied by some other kind of treatment would be sufficient to achieve significant recovery in any individual whose history with anorexia is severe or long-standing. While food restriction is the most obvious self-destructive behavior in anorexia, change in eating does not guarantee improvement in body image or resolution of the emotional problems which gave rise to the disturbed eating.

However, some Swedish researchers have recently revisited the role of starvation in inducing anorexic symptoms, and have suggested that a behavioral approach targeting anorexic *eating behavior*, as opposed to weight gain, can reverse anorexic symptoms. These researchers have noted that both anorexics and those who have volunteered in studies on starvation exhibit a reduced rate of eating as well as a smaller intake of food, as well as obsessive behaviors such as food rituals, and psychiatric symptoms including increased anxiety and irritability. In their view, starvation causes the abnormal eating behaviors of anorexia, which in turn lead to the psychological disturbances of the disorder. They have found that training patients to eat more food at a progressively higher rate reverses these symptoms, and that patients remain free of symptoms for an extended follow-up period (Zandian et al., 2007, pp.283–290).

In another study, members of a related group of Swedish researchers hypothesize that change in *eating behavior* in the treatment of anorexia can reset the disturbed neuroendocrine mechanisms involved in the origins of the disorder. The premise of this approach is that anorexia nervosa emerges as a result of a disturbance in neural mechanisms; it is this neurological disturbance which evokes the starvation behaviors and the subsequent psychological symptoms of anorexia. According to these researchers, the problem occurs when neural cues involved with reward and attention somehow overlap neural systems engaged in cues for eating. In other words, the mix-up in brain signals causes anorexics to feel rewarded by not eating rather than by eating. When patients are trained to re-learn normal eating habits, the new eating behaviors override the cues that maintain the disturbed eating pattern. Eventually, the anorexic's symptoms, including psychological symptoms, dissolve (Sodersten et al., 2008).

Retraining anorexic patients to eat differently in order to reverse their other symptoms is appealing in its apparent simplicity. However, from my experience, this would not suffice as treatment for anyone with a long-standing disorder. Nonetheless, the proposed approaches of training anorexics to increase their rate of eating and the quantity of food consumed, or to eat "normally," are relatively new hypotheses which have not been tested yet with any thoroughness.

More recently, behavioral methods combined with cognitive therapy in the treatment of anorexia address both weight restoration and the thinking distortions typical of anorexia in tandem. Currently, cognitive-behavioral therapy (CBT), which I discuss at more length in the next section, is frequently used in both inpatient and outpatient settings.

PERSONAL NOTE

Behavioral modification was among the therapeutic techniques used at Cathexis. When I entered Cathexis, I agreed to gain one pound per week as a condition of staying in treatment, and to maintain the weight once I had reached my target range. This was no small order: to gain weight at this rate, I had to significantly change my former eating patterns, tolerate the physical discomfort of eating more, and face my fears of being out of control, as I had to increase my body size by over 40 percent. Along with eating more, I was encouraged to change my previous negative associations with eating by choosing foods I liked, enjoying the qualities of those foods, and doing what I could to make eating enjoyable. So long as I maintained my weight increase — which was neither an unrealistic nor an unhealthy rate of change, despite my anorexic protestations to the contrary — I received verbal approval from my peers and therapists, and I could stay in the program and continue treatment. If I didn't meet the goal, I was required to be on "food supervision" until I gained the requisite pound. On food supervision, I was required to weigh, measure and eat all of my food while being observed by a staff person or a staff-approved peer. Making arrangements for food supervision was tedious and uncomfortable; being scrutinized while I ate was not enjoyable. Food supervision served as a definite deterrent to not gaining weight.

During the six to seven months that I was gaining weight, I was also participating in group therapy sessions for several hours a day. While it may be that I was not able to make much psychological progress until my weight was restored, evidently along the way I incorporated enough new information to convince me to stay in the program and to maintain my weight once I had reached my target. Gradually, the longer I remained within my new weight range and continued psychotherapy, the more I was able to tolerate my body at my new weight.

Behavioral modification was effective for me, but only because it was used in conjunction with daily group therapy in a supportive outpatient setting. Behavior modification for weight gain can probably be used in partial hospitalization or intensive outpatient settings, as well as inpatient, so long as staff can closely monitor behavior and provide consistent rewards and consequences. However, when used for weight gain, behavior modification must be part of a comprehensive treatment program; it cannot stand alone. Behavior modification can be useful in a very different way later in therapy. Most psychotherapists have an established policy of charging for missed sessions. Having to pay for a missed session serves as negative reinforcement. A cancellation policy serves, among other things, to encourage therapy attendance for the client who may be uncomfortable as she anticipates her session — which is not an uncommon occurrence for the anorexic in recovery.

Cognitive-Behavioral Therapy

Cognitive-behavioral therapy (CBT) is designed to help the anorexic identify and modify maladaptive thoughts and behaviors. Cognitive therapy helps the client develop an ever-increasing awareness of her beliefs and assumptions, how she processes them, the meaning she gives them, and how they reinforce unhealthy behaviors. Cognitive therapy relies on conscious experience and does not examine unconscious motivation. The cognitive therapist is active and directive, and primarily uses questions and education in conducting the sessions. Sometimes written or behavioral assignments are given to the client to do between sessions.

Unlike behavior modification, CBT does not use a reward-punishment system. Instead CBT works with the thoughts (cognitions) that precede the behaviors — when the client modifies a maladaptive belief, she can cease doing the harmful behavior which the maladaptive belief triggers. For example, an anorexic commonly believes that eating new foods will cause her to lose control and get fat. This belief triggers a behavior: she limits her intake to a small number of "safe" foods. The job of the therapist is to (very patiently) help the anorexic understand that the needs of her body will change when it is no longer malnourished and that she will lose the urge to eat uncontrollably; that she will be protected by eating new foods in pre-arranged amounts; that, in fact, control implies choice and she has no choice with her current eating regimen; that eating is about health needs, not gaining weight; and that her current limited food regimen is not serving her health. As the anorexic understands that eating new foods can actually increase her control, that there is protection built into making the change and that the consequences she dreads are unlikely to occur, she can experiment with eating different foods.

CBT is used with anorexics in both inpatient and outpatient settings. One of the earlier objections to cognitive therapy was that its focus on the content of the anorexic's thought processes did not take into account the impact of the interpersonal, therapist-client relationship on the therapeutic process. Failures in treatment were thus ascribed to the resistance of the client, rather than to a problem in the therapist-client relationship or to the client's possible mistrust of the therapist. However, with the recognition that anorexics may mistrust relationships in general, and may have significant misperceptions in interpersonal relationships, cognitive-behavioral clinicians have concluded that "establishing a strong therapeutic alliance is a key to motivating patients to confront dreaded eating behaviors and weight gain, as well as emotional and interpersonal predicaments" (Garner et al., 1997, p.100).

Psychologist and eating disorder specialist Dr. David Garner, along with Kelly Vitousek and Kathleen Pike, has provided a detailed description of the application of CBT to treatment of anorexia. In this application, treatment consists of three phases. The first phase, which is crucial to establishing the foundation of therapy, focuses on building trust and setting treatment parameters. This stage may continue for several months—or longer, for a client whose disorder is severe and long-standing—as it establishes the foundation for the remainder of the therapy. At this initial stage, the therapist has many tasks: to instill hope, be empathic, convey an understanding of the client's profound unhappiness, observe the client's reactions to the therapist as a window to comprehending her attitudes toward interpersonal relationships, learn the client's beliefs about weight and shape, find out about her life and functioning prior to developing anorexia, and communicate the rationale for restoring nutrition. It is important to educate the anorexic patient about the physiological and psychological consequences of starvation, as this information can help relieve some of the anxiety and guilt she feels about her distress. It further conveys that a minimum degree of physiological stability is necessary both to discern which of her emotional problems result from starvation, and to address those that do not. The therapist at this stage also clarifies for the client both the mortality rates for the disorder and the more optimistic outcome associated with receiving treatment (Garner et al., 1997, pp.98–103).

One tool that the therapist can use to help the anorexic understand the course of her illness is a generic visual diagram of the stages of weight loss in anorexia, with an explanation of what happens at each stage. This diagram helps to convey the way an individual uses anorexia to resolve certain life problems, although at great personal cost. The diagram shows that a girl gradually gains weight as she progresses from a pre-puberty stage to menarche, and then into adolescence. The therapist explains that, at that point, faced with the challenges of adolescence, a young woman may decide that weight loss is the solution to her social or personal problems. The diagram correspondingly shows a gradual decline in weight, to below the weight of menarche, resulting in amenorrhea. The therapist describes how, with this weight loss, the conflicts of adolescence fade. The diagram then shows the young woman's weight dropping to an even lower amount. The therapist points out that continued weight loss after this point becomes, in the anorexic's mind, like "money in the bank," a reserve against the previous negative experiences associated with shape and weight change. The therapist then discusses the possible trajectories, depending on whether the client engages in treatment, noting that "recovery" doesn't mean simply regaining weight, but also addressing the issues that made weight loss attractive in the first place. A client often appreciates the interpretation of her disorder as having psychological and developmental meaning (Garner et al., 1997, pp.106–108).

The first phase of CBT can also introduce the concept of gaining a small amount of weight in order to assess the client's beliefs about weight gain. Coupled with this, the therapist provides very specific eating guidelines designed to offset the anorexic's impulses to undereat and to minimize her fears about feeling out of control: Eating is to be mechanical, meals are both to be eaten at regular times and to consist of specific foods in precise quantities. These guidelines can relieve the anorexic of her obsession with constantly thinking and rethinking what, when and how much she is going to eat. The anorexic is also given some "distracting thoughts" to use to counter the urge to undereat, such as "Eating is protection," "I need food to keep me healthy," and "Regardless of what I feel, I am thin at normal weight." At this point, considerable cognitive work focuses on helping the client manage her fears—of getting fat, gaining weight "in the wrong places," and "losing control." It is also helpful to elucidate the "anorexic wish": to recover from the disorder without gaining weight. The therapist explains that these two desires are mutually exclusive, and assures the anorexic that if she chooses recovery, treatment can help her truly feel better about herself (Garner et al., 1997, pp.111–116).

In Garner and his colleagues' CBT protocol, the latter two treatment phases build on the foundation of the first phase. Phase two focuses on changing additional beliefs about food and weight, and broadening the scope of therapy to include interpersonal issues in the client's life. This phase also works on expanding the client's self-awareness through teaching her to label and express emotions and challenging her dysfunctional beliefs regarding self-evaluation and self-esteem. Other tasks of this phase include examining the client's beliefs and the assumptions under them — those attributions which tend to make the beliefs stick even if "on an intellectual level" the client recognizes that they are not valid. In this step, the anorexic learns to recognize her reasoning errors and to reframe the thoughts that she uses to keep her disordered eating patterns in place (Garner et al., 1997, pp.121–136).

The final phase of this cognitive-behavioral treatment focuses on relapse prevention and termination of therapy. The therapist reiterates the aspects of treatment that have helped with symptom improvement, and reinforces the need to maintain regular eating patterns and to continue holding an "anti-dieting" stance. The therapist and client discuss areas of vulnerability and warning signs of relapse. Also, the therapist encourages the client to keep an open mind about returning to treatment if needed and not view any need for further assistance as failure (Garner et al., 1997, pp.136–138).

This description of CBT with anorexia is of particular value because it addresses a wide range of common maladaptive beliefs in a course of outpatient treatment. CBT has also been used with inpatient treatment. Clinicians Wayne Bowers and Lynn Ansher used cognitive therapy in conjunction with a behavioral protocol in an inpatient setting to aid weight gain and improve mood and severity of eating disorder symptoms in anorexia. These researchers treated 32 hospitalized anorexics and concluded that this approach could significantly reduce eating disorder symptoms, depression and general psychopathology in anorexic patients. Follow-up one year later showed that many of the changes in weight, depression and other symptoms had been at least partially sustained (Bowers and Ansher, 2008, pp.79–86).

CBT has also been used to treat body image distortion in anorexia. Garner, Vitousek and Pike developed cognitive-behavioral strategies to address fears about weight gain and shape change. In this approach, weight gain is conceived of as "an experiment" to assess whether the client experiences gaining weight as having any advantages. Because the anorexic's entire belief system is wrapped around her body shape and weight, Garner and his colleagues tease out the specific beliefs that contradict the advantages of being thin, for example, "Being thin takes up so much time and energy," "People hassle me a lot about my weight," and "I don't like being cold all the time." They educate the client to help dispel her misperceptions and allay her fears regarding shape change. One of their goals is to introduce cognitive dissonance, or contradictory beliefs, into the client's views about her body shape and size (Garner et al., 1997, pp.111, 118–119).

Thomas Cash, a psychologist noted for his extensive research and numerous books on the psychology of personal appearance, has developed cognitive behavioral workbooks, CDs and texts on the subject of combating body image distortion. Many of his programs have been modified for use with individuals suffering from anorexia. His *Eight-Step Program for Learning to Like Your Looks* includes exercises such as writing an autobiography of body image development; keeping a body image diary in which to record occasions of distress around body image and the precipitants; behavioral strategies for altering avoidant behaviors related to body image; and identifying dysfunctional "appearance assumptions," such as "If I could look just the way I want to, I would be happy." His workbook also includes mirror-exposure protocols. For example, in one exercise the anorexic deliberately looks at her reflection. Initially she makes notes about thoughts that emerge. Later, she focuses on one body part that she doesn't like, and very gradually begins to create a new way to think about that part of her body (Cash, 2008, pp.63–69). Cash also coaches an individual to develop a positive body self-talk to replace the usual inner mantra of negative body thoughts. Most recently, Cash has added mindfulness techniques, including meditation, in combination with cognitive behavioral methods to address body image distortion (Cash, 2008, p.105).

Two British clinicians, Glenn Waller and Helen Kennerly, describe a form of CBT which addresses the many aspects of meaning that are evoked by a negative body thought. This multi-aspect meaning, termed a "schema," is a mental filter that has been shaped by previous experiences. A negative thought can activate cognitive, emotional, physiological and felt-sense responses. For example, for an anorexic, a trigger, such as someone saying, "You look good," leads to an immediate thought: "She thinks I look fat." This thought activates a cognitive response of "I'm unlovable," an emotional response of fear and self-disgust; a physiological response of increased adrenaline and flushing of the face; and a felt-sense of ugliness. This progression of thoughts then leads to a behavior: perhaps the anorexic goes for a run even though she is exhausted. Cognitive work directly addresses the schema, that is, the many different kinds of meaning evoked by the thought. These clinicians attribute a common refrain of most anorexics, "I feel fat," to the felt-sense, or internal mental representation, of the body. One goal of schema-focused CBT is to help clients recognize and restructure this distorted felt-sense (Waller and Kennerly, 2003, pp.244–248).

Many factors can affect whether CBT is successful, including the setting; the severity and duration of the anorexic's illness; her motivation and previous treatment history; the philosophy and skill of the therapist; and the client's degree of trust in the therapist. A cognitive-behavioral approach may have more usefulness with some populations of anorexics than with others. A study in 2005 compared three different treatment approaches—CBT, interpersonal psychotherapy and nonspecific supportive clinical management — with 56 anorexic adult women in an outpatient setting. The women receiving nonspecific clinical management fared the best, with the other two treatment approaches doing less well. In this study, the researchers concluded that the CBT might not be effective in an initial phase of treatment with more severely ill patients, because of their entrenched belief systems (McIntosh et al., 2005, pp.741–747). As with other treatment modalities, fitting the treatment to the client — and to the client's particular phase of recovery—increases the probability of effective treatment. CBT may be of particular value in addressing specific issues in anorexia, such as beliefs about food and weight gain, or body image concerns. It lends itself to use in combination with client education, for instance, about starvation and nutrition. The success of CBT in treating some anorexic clients in a variety of settings has certainly earned it a place in a comprehensive approach to the treatment of anorexia, whether or not it is the primary modality used.

Dialactical Behavior Therapy

Dialectical Behavior Therapy (DBT) was developed in the early 1990s by psychologist Marsha Linehan, who was working with clients challenged by intense emotions and suicidal impulses. Many of Linehan's clients suffered from borderline personality disorder, and manifested a significant degree of impulsivity, depression and emotional and interpersonal distress. DBT combined techniques drawn from several therapeutic disciplines including cognitive therapy, behavior modification, communication enhancement, and relaxation and meditation practices. Originally, DBT was used in group settings, but clinicians have found that it is also effective in individual therapy with clients who have difficulty managing intense feeling states. Recently, some clinicians have used DBT in treating eating disorders because they have found that it can address the emotional and relationship distress common among those with eating disorders. Anorexics in the throes of starvation may suffer severe depression or intense anxiety. In addition, the onset of anorexia generally coincides with a phase of heightened emotionality. As the anorexic succumbs to food- and body-related means to handle life, her previous emotional deficits are compounded by missing out on the emotional learning of adolescence. Then, in recovery, the anorexic's feelings begin to surface and she may feel overwhelmed. She has few emotional resources with which to navigate this new resurgence of feelings.

DBT has four main skill areas and teaches methods for learning distress tolerance, mindfulness, emotional regulation and interpersonal effectiveness (managing relationships). This approach depends on balancing *acceptance* and *change*—acceptance of oneself and one's situation, and at the same time, change in one's behavior to better adapt to the necessities of the moment.

Acceptance is a tremendous challenge for an anorexic, who is never satisfied with herself and blames herself for many things beyond her control. Nonetheless, it is exactly this challenge which makes DBT a good fit with anorexics, because the perfection the anorexic seeks is unattainable, and continuing that pursuit prolongs her pain. Non-acceptance and distress have led the anorexic to avoidance activities including restricting food intake, performing food rituals and narrowing her life. Generally an anorexic thinks obsessively about past situations and future events, running them over in her mind, reassessing what she should have done and contriving how to manage a future event. Linehan's concept of "radical acceptance" is fundamental to DBT, and to tolerating distress, and can be summed up as an acknowledgment that the present simply is what it is (Linehan, 1993, p.28). This means accepting something completely without judging it or oneself (McKay et al., 2007, p.51). Affirmations and coping statements can help the client focus on accepting the present; she can repeat to herself phrases such as "It's no use fighting the past. The present is the only moment I have control over. The present moment is perfect, even if I don't like what's happening" (McKay et al., 2007, p.11). Accepting the present is not easy, but learning to do so can forge a fundamental shift in attitude. To alleviate distress, the client also learns relaxation skills and distraction techniques. As the anorexic implements these coping skills, she finds that her discomfort dissipates.

The second aspect of DBT, mindfulness or meditation drawn from millennia of Buddhist,

Islamic and Judaic-Christian traditions, helps reinforce distress tolerance. Meditation has found therapeutic application for stress reduction, easing chronic pain and reducing anxiety. In the words of psychologist Jon Kabat-Zinn, who pioneered use of meditation with chronic pain patients, mindfulness is "the awareness that emerges through paying attention on purpose, in the present moment, and non-judgmentally to the unfolding of experience moment by moment" (Kabat-Zinn, 2003, p.145). Mindfulness requires practice, but with repetition it can help an individual focus attention, soothe strong emotion, identify judgmental thoughts and separate fact from judgment. The ability to discern fact from judgment is an important cognitive skill for anorexics who are highly critical, particularly of themselves, but believe their judgments are truth. Also, anorexics generally lack much capacity for self-soothing, except through the self-destructive food rituals they have developed. This inability of the anorexic to find internal comfort reflects a core self-deficit. When a child's sense of self has been nurtured, he "can turn to a place within his body for a grounding, supporting feeling of well-being from which he can return, strengthened, to the world" (Rosenberg et al., 1991, p.163). Thus, mindfulness can build a foundational piece of self-structure.

Emotional regulation, the third DBT principle, is a key concept for a recovering anorexic who is just beginning to develop a new awareness of her feelings. Identifying emotions is the anorexic's first step; then she must develop ways to handle those emotions. Mindfulness skills, radical acceptance and distress tolerance are aspects of emotional regulation. So, too, is recognizing physical or cognitive vulnerability and being prepared to take precautionary measures as discomfort arises (McKay et al., 2007, pp.136–145). For example, when the anorexic knows she will be attending a family gathering, she can prepare for the event by planning to call someone for support before and after, giving herself plenty of time to get there, figuring out what she will wear well in advance of the event so she can be less obsessive about her wardrobe close to the time of the gathering, and reminding herself to stay in the present and neither jump to the future or revisit the past — in other words, to not obsess about previous family gatherings *or* about the one that is coming up. Before going, she can take a soothing bubble bath or do an extended body-relaxation exercise. Once at the gathering, the anorexic can use relaxation tools to stabilize her mood: she can recite self-encouraging coping thoughts in her head, such as "This situation won't last forever. I've survived other situations like this before"; use word-linked relaxation skills to focus on a calming word, such as serenity; carry something soft in her purse or pocket that is soothing to touch. At any point before or during the event if the anorexic begins to feel distressed, she can focus on her breath. As the anorexic develops a repertoire of constructive, problem-solving behaviors to manage difficult feelings, not only is she less vulnerable to the force of negative events and negative emotions, but she feels more in control without resorting to self-harm.

Interpersonal skill building is the fourth principle of DBT. Generally the anorexic has a paucity of interpersonal skills, and those she has are founded on pleasing the other person. People-pleasing, of course, precludes the anorexic's building an identity of her own. Much of her energy is directed at deciphering what she perceives as the expectations of others. For the anorexic, learning to separate "shoulds" from "needs" and "wants" is critical; "shoulds" have been her guideposts. The anorexic also lacks conflict-resolution skills; indeed, she goes to great lengths to avoid conflict. Effective interpersonal interaction demands self-knowledge. DBT skills can contribute to the anorexic's base for self-development and help equip her to manage her emerging feelings, interpersonal difficulties and life situations.

Because DBT provides a large variety of skills, it is possible to draw from its vast repertoire and use some very basic tools, such as methods for self-soothing, early in treatment and to slowly build on those. Although DBT is usually taught in four discrete skill areas, in fact, there is sufficient overlap in the skill sets, and wide enough application for their use, that they can be learned and used in much smaller units. Given the level of distress that many anorexics experience, combined with the paucity of self-regulatory skills they often possess, acquiring just a few techniques can be very helpful. Learning very basic DBT skills does not demand a lot of psychological or cognitive ability, which makes them accessible even to the anorexic whose physical and psychological capacities are compromised. Furthermore, these skills can be integrated into a variety of other therapeutic approaches, giving them broad application during the remainder of treatment, and provide the anorexic with means of coping that can benefit her throughout her life.

Psychodynamic Psychotherapy

Unlike behavioral and cognitive-based therapies, psychodynamic approaches to psychotherapy focus on the role of the unconscious in creating and sustaining symptoms. The work of cognitive and behavioral therapies resides in remolding reality; psychodynamic psychotherapy attends to the client's internal world. There are a number of different theoretical orientations within psychodynamic psychotherapy. In considering the origin of psychological problems in general, and anorexia in particular, different schools of psychotherapy vary in their view of the psychic structure, or internal world, of the newborn infant: what kinds of good or bad "objects," or representations of another person, the infant internalizes; what internal dynamics, or interrelationships, exist among the parts of the infant's mental structure; and what kinds of disturbances in the development of these internal structures give rise to psychological problems. Some theoreticians focus on internal conflicts; others on distortions in internalized representations. Rather than differentiating among various theoretical orientations—among them object relations therapy, self psychology, intersubjectivity and interpersonal therapy—I focus here on some of the underlying principles common to most psychodynamic psychotherapies in their approach to the treatment of anorexia.

In general, psychodynamic clinicians agree that the work of psychotherapy is to clarify and interpret the client's internal misalignments or misattunements in favor of a perspective that offers the client relief from the struggles causing or maintaining her symptoms. Psychodynamic psychotherapies explore the internal representations of the self and others from past experiences that get reenacted in present relationships and interactions. These therapies are particularly interested in how these past relationships show up in the present relationship between therapist and client—a phenomenon known as transference. As psychotherapist Deborah Luepnitz writes, "The concept of transference turns on the fact that we don't meet other people as much as we construct them based on previous experiences going back to childhood" (Luepnitz, 2002, p.12). In psychodynamic therapy, the therapist is an empathic listener, attuned to the client's experience and emotions in the present. The therapist seeks to clarify and understand how the therapist-client interactions relate to the client's difficulties, and to educate the client about these dynamics. In other words, the therapist-client relationship becomes the arena in which the client can work out internal and interpersonal issues.

In working with the anorexic client, however, the therapist cannot simply ignore eating behavior while attending to intrapsychic issues. Instead, psychodynamic psychotherapy with an anorexic demands delicate shifts between the two areas. Clinician Judith Brisman describes this work as "a mixture of direct intervention with the symptom (speaking the patient's language) while at the same time exploring what that very intervention means to the patient and what purpose the symptom plays in the patient's intrapsychic and interpersonal world (speaking the therapist's language)" (Brisman, 1996, p.45).

Most clinicians agree that psychotherapy is of little value with a starving patient. Many aspects of "anorexic behavior," including the constant concern with food, food rituals, hoarding food, depression, and apathetic demeanor, are the direct effect of starvation; nutrition must be restored before effective treatment of underlying issues can be conducted (Bruch, 1973, p.349). Other clinicians have observed that "when psychotherapy directed at uncovering unconscious motivation for self-starvation and removing defenses against anxiety is the sole mode of treatment, the eating behavior will very likely remain unchanged or even worsen" (Lucas et al., 1976, p.1034).

Psychotherapy offers an opportunity for the anorexic to understand herself. It is a venue for her to be listened to intently and thoughtfully, and responded to empathically; to develop autonomy as she voices her own thoughts and feelings; to have her self-destructive behaviors noted and her ambivalence about recovery explored and understood; and to grieve the losses that accompany change, growing up, becoming her own person, and letting go of her childlike persona.

Hilde Bruch was among the earliest of psychotherapists to work effectively with anorexic patients. She believed that most interpretations, or suggestions to the client of the psychological meaning of what she is saying, particularly in terms of the therapist-client relationship, were too intrusive with this kind of client and that psychotherapeutic intervention should limit itself largely to clarification, or asking questions to help the client talk in more detail about herself and whatever topic she has brought up. Bruch held that anorexics are unresponsive to traditional psychoanalysis because the interpretive approach resembles the interactions the anorexic had with her parents, who told her how she felt and what she thought, rather than allowing her to develop and trust her own feelings and thoughts. This form of treatment reinforces the anorexic's sense of inadequacy, lack of selfhood and overdependence (Bruch, 1973, p.336). Instead, Bruch advocated a modified form of psychotherapy in which the client is encouraged to become aware of her own needs, impulses and feelings and to initiate her own behavior based on her new self-awareness (Bruch, 1973, p.341). The role of the therapist is to consistently confirm or comment on the client's self-expressions and self-initiated behavior. The client takes an active part in her treatment process, which serves as a foundation for her assuming responsibility for her own life (Bruch, 1973, p.335).

Bruch further notes that if issues develop in the therapy which need to be uncovered and interpreted, it is important that the client make the discovery on her own and have a chance to say it first (Bruch, 1973, p.338). Rather than dealing with the relationship between internal conflicts and disturbed eating, this therapeutic approach seeks to repair the anorexic's underlying sense of incompetence and to correct her conceptual distortions.

Bruch's method was a definite step forward from psychoanalytical approaches to anorexia which suffered from excessive interpretation. However, psychotherapist William James Swift voiced a concern that Bruch, in discarding interpretation altogether, overlooked that "transference phenomena are ubiquitous in treatment, no matter how empathic the approach" (Swift, 1991, p.55). In other words, there is *always* something happening in the moment between the therapist and the client which has relevance to how the client is using, distorting or dismissing the therapist's words. In fact, since the anorexic client has chosen an oppositional stance with respect to food, it is valuable to know whether and how the client is hearing and taking in what the therapist has to offer her. However, Swift notes that Bruch made many valuable contributions to the psychodynamic treatment of anorexia, including establishing that interventions should be based on the clinical encounter, not on theory, and that the therapist should make the patient an active participant and true collaborator in the process. Bruch also stressed key treatment principles such as empathic listening, supportive helpfulness, non-intrusive concern and the need to confirm the inner reality of the client (Swift, 1991, pp.63–64).

Probably of more significance than any actual "technique" in psychotherapy is the establishment of a sound therapeutic alliance between the therapist and client; this alliance is particularly critical in working with an anorexic client. Anorexics in general are mistrusting; they tend to be introverted, private and parsimonious in their disclosures. The language of feelings, so central to psychotherapy, is foreign, unfamiliar, and frightening; and the work of psychotherapy with an anorexic is not a short-term process. Patience on the part of both the psychotherapist and the client is required for effective therapy with an anorexic.

The psychotherapist working with an anorexic needs to possess the attributes of any attentive, well-attuned, empathic psychotherapist who is capable of being present, respectful and non-judgmental. However, the psychotherapist in addition needs to be able to support the gradual unfolding of the fragile Self of the anorexic torn between growing up and staying a child. Psychologist Steven Stern notes that early psychotherapy with an anorexic hinges on the "management of contradictory interpersonal currents." Anorexics are caught between legitimate needs of the Self—for emotional nourishment, empathy, and support for separation-individuation—and the self-denial and self-sacrifice that have become their safe haven. The task of the therapist is to support whichever theme is prominent in the client's current interactions with the therapist (Stern, 1991, pp.86–88).

The psychotherapist must be—or at least appear to be—solid, unflappable and a person who the client believes can tolerate her issues and her pain, lest the client reenact her old caretaking, people-pleasing role. Psychotherapy with an anorexic requires that the therapist provide a stabilizing, mood-regulating function for the anorexic; this, too, may require more than usual patience on the part of the therapist. Plus, more than in working with any other population, the therapist working with an anorexic needs to know that the therapist's own body will be under scrutiny and that body image—both hers and the client's—will be an unspoken, constant concern for the anorexic client.

"From the patient's point of view psychoanalysis does several things you can't get any other way.... It maintains a sense of being listened to intently by a thoughtful person" (Daniels, 2001, p.240), says novelist and clinical psychologist Lisa Daniels, who struggled with anorexia for many years. Building on this idea, psychiatrist Kathryn Zerbe explains that as the therapist listens, attentively and respectfully, the client develops a sense of her own value, and a sense that this is a safe place to speak, undirected, "gradually revealing new facets of herself as she engages in the work and overcomes her difficulties (e.g., resistances) to telling more about herself" (Zerbe, 2007, p.313). Psychotherapy becomes the arena in which the anorexic can gradually grow and expand, from an almost invisible shadow to a solid being of dimension, affect and cohesion.

Daniels also speaks of the psychotherapist "who will not let you be self-destructive without at least asking a question, but who will also, unblamingly, let you accept the consequences of your mistakes" (Daniels, 2001, p.240). Addressing self-destructive behaviors is central to psychodynamic psychotherapy, and speaks to the issue of ambivalence about getting better—not only for the anorexic, but for all clients. Consciously, the anorexic wants to "improve" and "feel better," but the symptoms play significant roles in holding her world together; limiting her food intake gives her the illusion of control on which her very identity depends. The anorexic does not want to be in pain, but the cost of recovery is to face separation from her family—the developmental task her disorder halted. That separation process may be fraught with guilt and conflicts in loyalty. She may worry what her achieving autonomy means to and about her, and for her family. Plus self-destructiveness manifests in ways other than food restriction. Missing appointments with a nutritionist, or "forgetting" to reschedule them, coming late to therapy sessions, omitting self-care, allowing the "eating disorder voice" or "inner critic" to direct her choices, assuming the therapist does not want her to live her own life—all of these undermine the anorexic's forward movement. And all of them pose a bind for the psychotherapist: how to point out the behavior, and its consequences, without the anorexic's internalizing the comment as evidence of her "badness," her failure or inadequacy. The therapist wants to help the client develop better coping mechanisms but without the risk of being directive, as a central function of the work is to help the client's own sense of efficacy and autonomy. However, Zerbe points out that "repeatedly raising questions about the meaning of the patients' progress and relapses helps set the stage for mastery, ultimately leading to an enhanced sense of autonomy" (Zerbe, 2007, p.315). Also, as the anorexic recovers, she develops a capacity for gratification beyond what her eating disorder provides and can work though the guilt that accompanies her becoming her own separate person.

Psychotherapy, as Daniels points out, "provides support during the process of working through conscious and deeply unconscious separations and for bearing the pain that such losses entail" (Daniels, 2001, p.240). The anorexic may bear ungrieved losses from life's earlier misattunements; in general, her emotional capacities were limited and overstretched in some ways prior to puberty or the onset of her disorder. At the developmental juncture of adolescence, the girl whose coping abilities have begun to crumble in the face of coming challenges may choose regression to pre-adolescence as the safer alternative to growing up. In the process of recovery, although chronologically older, she revisits that juncture. To move forward into adolescence and beyond, she must grieve not only the childhood losses that accompany puberty, but in addition, the loss of the identity that she assumed to shield her from the pitfalls of adolescence. She must mourn the role of her eating disorder as the cornerstone of her self-concept.

Dreams are also the province of psychotherapy; dreams are windows to the unconscious and operate as nighttime metaphor for daytime struggles and deeper issues. The client's internal world becomes available symbolically and the symbols and feelings from dreams can offer psychotherapist and client another avenue for exploring the anorexic's inner conflicts. The job of the therapist is to listen attentively as the anorexic describes and construes the meaning of her dream, to respond empathically and then perhaps to ask clarifying questions. When the anorexic interprets her own dreams, it encourages her to own and value her perceptions; it also fosters her autonomy and builds her respect for her inner world

Psychodynamic psychotherapy delves into the meaning of an anorexic's eating disorder, and into her internal world of relationships that manifests in the outer world. It addresses the complexities of her struggle to become separate: what it would mean to her and what she believes it would mean to her family for her to become more autonomous; her difficulty with owning her own needs and wants; her self-destructive behaviors and their role; her fear of rejection or abandonment and her need to please; her loyalty toward her family; her terror of growing up — her fears, fantasies and concerns about being female and being an adult. In sum, psychodynamic psychotherapy helps the anorexic transform the conflicts, internal struggles and unconscious motivations that she has manifested through her body into a narrative about herself; it can help her both to make sense of her history and to forge a future that is not dependent on her former coping mechanisms. Learning to trust herself, her own sensory awareness and intuition, and her own capacities is a long-term process for the anorexic in recovery. So, too, is dealing with the guilt and loyalty that have stifled her earlier growth.

In the treatment of anorexia, psychotherapy is integrated with appropriate medical and nutritional guidance in order to safeguard the individual's health. However, psychotherapy may continue long past the point where the anorexic has become physically healthy and medical involvement is no longer required. Psychotherapy has no specific discernible "end point," as recovery, along with life itself, continues to unfold.

Nonetheless, therapies do end, and a termination that therapist and client agree is well-timed is a measure of the growth and maturity of the client. The therapist reminds the client that she is welcome to return to therapy if she encounters stressors that tax her coping abilities. Readiness to leave therapy means that client is well beyond simple management of food behaviors. It means that she has effective coping strategies, has internalized a sense of her own value, has some measure of self-confidence and self-acceptance; that she possesses a solid support system, meaningful friendships, some ability to manage conflict, and a capacity to manage the stressors of daily life; that her life functioning and life goals are stable and age-appropriate; and that fun is a regular and frequent part of her life. If the client is ready to terminate therapy, she has managed to build some sense of a core Self.

Psychotherapy is an essential ingredient in recovery from anorexia. It seldom stands alone, because nutritional needs must be addressed, and adjunctive therapies can be valuable; furthermore, it is not useful with an anorexic whose health is compromised. But once the anorexic has achieved a foundation of physical strength, psychotherapy provides the arena for her to explore, evaluate and change her inner world. For an anorexic to achieve lasting recovery, she must develop a different view of herself and of others. She must develop a Self: a sense of herself as an autonomous being, a person of value, who is entitled to her own needs, wants, thoughts and feelings. She must believe in herself, feel competent and capable, and possess the capacity to soothe herself. She must also grieve the identity she created as an anorexic, the persona that served her as she tried to cope but that eventually caused her harm. Psychotherapy works through the relationship of therapist and client; it is in this powerful dyad that the anorexic receives the attention, empathy, compassion, encouragement, feedback and guidance she needs in order to reconstruct her inner and outer realities. It is within this relationship that the anorexic can reveal and develop the aspects of her being that her disorder has thwarted: her capacity to cope with feelings, relationships, and life. It is within this relationship that the anorexic can develop her Self.

PERSONAL NOTE

After my treatment at Cathexis Institute, and my initial outpatient therapy with a cognitive-behavioral therapist trained at Cathexis, I entered therapy with a psychodynamically-oriented psychotherapist. Since then, I have been in therapy with several psychodynamic therapists, and have grown and changed significantly through the years of work.

One of the most important lessons I learned from one therapist was actually a byproduct of the therapy itself. I had worked with a female therapist for a couple of years, mostly focusing on leaving a romantic relationship I had been involved in. When I finally left the relationship and became happily single, the focus of my therapy sessions turned to my shyness in certain work or social situations. My therapist, who in general was empathic, responsive and non-intrusive, in these discussions veered onto a different track and gave me examples from her mastery of riding a horse. At first I was annoyed. But she persisted in offering examples from riding despite my telling her I felt unheard when the conversation turned to what had worked for her. Not only was my internal world not comparable to hers, riding a horse did not interest me. Our conversations went back and forth. I insisted her examples not only were not helpful, they were offensive; she sometimes backed down, other times became defensive, and still other times seemed irritated that I wasn't making better use of her information. Eventually, we came to an impasse; I sought consultation about the situation from another therapist, then returned to my therapist and discussed the deadlock and the consultant's suggestions. My therapist and I were able to talk in more depth about the impasse and to heal some of the pain it had caused, but the rupture was never fully repaired and I soon initiated termination of the therapy.

Working through most of my conflict with my therapist, it turns out, facilitated my autonomy. I generally avoided conflict; I was accustomed to comply and grant power to the person in authority, tending to believe the other person knew what was best, even for me. The discomfort of my predicament with this therapist forced me to take a new stance. I was impelled to assert what felt right for me, even in the face of my therapist's disagreement and disapproval, and despite my feelings of fear, anger and disappointment. Inadvertently, our conflict re-enacted an old dynamic for me — when I would give in to whatever my mother decreed was right — and gave me a chance to respond in a new way.

Psychotherapy has helped me change and grow in many other ways; I mention only a few examples here. While cognitive-behavioral tools have helped me to tame and quiet my ruthless inner critic, psychodynamic therapy has helped me to understand the role the critic plays in my life and why it has persisted despite my best cognitive attempts to dismantle it. I grew up a twin, always the last-born, least smart and only female among three children. My mother was critical, distant and unhappy. Perfectionism was my attempt to win her love; "not good enough" was the mantra I internalized from my failures. My inner critic kept me believing that my mother's inattention was my fault, and incited me to keep trying to win her — and ultimately, everyone else's — approval. My critic had squelched my self-development: so long as I felt ineffective and inadequate, I could not believe I had the right to take charge of my life.

Psychotherapy has fostered my self-development by helping me develop and strengthen inner voices that speak with more force and authority than my critic: a competent adult voice that can coach me in being effective and resourceful; a compassionate, wise-woman voice that can guide me in living from my heart and soothe the pain that life events evoke. I used to beat myself up for misplacing anything or for making minor — as well as major — mistakes. I knew that self-criticism did not help me to repair the situation, and gradually I was able to better tolerate my mistakes, learn from them, fix what I could, and move on. I also learned that criticizing myself reaffirmed my family role as "the incompetent one." Psychotherapy has helped me to let go of and grieve this internal connection to my family, and the feelings arising from realizing the impact this self-view has had on my life.

Furthermore, psychotherapy has helped me know and trust my feelings, and those feelings in turn have given me a "center," a way to feel grounded and whole, and a core foundation of Self. Week after week, hour after hour, talking with an attentive and non-judgmental therapist about *my* thoughts and feelings, being questioned, thinking in more depth about the nuances of why I thought what I thought and how I put it together: this is the process that helped me recognize my own internal knowing and the wealth of inner resources on which I can rely.

It is through psychotherapy that I have learned how to operate as a separate person in relationships, to be my own Self rather than to fade, chameleon-like, into the agenda of the other. Without that solid grounding in my Self, my relationships were exercises in frustration. Caretaking was my forte; my attempts at self-care and self-acknowledgment were abysmal. My therapist's mirroring my nascent thoughts, nuances of feeling and persistent struggles has helped me grow. The process of psychotherapy — the slow, step-by-step exploration of my inner world — has helped me build a strong, cohesive Self.

Experiential Modalities

In experiential therapies, clients communicate symbolically through non-verbal forms of expression such as movement, music and art. Because experiential modalities offer a variety of avenues for self-expression, many of which can serve as a bridge to verbal communication for those who are uncomfortable talking about their feelings, they provide a wealth of tools for adjunctive treatment of anorexia. Although anorexics may at one time have been verbally facile and communicative, at the height of their disease they tend to be introverted and reticent. Furthermore, they have limited awareness and understanding of their feelings. Often anorexics are regarded as alexythymic, which translates literally as "warding off feelings" and generally means out of touch with emotions. The anorexic has a language for her thoughts and feelings, but it is a language of self-harming behaviors; the anorexic's food behaviors and body condition communicate her pain, although the actual meaning of her message is unclear, and its intended recipients are not identified.

Psychologist Hilde Bruch characterized anorexics as suffering from "a paralyzing sense of ineffectiveness" (Bruch, 1973, p.254). This sense comes, in part, because anorexics tend to lack a feeling of mastery; they rarely acknowledge their accomplishments, which to them are never good enough. Many forms of experiential therapy provide an opportunity for the anorexic to create something that symbolizes her inner world — a poem, a drawing, or a movement, for instance. With appropriate recognition from her therapist, this creation can be framed as an accomplishment, and can give the anorexic a sense of mastery of the medium in which she has worked. In addition, expressive therapies can sometimes bypass the anorexic's critic, which otherwise can both stifle her expression and undermine her accomplishment. The symbolic nature of these therapies provides a greater freedom of expression for the anorexic. Also, because the creative process is subjective, her creation is not quite so vulnerable to the harsh measurements with which she grades other tasks. Depending on the medium, perfectionism and the fear of judgment and disapproval can all be discouraged if the anorexic is instructed to focus on the process, not the result.

What most of these therapies have in common is a guided activity which results in an experience or creation. By respectfully and thoughtfully acknowledging the anorexic's creation — or creative process — the therapist mirrors and validates the anorexic's internal experience. If the anorexic is coaxed to interpret her creation, perhaps prompted by the therapist's questions, she can begin to communicate verbally about her experience and to deepen her connection to her internal world. For example, an art therapist might suggest an anorexic use colored pens to draw a picture of her family, and then ask her to describe the picture. The drawing provides something specific for the client to talk about. Both through the symbolism of the picture itself — which colors are being used, where the figures are placed on the page — and her own explanation, the client communicates her feelings about her family. Thus, expressive therapy offers a way for the anorexic to externalize and represent her internal experience metaphorically, and then to translate her experience into words.

I include here synopses of eight approaches which can be or have been used in adjunctive treatment of anorexia: Hypnotherapy; Guided Imagery; Art Therapy; Music Therapy; Poetry Therapy; Movement Therapy; Psychodrama and Gestalt; and Therapeutic Bodywork. There are many other experiential approaches that neither space nor time allowed me to include, among them Sand Tray, Dance, Drama and Writing Therapies. As research continues and our understanding of effective treatment for anorexia grows, there may be room for even more use of experiential therapies. Death rate from anorexia is high and many therapists are frustrated by the difficulty of working with anorexic patients. Clearly, more and better treatment tools are needed, and the metaphorical approach of experiential therapies holds promise in working with this population.

Hypnotherapy

Hypnosis has a checkered past. In use for thousands of years, hypnosis has mostly been the province of magicians, priests and shamans. In the eighteenth century, a German physician, Mesmer, introduced "mesmerism" — using magnets on patients in a suggestible state to cure the sick — but his treatments were eventually ridiculed and used theatrically. Others took up Mesmer's work and developed hypnosis, which induces a trance-like state. In some quarters, hypnosis began to be used medically for improving ailments with a psychological origin, but elsewhere it was still vilified as snake oil.

In reality, hypnosis cannot "make" someone do something. In using hypnosis, the modern practitioner induces a mild trance state in the client; this state relaxes the defenses of the conscious mind. The therapist then gives suggestions to the client's less-resistant subconscious mind. These suggestions can continue to influence the person when he returns from the trance state.

In the past century, hypnosis has gained recognition in the medical field and been used therapeutically, as "hypnotherapy," for anesthesia, pain reduction, and increasing immunity, as well as for stopping habits such as smoking or nail-biting. Hypnosis has also been used to address numerous psychological problems. As Canadian hypnotherapist Reuben Pecarvé explains, the hypnotherapist "sets out to try to break up the self-sustaining fear-tension-ailment feedback loop within the patient's mind and body" (Pecarvé, 2002, p.101). In other words, hypnotherapy seeks to resolve the fear or anxiety which has both caused and maintained physical problems. Since many anorexics experience anxiety or hyperactivity, some clinicians have reported using hypnotherapy to help anorexic patients relax. Hypnotherapy has also been used with anorexics to help them regulate weight gain; lessen body image distortion; recognize sensations of hunger and fullness; overcome feelings of ineffectiveness; stimulate appetite; and reinforce images of themselves as healthy and vital. In the treatment of anorexia, hypnotherapy is generally used in conjunction with other therapeutic methods.

In 1981, Dr. Meir Gross, chairman of the Child and Adolescent Psychiatric Department at the Cleveland Clinic Foundation, reported success in using hypnotherapy to treat 50 adolescent anorexics. Gross points out that because the anorexic fears loss of control it is important to show the client that a trance cannot be induced against her will. Gross found that self-hypnosis, in which the client is shown how to put herself into a trance state, is particularly valuable. Self-hypnosis helps the anorexic feel that she can control her own level of calmness, as well as take charge of the issues she wishes to address without having to please a practitioner. The anorexics in this study learned to use self-hypnosis to regulate weight gain and to limit weight increase once having reached target weight. In addition, Gross noted that when the anorexic understands she can use self-hypnosis to achieve what she wants, her motivation to use this technique increases (Gross, 1981, pp.97–99).

One of Gross's anorexic patients was distressed by the level of anxiety she felt when playing golf, although it was a sport she enjoyed and played well. When she was given the hypnotherapeutic suggestion that she could hit the ball with more force if her arms were stronger, she began to improve her eating to make herself stronger and healthier. By using self-hypnosis to suggest to herself better golf performance, she indirectly suggested to herself the better eating habits necessary for her to get stronger so she could play better golf (Gross, 1981, p.99).

Gross reports that during both regular hypnotherapy and self-hypnosis sessions he also has taught anorexics to relax and to reduce their usual hyperactivity. The anorexic chronically pursues vigorous physical activity, both to burn calories and to alleviate anxiety and emotional distress. Hyperactivity is a substitute for learning other ways to cope with a troubling situation or disturbing sensations. However, the anorexic generally finds her restlessness and agitation uncomfortable, and may frequently be bothered by the obsessive thought, "I wish I could just relax!" By learning how to use self-hypnosis to relax, the anorexic experiences physiological, emotional and cognitive benefits. Relaxation helps reduce the chronic muscular tension anorexics typically experience, and can also decrease both heart and respiration rate — both of which can be problems in anorexia. It can bring on an increase in slow alpha brain wave activity, another sign of a more tranquil state. One anorexic reported that by using self-hypnosis to relax and feel calm, she was able to think about herself and the conflicts that made her start dieting. Self-hypnosis also enabled her to be aware of her body, and of her feelings and sensations (Gross, 1981, p.97).

Gross has also used hypnotherapy to effectively treat body image distortion. By combining the use of photographs of the anorexic client as she appears in her emaciated state with hypnotic suggestions to make her aware of her extreme thinness, he found he could help her see herself objectively. In this case, he then urged the client to find pictures in magazines of females whom she found attractive and to paste a photograph of her head onto the picture of a body she liked. While the client was in trance, Gross used verbal suggestions of this image in future situations and presented this as a goal for the client to achieve. In addition, the client was encouraged to practice self-hypnosis and to touch and feel parts of her body during trance, such as her stomach, her legs, and where her heart beats. This helped improve her accuracy in both her cognitive awareness of the size of her body and her perception of the physiological sensations emanating from her body. In the end, the client was able to achieve a more realistic body image and was also better able to conceptualize the physical location of her internal sensations (Gross, 1981, p.97).

Anorexics commonly lack a realistic awareness of what it means to be either hungry or full, and Gross also used hypnotherapy to unblock perceptions of hunger and fullness (Gross, 1981, p.98). The anorexic exercises or denies being hungry to avoid feeling hunger, and will claim to feel full after a few bites, when in fact she is actually using exquisite control so as not to eat more. In addition, the anorexic sometimes stops using control and binges, with no awareness of when she is full. Gross helped an anorexic client in trance to imagine feelings of hunger, and then eat only until she felt satisfied. The client was then encouraged to notice the feelings of fullness and to stop eating.

A sense of ineffectiveness and a need for control are two more aspects of anorexic pathology which Gross addressed. Initially, just giving the anorexic the tool of self-hypnosis and the insight that she can use this technique for her own benefit is useful and empowering for her. In addition, hypnosis has several specific applications with these issues. In one case, an anorexic client was distressed because she was powerless to change her home situation and the fact that her parents were on the verge of separation. Gross used hypnosis to show the client to look to a time beyond her current familial entanglements. Projection into the future during trance helped her to separate herself emotionally from her parents. The client was able to achieve an awareness of the control she had over her own life and to create a positive image of her own future (Gross, 1981, p.99).

The clinicians William Kroger and William Fezler, authors of *Hypnosis and Behavior Modification: Imagery Conditioning*, used hypnotherapy to treat two anorexic clients. One of the two clients benefited; the other, unfortunately, did not attend her appointments and died. Kroger and Fezler term their approach "hypnobehavioral," meaning they use hypnosis to induce a relaxed and focused state in the client, who then is responsive to the behavioral suggestions of the hypnotherapist. While the anorexic was in a hypnotic trance, they suggested she create a vivid, appealing image of a sunset or an ocean scene. Then, the hypnotherapist suggested that she associate the appealing image with the behavior that she wanted to change. Next, he suggested she modify the image somewhat—change the color of the sunset, or add a boat to the ocean scene—in order to transform the old behavior, and then associate the *new image* with good feelings. This exercise reinforced the new image and helped the client replace the old behavior with the new one. Kroger and Fezler also taught their client to recreate the hypnotic state on her own and to practice visualizing by herself the images created in therapist-induced trances (Kroger and Fezler, 1976, pp.85–92).

Kroger and Fezler used hypnotherapy to stimulate appetite and to help clients relearn the feeling of hunger. They did this by creating images in which delicious food and feelings of hunger were associated with pleasant settings of gardens, seashores and idyllic landscapes. They found that hypnotic recall of cliffs and skies in particular was valuable in creating a sensation of lightness or emptiness in the stomach and in generating a realistic sense of hunger (Kroger and Fezler, 1976, p.287). Other therapists, including clinician Michael Yapko, have applied similar techniques in working with anorexic patients (Yapko, 1986, pp.224–232).

More recently, clinician Moshe Torem has also found a variety of hypnotherapeutic techniques to be effective in working with anorexic patients. He, too, has helped clients relax through hypnosis, and to use self-hypnosis to recreate tranquil feelings for themselves. He has also used hypnosis to give suggestions for healing and recovery. Torem reports having had particular success with a technique called age progression. With this method, Torem directs the client, while she is in trance, to go forward in time and to imagine herself as a healthy person. He introduces images of her as a strong and vibrant individual, being successful and happy in various aspects of her life, of enjoying activities that had been pleasurable to her before she became anorexic (Torem, 1992, pp.105–118).

Another hypnotherapist, Canadian Reuben Pecarvé, has used hypnotherapy with anorexia and bulimia (Pecarvé, 2002, pp.127–132), though he stresses that a hypnotherapist must work closely with the psychotherapy professionals when treating an eating disordered client. Eating disorders are serious mental disturbances, he notes, and while hypnosis can play a role in facilitating recovery, it cannot be the sole treatment. Pecarvé also notes that in anorexia, it is frequently necessary to regress the patient to early childhood to seek the root causes of the disorder, and that hypnosis can do this regression quickly and effectively (Pecarvé, 2002, p.132).

More recently, clinician Bart Walsh has commented on the fact that anorexics sometimes exhibit trance-like states such as dissociation, hallucination, catalepsy and time distortion, and has suggested that this propensity can make those individuals more readily hypnotizable (Walsh, 2008, pp.301–310). Others have suggested that hypnotizability may be involved in maintaining self-defeating eating behaviors. Australian clinicians Susan Hutchinson-Phillips, Kathryn Gow and Graham Jamieson also advise caution in interpreting the effectiveness of hypnosis in treatment because there is a lack of uniformity in measurements. (Hutchinson-Phillips et al., 2007, pp.84–113). Clinician Marianne Barabasz echoes this caution and says that replication of methodology is difficult and hence evaluation of results is problematic (Barabasz, 2007, pp.318–335). Nonetheless, Walsh has devised several hypnotic approaches for eating disordered clients to "inspire the establishment of a reality-based body image" (Walsh, 2008, pp.301–310).

It appears that hypnotherapy can have a place in the treatment of anorexia. However, some clients are more hypnotizable than others, and hypnotherapy is best used with specific problem areas and as a part of a comprehensive treatment plan, rather than as the sole tactic. Hypnotherapy can be a valuable tool for relaxation, particularly when an anorexic learns self-hypnosis and is able to calm herself; it also appears useful in helping an anorexic become more familiar with and comfortable in her body and more at ease with her body's sensations, as well as helping her correct distorted body image.

PERSONAL NOTE

I had the opportunity to experience hypnosis while I was at Cathexis. During these sessions, a skilled hypnotherapist on staff helped me develop a positive image of myself as a female and as a grown-up. At that time, I was disturbed because I was having difficulty imagining myself as having a job or a career or even a life in the future. Initially, the therapist taught me to become calm and peaceful. He guided me to become deeply relaxed and to create a detailed image of myself floating in a tranquil lagoon bathed in sunlight. I used the image afterwards to help me relax at times that I felt agitated. In another session, he asked me to recall a time when I was a young child and there were things I didn't know yet, and even things I didn't know that I didn't know. I don't recall what specific scene I used, but I came out of the session feeling more relaxed about not yet knowing what I wanted to do in the future. I felt I had received permission to experiment and take time to find out what I enjoyed and wanted to pursue, without the pressure of "finding the answer" immediately.

Since leaving Cathexis, I have experienced hypnosis on a couple of occasions. I've acted as a guinea pig for some of colleagues when they were training in hypnotherapy. Each time I have found the experience has produced a gentle feeling of relaxation and calmness that has continued for many hours after the session ended. Several years ago, I learned self-hypnosis, and I still use it to calm myself during anxious times.

Self-hypnosis seems particularly useful in the treatment of anorexia because it allows the client to maintain control of the process. Pecarvé reports that self-hypnosis can be applied to many, many issues, including increasing self-esteem, self-confidence, self-worth and assertiveness (Pecarvé, 2002, p.104). Growth in any of these areas can benefit an anorexic's development of her Self.

Guided Imagery

The relaxed but awake mind operates differently from the normally awake mind, allowing the emergence of feeling states, images and answers to which we may not be privy while in our usual awake state. Guided imagery makes use of this state of mind, and works with mental imagery for self-exploration. Because of its focus on images, guided imagery lends itself well to working with the core issue of anorexia: body image distortion.

Clinician Marcia Hutchinson has used guided imagery extensively to help women modify their body concept. She explains, "Body image is itself an image, and controlled imaging is an appropriate tool for entering the realm where the subjective experience of the body can be accessed and altered." She further elaborates that "image is the language of the unconscious and of feelings" (Hutchinson, 1994, p.157). Guided imagery can be a path into this "language" of mental images and feelings that both houses and comprises body concept. Guided imagery is a powerful tool, yet it is non-intrusive and tends to provoke less resistance on the part of the client than cognitive work or psychotherapy. Simply entering a relaxed state can be therapeutic for the anxious anorexic. Thus guided imagery is helpful in addressing both body image distortion and body tension in anorexia.

Another way that guided imagery can be valuable in working with eating disorders is by helping the client to develop a sense of Self. As Hutchinson points out, mapping the internal world of feelings, sensations, images, and memories is an antidote to feelings of emptiness (Hutchinson, 1994, p.158).

Clinician Ann Kearney-Cooke has developed a guided imagery program to treat body image disturbances in bulimic women. Several of the exercises can be used equally well with an anorexic. One exercise, called "Beginnings," can be used to explore the origin of the client's negative body image (Kearney-Cooke, 1989, pp.18–20). The client, in a relaxed state, is asked to consider the delivery room scene at her birth. Then the therapist suggests that the client imagine herself being born and visualize the birthing scene in vivid detail, and particularly to note the reaction of each parent to her birth. The therapist further guides the client to consider what each parent might have been dreaming at that point about their daughter now, at her current age. The therapist then leads the client out of her past images and into present time, and they discuss the images that emerged for the client during the session. For example, the client may say that her father looked disturbed because he had wanted a boy, or her mother was upset because she was scared and the baby was premature. The therapist can help the client process any uncomfortable thoughts or sensations that arise from these images (Kearney-Cooke, 1989, pp.19–20). As discussed earlier, a child internalizes attitudes about her body from her emotional and physical interactions with her caretakers in infancy and later. Neurologist Paul Schilder noted, "The building-up of the body image is based not only upon the individual history of the individual, but also on his relations to others" (Schilder, 1935, p.138). The birth scene can therefore help elucidate some of the anorexic's earliest interactions with her parents that may have influenced her internal perception of her body.

Hutchinson uses a different guided imagery exercise to further explore origins of body image disturbance and help modify the detrimental feelings that came from an earlier time. She has the relaxed client scan her life for a memory of an incident that was damaging to her feelings about her body, such as when classmates teased her in seventh grade and nicknamed her "Big One" while calling her smaller best friend "Little One." The client visualizes the incident in detail, and then imagines herself as an older adult observing the scene involving the younger her. Hutchinson helps the client rewrite her history by asking her to consider what she might have needed at the younger age and what resource she can bring into the picture to help the younger her feel okay about herself. Perhaps she imagines herself feeling strong and reciting to herself, "Sticks and stones can break my bones but words can never hurt me." She then has the client visualize a time recently when she used that resource, and the client recalls that she felt strong and used that phrase silently once when a co-worker was unpleasant to her. Hutchinson next moves the client into the future, asking her to imagine a situation in which she can call upon the sense of feeling okay (Hutchinson, 1994, pp.161–166). Through repetition of similar exercises, the client slowly builds a repertoire of positive feelings about her body.

In a variation on this technique, Ann Kearney-Cooke and clinician Ruth Striegel-Moore also use imagery to help clients rewrite the script of earlier body-related life scenes. In their view, negative body image is held in place by a schema, or complex web, of negative body perceptions, cognitions, feelings about the body and compensatory behaviors. Rewriting the script entails developing an alternative schema, meaning new perceptions, cognitions, feelings and behavior. The therapist guides the relaxed client to recall an early life scene that evoked the current body image distortion, then asks questions to explore in depth the client's feelings, thoughts and behaviors associated with that event, and the conclusions she drew about her body from the experience. Then, as in Hutchinson's work, the client imagines herself in the childhood scene, but with new resources or powers. Finally, the therapist engages the client in developing a new script with a detailed and complete schema that empowers the client both to respond to the original situation in a positive way, and to internalize a positive schema (Kearney-Cooke and Striegel-Moore, 1997, pp.301–302).

Kearney-Cooke and Striegel-Moore use another type of imagery to help the client let go of negative body image and create an alternative body schema. In this sequence, the therapist guides the relaxed client to imagine herself walking down a beach and encountering a wise and compassionate figure. The client begins to see all of the negative images of her body and to hear all of her negative body thoughts. The wise figure reaches out a hand which works like a magnet and absorbs all the negative images and thoughts. Then the client looks up and sees a screen in the sky where she can see new images of herself. In these new images, she experiences herself in a more positive way, treating her body well, eating when hungry, stopping eating when full, resting when tired, wearing fabrics that feel good next to her body, feeling empowered, and being supported by the wise and compassionate figure. The therapist also asks the client questions about what she sees, so that her new images may be incorporated into future visualizations. The clients imagery is then repeated during the first part of future sessions; repetition serves to strengthen the new images as well as to develop a broader repertoire of positive body images. In the words of these psychologists, "Guided imagery is an especially powerful tool, because body image is an image that clients have the potential to change. It is a powerful technique for psychic reconstruction, as well as for the creation of alternate images of the body" (Kearney-Cooke and Striegel-Moore, 1997, p.303).

While most people have strong visual sensory abilities, some people are more attuned to auditory than to visual cues. Guided imagery does not work as well for these aurally-inclined individuals, but it can still be used because auditory representations—words, thoughts, and verbal associations—may emerge for the client. The therapist and client can then process these sound elements and their meanings as if they were exploring visual images.

Like other experiential modalities, guided imagery affords the anorexic an indirect and non-threatening way to approach her feelings. It works well in conjunction with psychotherapeutic modalities precisely because it offers an alternate avenue to work with the body image distortion central to anorexia. While specialized training in guided imagery is available through classes and through schools of imaginal studies, there are no certification requirements for use of guided imagery. Some therapists combine psychotherapy and guided imagery, and find guided imagery particularly useful in the early phases of psychotherapy in anorexia when clients tend to be anxious, reticent, and unfamiliar with their feelings.

PERSONAL NOTE

As a therapist, I was introduced to the tool of guided imagery many years ago, when I was training to lead groups for women with body image concerns. I liked the process—and still do—because it is relaxing and soothing, but also because it can be a gentle but powerful change agent. At one time during a guided imagery session in the training, I was picturing myself as a young baby and imagining what that young baby needed in the moment. I saw myself as a nine-month-old little Gerber baby, looking happy and bubbly but wanting to be nurtured and held. Self-nurturance was still difficult for me at that point in my recovery; I felt more comfortable taking care of people other than myself (and hoping, not quite consciously, that someone else would take care of me). Something about that particular image left me with the feeling of *wanting* to nurture and take better care of myself. The image stayed with me, and comes up for me occasionally now in times of particular stress, reminding me to soothe and nurture myself.

Art Therapy

"Essential to art therapy is that it partake of both art and therapy," wrote Elinor Ulman, founder in 1961 of the *American Journal of Art Therapy*. Art, she continued, is the meeting ground of the individual's inner and outer worlds, while therapy aims to create positive change in personality or in life that "endures beyond the therapeutic session" (Morenoff and Sobol, 1989, pp.145–146). Non-verbal expression is the anorexic's forte, though she uses this skill self-destructively. Meanwhile, her capacity to use spoken words to express emotions is limited. Art therapy provides the anorexic with a bridge between non-verbal and verbal expression. As the anorexic talks with her art therapist about what she has produced, she can eventually learn to describe in words what she has represented in her artwork and develop a verbal language for her emotions.

The prospect of putting an image on a blank piece of paper, or forming an object from a solid lump of clay, can be immobilizing to a perfectionist. The anorexic's inner demons may be crying: "I don't know how to draw! I've never made anything out of clay. How should I begin? Then what should I do? What if I can't think of anything?" Initially, the art therapist may need to coax the client gently to enter this unknown world and to reassure her that there is no expectation, no anticipated outcome, that whatever she creates is sufficient, that she will not be judged for what she makes, or how much or little she produces.

Art therapy can be used to foster recovery from a number of the developmental deficits of anorexia. Anorexics lack the capacity to comfort themselves, except through food-related activities; the art process can help the anorexic learn to self-soothe. As the anorexic engages in her creative process, she becomes absorbed both in being with herself and in representing what is going on in her inner world through the medium before her. Anorexics must confront their imperfection when a painting or art project does not turn out the way they hoped it would. The art therapist can then guide the anorexic to talk about, or represent through another project, what imperfection means. Creating an art product can also play a role in helping the anorexic internalize an authentic self and develop inner cohesion: the art product is a representation of her inner world, and by talking with her art therapist about it, the anorexic takes ownership of this aspect of herself. Anorexics feel ineffective and incapable of influencing the environment beyond their bodies; the process of creating art confers a sense of accomplishment and a means to influence something external — what they have produced — instead of controlling their bodies or their lives in unhealthy ways. The anorexic can gain a sense of self-efficacy and mastery by making something that has meaning for her.

Furthermore, art materials resemble food: they can be handled and held; they have texture, shape, weight, consistency and color. Initially, the anorexic may handle the art materials as she would food, in a restrictive, limiting and cautious way. However, as she experiments with more media and her use of materials becomes more expansive, it can have an impact on her negative beliefs about her own internal sense of smallness and the restrictions she imposes in many arenas of her life, including food (Betts, 2008, p.15).

Art therapist Mari Fleming describes how she views art therapy with an anorexic as a developmental process in which the anorexic slowly builds more internal structure and strengthens her sense of self through three distinct phases. The nature of the art therapy work, and the kind and type of involvement of the therapist, changes at each phase. Initially, the art therapist provides a non-threatening holding environment; she is empathic in understanding the client's experience and actively mirrors the anorexic's artistic expression. The therapist's goal at this phase is to provide a safe place for the anorexic, an environment where she feels enough at ease to express herself in imagery. Familiar art materials such as crayons and pencils are reassuring and calming for the client. Initial activities focus on images that are comforting and represent safety for the client. The therapy then progresses to depicting the client's concerns. However, if the client becomes apprehensive, the therapist encourages her to return to safer topics, materials or activities (Fleming, 1989, pp.283–284).

In the middle phase, the art therapist introduces materials such as soft pastels, oil pastels and paint to encourage expression of feelings and to promote self-investigation. The therapist assists the client in overcoming frustration, and models and encourages self-soothing. At this phase, the art therapist supports the client's self-esteem and mastery, demonstrating an investment in the client and the client's artwork, and confirming and mirroring the client's artistic expression. When feelings and memories emerge, the therapist is empathic and responsive, helping the client to achieve greater self-awareness and self-acceptance of her inner world. As the anorexic internalizes more of the therapist's responses, she integrates more of a Self. The therapist always defers to the client's authority on the meaning of her work, which further strengthens the client's sense of accomplishment and autonomy. As the client progresses, the therapist acknowledges her growth. In later art activities, the client depicts aspects of her Self and is encouraged to integrate the different aspects by placing the various images she creates in a container or in a shape such as a circle (Fleming, 1989, pp.284–285).

The final phase, with the approach of termination, focuses on issues of loss and the feelings of rage, guilt and anxiety that accompany separation. The therapist encourages the client to portray her memories of early losses. Often feelings of childhood abandonment emerge at this time, and the anorexic depicts these powerful feelings in her artwork. In this phase, the client is allowed to choose her art materials, which is both calming for her and encourages her autonomy. Also, taking control of art materials provides a substitute outlet for the anorexic's wish for control, which formerly manifested itself with food. At any point that the client becomes anxious and uncomfortable in doing this work, she may return to using materials from the earliest stage in her therapy — the familiar crayons and pencils. The consistency and stability of the therapist and the deepening relationship between the therapist and the client continue to reinforce the anorexic's accomplishment and sense of self as she prepares to terminate therapy (Fleming, 1989, p.285). Thus Fleming's model of art therapy with an anorexic corresponds to normal child development, and parallels the process of psychotherapy, in which the anorexic gradually builds and strengthens her internal Self structure and progresses from immaturity and dependence to individuation and being her own person.

Another approach to art therapy in anorexia is to suggest the anorexic do a specific art exercise to address a particular problem or issue. For example, in order to reinforce a client's progress and to help her acknowledge the changes she has made, an art therapist might suggest that the anorexic use drawing and painting to differentiate "how she feels now" from "how recovery feels"; or to use imagery to separate her "true self" from her "eating disordered self"; or to create an "inner image" of her body that is different from her distorted body image (Betts, 2008, pp.17–18). Many of these exercises can be done in any of a number of media, offering the client a broad range of artistic forms of expression. Art therapist Donna Betts has formulated exercises to enhance the anorexic's capacity to identify and acknowledge her feelings. At the beginning of each session, she asks a client to use one word to describe how she is feeling physically and one word to describe how she is feeling emotionally. Through this exercise, the anorexic learns to distinguish between body sensations and emotional states, and discovers how the two are related. Next, Betts instructs the client to draw how she is feeling physically and emotionally using lines, shapes and colors. She encourages the client to verbalize the meaning of what she has drawn by asking questions such as "What do you like and not like about the image? What would you like to change? Does the image have anything to say? Invite the parts to talk with each other — what do they say?" Gradually, the client uses words to describe the internal feeling states she has represented on paper (Betts, 2008, pp.21–22).

In the treatment of anorexia, art therapy is generally used in conjunction with psychotherapy. The two modalities together can be very effective; psychotherapy can provide a venue to explore images and feelings that may first arise in art therapy, and art therapy can provide a means to represent through imagery topics discussed in psychotherapy. Art therapy fosters expression of feelings that either get censored by verbal defenses or remain inaccessible through words alone. Thus art therapy can provide access to deeper feelings and earlier memories than talk therapy. As Fleming notes, "Art used in therapy may provide both the first experiences of safety and the first expression of pain" (Fleming, 1989, p.303). The creativity fostered by art therapy provides tools for handling difficult feelings and a method for building and internalizing a self-structure. Supported both by the art process and by the relationship with her art therapist, the anorexic can progress on the path toward developing a cohesive, authentic Self.

Personal Note

While I have never worked with an art therapist, I was exposed to the draw-a-person exercise at Cathexis, as I mentioned earlier in discussing body image. The first time I did this exercise, it was early in my treatment and I probably weighed 75 percent of normal. My therapist handed me pencil and a sheet of plain white paper and instructed me to simply draw a picture of a person. I was pretty clueless, and didn't have any suspicion that I was sketching a representation of *me*. I drew a figure that looked more like my father than myself: a stick-like man with an oval head, but no face, wearing a fedora like the one my father wore on rainy days, a straight body in a long overcoat with little, rectangular legs protruding out underneath; the figure had tiny, barely formed hands and no feet.

When my therapist told me that the picture I had drawn revealed some things about me, I remember first feeling tricked — why hadn't she told me that before? But as she interpreted my drawing, I was intrigued by her comments and by how well her conclusions fit how I felt inside. That I had drawn a man suggested I thought of myself as more male than female and that I certainly didn't feel very feminine. Without a face, I was expressionless: not only did I exhibit no feeling, I lacked any awareness of feeling. The absence of feet indicated that I was not grounded; without well-formed hands, I could not reach out to others; with no eyes, ears, mouth or face, I was disconnected from people. The hat and overcoat kept me covered — hidden — and gave me protection.

The accuracy of my therapist's insights startled me. At that time, I felt more sexless than female or male, more like a child than an adult — though I was 30 years old. I don't think I knew what feeling grounded meant, and I had no real sense of emotions except for the numbness of depression alternating with the tension of anxiety. I had very little connection to any person. I felt vulnerable and alone, and the idea of wrapping myself in a big overcoat and hat felt safe.

I did the draw-a-person exercise again about a year later. This time, my drawing depicted a person who was more female than male, but not exactly feminine. The figure looked like a chubby girl, had long hair, and was wearing a skirt and no hat. She had little eyes, but no nose, ears or mouth. She had little feet and slightly defined hands. My therapist commented on the change since the first drawing. I thought the drawing was ugly; but at that point I felt ugly, inside and out. I had gained weight, but didn't like how I looked, or how the weight had distributed itself. I felt fat. I didn't feel feminine and was having trouble with simply owning my femaleness. I didn't feel like a man, either. I hated the drawing and actually wished I felt more like I had when I'd made the first drawing. At that point at least I had felt independent and disconnected from people, instead of being in this difficult transition where I knew I needed people but hated feeling dependent.

This exercise gave me respect and awe for the depth of meaning that can be gleaned from a seemingly innocuous drawing. It made me realize the potential power of experiential exercises. Had anyone asked me to simply describe how I felt about myself, I would not have been nearly so eloquent as my drawings were. Despite my love of words and their descriptive power, I understand how much they can omit.

Music Therapy

Music therapy, like other experiential therapies, allows the anorexic a medium through which to practice self-expression and to expand her self-knowledge. Music therapy can include listening to music, having music in the environment and making music. The client in music therapy engages in a musical activity, evaluates the activity, and then arrives at some conclusion or insight which she can use outside the therapeutic setting. As the anorexic talks with the music therapist about the musical activity, she gradually learns to expand her emotional vocabulary and to develop more ability to communicate about her feelings.

Music therapists, working either with groups or with individuals, are more commonly found in residential or inpatient settings, but some work in outpatient private practice as well. For anorexics, music therapy can help develop more healthful, constructive and pleasurable activities to supplant their negative, obsessive and self-destructive patterns. In the view of music therapist Alice Ball Parente, music therapy provides three basic processes to enhance positive behavior: experience within structure, in this case the structure of music; experience in self-organization, which leads to stronger self-identity; and experience in relating to others. Each of these processes can address specific developmental deficits and dysfunctional behaviors that are common in anorexia (Parente, 1989, p.307).

"Experience within structure" refers to the fact that music itself has structure — harmony, rhythm, melody, style — and that these parts all work together to create a particular piece of music. One issue in anorexia is the misplaced use of control; that is, the anorexic is at all times attempting to control her body and her food. In a music therapy setting, the therapist points out that the client can commit herself to the process only as much as she chooses — that she can *control* her environment. In time the client can tolerate the expansion from listening to or creating a small musical phrase to a measure to an entire piece; always she remains in charge of her own pace. Music therapy also offers experience in structure by assisting the anorexic with reality acceptance. The client can be encouraged to listen to a piece of music and clap her hands with an intensity appropriate to the piece. She will recognize that varying tempos and types of music are more dramatic than others, and learn to respond accordingly. Furthermore, by hearing or playing different kinds of music, and discussing their impact on her, the client can choose music according to her mood and her need in the moment. Soft, soothing music can be comforting; songs with upbeat lyrics or lively tempos can be used in times of sadness to lift her mood; with music she enjoys, she can create an experience of pleasure. The anorexic can then use music as a tool if she begins to obsess or get caught in a negative spiral of thinking or feeling (Parente, 1989, pp.307–311).

Parente's second process, "experience of self-organization," refers to the client's attitudes, interests, and values and the establishment of personal identity. Anorexics tend to look outside of themselves for approval; they have an underdeveloped self-concept, an external rather than an internal orientation, and often do not know their own likes and dislikes. Parente explains that the music therapist helps the anorexic's slow discovery of her own opinions and perceptions through honoring the client's choices of music and mirroring her reactions to what she hears. In addition, the client can use specific songs with positive, self-reinforcing lyrics as affirmations, both by listening to a song repeatedly and by writing the lines out on paper. Songs such as "I am Woman" or "I've Gotta Be Me," or lines about learning to love yourself from "The Greatest Love of All" are examples of self-affirming lyrics. Music therapy can further offer the anorexic a venue for safely learning to identify and express negative feelings. She can choose pieces of music to share with her music therapist that represent specific uncomfortable or "unacceptable" emotional states. By responding empathically to the client's choices and what they represent, the music therapist creates an environment in which the client can feel safe to talk about what the music evokes in her. The anorexic can share her fear of revealing the feelings elicited by the music and can learn to tolerate and accept these "bad" feelings (Parente, 1989, pp.311–314).

Another music therapist, Marah Bobilin, supports Parente's view of music as a way for the anorexic to strengthen and expand her sense of self. Just as psychotherapy allows the anorexic to develop more emotional space, expanding the dimensions of her internal world, music therapy can help a client to grow and take up more "musical space" (Bobilin, 2008, p.146). In other words, when a client gradually takes a larger role in asserting her musical preferences, using music for emotional expression or mood management, and valuing her own musical expression, she owns her musical tastes and capacities. This expansion and strengthening of her sense of self in the sphere of music can generalize to other areas of her life.

Parente's third process, "experience in relating to others," is sometimes best provided when music therapy is conducted in a group setting — often by several clients playing music together — although some of the same goals can be achieved in a less dynamic way when the client meets individually with a therapist. In a group, if several members are singing or playing a piece together, each member's participation is important to the whole. The anorexic can thus learn that her involvement has value. Plus, a music therapy group can be an arena for learning to tolerate mistakes in oneself and in others and for recognizing that imperfection does not lead to rejection. As the group practices a piece over and over, the strengths and weaknesses of each participant become evident. But the anorexic is encouraged to view the group not as an opportunity for comparison but as a space for co-creating. She is also encouraged to see herself as an integral part of the whole, bringing something that is essential to the group. In addition, when a group selects a specific piece of music, the anorexic can express through musical preferences feelings that she otherwise refrains from voicing (Parente, 1989, pp.316–317).

Bobilin addresses in more detail the way in which music therapy can aid the client in developing her capacity for interpersonal relationships. She speaks of the improvisational nature of music-making in a group setting for eating-disordered clients. The music therapist facilitates the minimum amount of structure required, and the clients are encouraged to take as much responsibility as possible for creating the music (Bobilin, 2008, p.148). This process requires the individuals to communicate, voice preferences, negotiate, compromise, and cooperate in making decisions. Later, the music therapist leads discussions about their interactive process—what worked, what didn't, what each person learned, how they came to make particular choices, and how the process felt. This kind of group provides the anorexic with a laboratory for learning from others about herself in relation to others, and learning skills which she can take to other interactions.

In sum, music therapy offers the anorexic opportunities for creativity and choice, learning and expressing her own preferences, and building interpersonal skills. Because each aspect of music therapy requires the anorexic to *refer to herself* to discover her own likes, dislikes, perceptions and preferences, music therapy provides a valuable venue for self-knowing and self-development. In addition the anorexic learns she can influence her own mood through the music she chooses, and that she has some capacity to control and make choices based on internal cues. The music therapist honors the anorexic's choices—by mirroring and empathizing with her preferences and reactions. If the anorexic plays music or sings, this expands her use of music therapy to include all the choices and nuances involved in musical expression. If the client creates a musical measure or line or piece, the therapist can mirror her accomplishment as well as her process, which can help build the client's self-esteem.

Poetry Therapy

Developmentally, the experience of feelings and the body sensations from which they emanate are preverbal in origin, and not always conscious (Woodall and Andersen, 1989, p.193). Poetry, which works with emotion and image, can help the anorexic develop a voice and a metaphorical language with which to describe her internal experience. In time, metaphor can create a bridge between the anorexic's internal world and verbal dialogue. Some therapists have found poetry therapy to be a useful adjunct in the treatment of anorexia because it can provide the anorexic with an avenue to express indirectly what she has trouble speaking about directly. Also, writing a poem builds a bridge between the anorexic and her therapist; it allows her to put into words the pain that she otherwise conveys through her body and behavior (Woodall and Andersen, 1989, pp.204–205).

Anorexics suffer from a sense of ineffectiveness and a corresponding difficulty with self-assertion. When the client is asked to write, her "reticence gives way to the interest in a cognitive task (which ends up full of feeling), and the spontaneous poem itself becomes an emergent self-assertion" (Woodall and Andersen, 1989, p.194). An anorexic may have trouble talking directly with her therapist, or indeed, knowing what to talk about. However, writing a poem — which is a concrete task she is likely to accept doing — provides considerable material for discussion and interpretation by the therapist. This both builds the alliance between the client and her therapist, and provides a glimmer — to both client and therapist — for the anorexic's inner experience.

Initially the therapist may read a published poem with the client. For use in poetry therapy, a poem should be concise, the subject matter about deeply personal issues, and the tone empowering. The works of Emily Dickinson and Robert Frost are among those that fit these criteria. Furthermore, aspects of Emily Dickinson's life may resonate with the anorexic, and Dickinson's poetry may evoke some recognition and even identification. Dickinson was reclusive, and after college returned to live at her parents' home, where she stayed for the remainder of her life, corresponding with friends and writing poetry. She is described as very self-controlled and a perfectionist. Dickinson wrote about isolation, depression, fear, loss, and feeling ineffectual. She even wrote a couple of poems about food restriction, and one poem that psychologist Camay Woodall suggests "seems to be about Dickinson's experience with anorexia nervosa" (Woodall and Andersen, 1989, p.194).

Early in therapy, the therapist may choose a published poem about loneliness or sadness. Later, the therapist may pick a poem about anger — which is often a more threatening feeling to an anorexic than loneliness or sadness — or about more complex feeling states, such as disappointment or guilt. Initially, the therapist has the client read the poem, first out loud and then to herself. The therapist asks the anorexic to describe what the poem is about. As the client interprets the poem, she has an opportunity to verbalize an internal reaction to something that is not related to herself. The therapist also interprets the poem. The client is asked to write a four- or five-line poem in response to the one that was read, either about the same theme or about her reaction to the poem. The therapist carefully instructs the client that there are no expectations about the content of the poetry, that words do not need to rhyme, but that poetry has a natural rhythm which will emerge from her own feeling (Woodall and Andersen, 1989, p.203).

The attitude of the therapist in receiving the client's poem is probably as important as the content of the poem itself. Whatever the client writes, the therapist welcomes and acknowledges as the client's self-expression. The therapist's appreciation helps the anorexic feel understood, an essential step in building a trusting alliance between the two individuals. If the client is shy about reading her own poem, the therapist reads it, slowly and respectfully. If the client reads it, the therapist also reads it out aloud, which allows the client to experience her poetry in a different way. Then the two discuss the client's poem, which reveals more than just her reaction to hearing a published poem; it also describes metaphors for her own internal experience. The client is asked to talk about what her poem means, and each phrase or line of the poem is discussed in detail. Then the therapist offers her interpretation of the poem, phrasing her comments as questions, so the anorexic can remain in charge of her truth about the meaning of the poem. In this way, it is established that the client is both the author and the authority on her poem (Woodall and Andersen, 1989, pp.203–204).

In individual therapy, this process can be repeated with additional poems; alternatively, the client may sometimes write a poem to express her feelings about something that comes up in a session. At all times, the therapist's respect and appreciation of the client's poem is critical. As the client goes through the experience of having something she created being valued, it can help with her own process of self-valuation.

Poetry therapy also lends itself to group work. In one format, a poem by a published author is read and interpreted by the therapist, and then discussed by the group. Then each group member writes her own poem in reaction to the one that has been read. In a different approach, after introducing a published poem, the therapist leads a group poem-writing exercise. First she writes one line of a poem. Then each member contributes a line or two to the poem, and then the therapist reads the final poem and leads a discussion about it. Of course, each group member is revealing something about herself and her feelings in the line or two she writes (Woodall and Andersen, 1989, pp.195–196).

There are several advantages to using poetry in working with anorexics. Reading a published poem provides initial contact with a person who is not present — the poet — and therefore is non-threatening. Also, a poem may bring up feelings or a conflict that the anorexic can identify with. This identification can provide vicarious relief, as well as introduce an opening for the anorexic to put her own struggle into words. When the anorexic writes her own poem, it is a concrete accomplishment and can be a source of pride and self-esteem. Any poem the anorexic writes is a form of expression, albeit metaphorical, of her own experience. In the words of British psychoanalyst D.W. Winnicott, "A poem is layer upon layer of meaning ... and always about the self" (Winnicott, 1971, cited by Woodall and Anderson, 1989, p.204). Writing poetry, therefore, can be a helpful, if oblique, way for the anorexic to approach her inner Self.

Movement Therapy

Movement is key to development of healthy body image in infancy. Along with the sensory stimulation provided through being held and touched, movement helps the infant give and receive vital sensory information. Movement also provides a process of internal feedback through which to interpret and integrate physical sensations. Basically, *movement therapy* mimics for the client what *actual movement* provides for the infant: it helps to integrate physical movement with mental awareness of the sensations accompanying the movement so that the individual can develop a more accurate perception of her body in space. Given that distortion of body image is central to anorexia, movement therapy offers an avenue for helping the anorexic to increase her body awareness and thereby modify her body concept. When individuals have missed some of these important developmental experiences in infancy, movement therapy later in life can help them to reinhabit their bodies.

Movement therapists Julia Rice, Marylee Hardenbergh and Lynne Hornyak have identified six body-mind issues that are core to an anorexic's body image disturbance. These include experiencing pleasure; sensory awareness; differentiation from the environment; perceiving the parts of the body as a whole, or integration of body parts; initiating movement in space; and developing an internal locus of control, or sense of centeredness, which is essential to the process of individuation (Rice et al., 1989, p.257). Furthermore, these authors have made a number of observations about the movement patterns of anorexics, and found that typically, anorexics move in a rigid and controlled way, with little fluidity. Their breathing is shallow, which reduces their awareness of both physical sensations and emotions. Anorexics tend to initiate movement from the limbs, not from the trunk, which can contribute to their experience of disconnectedness between body parts. They also have very constricted movement, as though they have little concept of personal space. Anorexics often exercise in a rigorous, compulsive and punitive way that also contributes to the lack of integration of body parts. When an anorexic moves one side of her body, she usually repeats it on the other — unilateral movement is rare. This lack of unilateral movement further suggests the anorexic's rigidity and control (Rice et al., 1989, pp.259–261). The anorexic's constriction in body movement correlates with a constriction in self-development, as anorexics tend to be rigid, controlled, careful and contained.

Movement therapy is highly compatible with the changes in the self that are requisite to the anorexic's recovery. The anorexic's development is stunted both physically and emotionally. Movement therapy relies on the reciprocal body-mind process, a bi-directional feedback loop in which movements are influenced by thoughts and feelings, and changes in internal perceptions in turn alter movement patterns. The basic components of movement therapy — attention to movement, experimentation with movement, exploration of the sensations associated with movement — can address the core deficits in anorexic movement patterns. Also, movement is a process activity — the body is the vehicle of communication, with no need for verbal translation. In addition, the body is the center of the work, giving the client a heightened sense of her physical reality. Furthermore, movement therapy offers corrective body experiences. It can create sensations that the anorexic can identify as positive, which is a very different way for the anorexic to experience her body (Rice et al., 1989, p.261).

Rice and her colleagues propose a model for treating body image disturbance with movement therapy that proceeds through three stages, mimicking the progressive nature of body image development in a growing baby. During each stage, the therapist conducts a series of specific exercises with a client. Exercises in the early stages involve more *noticing* than *moving*. The first stage — which Rice and her colleagues call "What Body?"—focuses on helping the client increase her body awareness. At this stage, the client also learns to identify body reactions, such as discerning if she likes or dislikes certain movements. The therapist will guide the client in making small gestures, such as raising her arm, and indicating whether or not the movement is pleasurable. To facilitate noticing and observing spatial proportions, the therapist asks the anorexic to arrange two chairs the same distance apart as the width of her body. Then the therapist asks her to stand between the chairs and encourages her to talk about her reaction to any size differences between her imagined body width and her real body width. Another exercise is the Body Map, in which the client lies on a piece of paper and the therapist draws a line around her whole body. The client "personalizes" the body map by drawing and writing on it. The therapist may ask her to make notes on parts she likes and dislikes, or parts that have particular significance to her. To encourage a client's expression of self-care, the therapist may instruct her to hang the body map in a safe place and to touch and care for it as she would like to care for herself (Rice et al., 1989, pp.261–265).

The next stage is "Who Owns This Body?" It teaches the client about boundaries and making choices. In one exercise, Proximity, the therapist instructs the client to tell the therapist where to sit. The client then approaches and moves away from the therapist, noticing what distances feel comfortable and what distances make her feel anxious. The client then repeats this exercise, imagining that the therapist is each member of her family or any other significant person in her life. From this, the anorexic learns that she can control her distance or closeness from each person. In another exercise, Safe Space/Bubble, the client finds a safe space to sit anywhere in the room, closes her eyes and molds an imaginary bubble around her with her hands. She describes the perimeter of the bubble around her and also what it feels like to be inside the bubble. This exercise helps the anorexic establish an external boundary beyond her skin that can make her feel less vulnerable. It also gives her permission to take ownership of the space that she occupies (Rice et al., 1989, pp.265–267).

The third stage is less structured than the earlier stages. In "What Can My Body Do?" the therapist may suggest that the client explore a theme through movement, such as the concepts of "open" and "closed" or "active" and "passive." The therapist acts as witness to the client, who is the mover, validating the client through observing her actions, and acknowledging her expressions through movement. The therapist also explains to the client that her movements demonstrate her creativity and capacity for self-definition, thus reinforcing the client's sense of competence. In addition, at this stage the client can use movement metaphors to express real-life situations that are uncomfortable or problematic for her, such as an interaction with a difficult co-worker. In this way, the client uses movement almost like drama or pantomime. Exploring the situation through movement can help the client work out a movement-based resolution which she can translate into a real-life resolution that she can then apply. Work at this level requires that the client already have developed a degree of connection with her body, which she has gained in the first two stages (Rice et al., 1989, p.268).

Rice and her colleagues stress that a movement therapist needs to be very sensitive to each client's particular body issues and body sensitivities, and to monitor the process of the therapy carefully, gauging the pace to accommodate the client's capacities. Initially, some clients may be extremely fearful of using their bodies as vehicles for therapeutic change. They have safeguarded their bodies as bastions of control. Also, it is helpful if the movement therapist working with an anorexic client values and is comfortable with his or her own body; personal body discomfort can be communicated unwittingly by the therapist and undermine the work with the client. When conducted with care and compassion, movement therapy can be a useful adjunct in the treatment of anorexia.

Movement therapy, as well as dance therapy, is generally conducted by registered dance therapists. Dance therapy and movement therapy overlap — dance therapy *is* movement therapy, and dance therapy sometimes extends the concepts and functions of movement therapy. Frequently, the modality is referred to as dance/movement therapy (Stark et al., 1989, p.122). However, dance therapy generally incorporates more free-style gestures and sequences than movement therapy. Dance therapy also makes use of natural energy and rhythm. For the anorexic, dance therapy can be a helpful adjunct later in therapy. In early recovery, the anorexic is likely to feel threatened by the more spontaneous, free-style motions typical of some dance therapy exercises. That said, it is also the case that some anorexics *are* dancers, and that students of some dance modalities, particularly ballet, are prone to developing anorexia. However, just as those with anorexia may move their bodies during exercise but still be out of touch with their body feelings and have a distorted body image, so it is in dance: dancing does not automatically confer a mental connection with internal emotional cues or a realistic body image. Dance therapy is different from dance, however, just as movement therapy is different from rigid repetitive exercise. Dance therapy, like movement therapy, helps the individual focus on her internal sensations connected to movement rather than on her external precision of movement.

Dance/movement therapy can be invaluable in treating anorexia because its medium — the body — holds so much meaning for the anorexic. Dance and movement therapy help the client strengthen her awareness of body sensations, develop healthy boundaries and build trust in her body. Dance/movement therapy also cultivates a consciousness of the Self. As the anorexic opens to experiencing her sensations, and then to communicating these through movement, she gradually becomes aware of her sensations as intimations of who she is. In addition, she can develop a sense of pleasure in her body. Movement therapy also offers the anorexic the opportunity to experience her body, and to use her body as a nonverbal form of expression, in ways which are not self-destructive. For the anorexic to inhabit the body she has viewed as a prison, to identify internal signals and to actually derive pleasure from physical sensations instead of fearing, ignoring and overriding them, fosters growth of her Self.

Psychodrama and Gestalt Therapy

In the therapist's office, an anorexic client is arguing with her eating disorder, moving back and forth between chairs as she alternates between speaking for herself and speaking for her eating disorder:

EATING DISORDER: *"You shouldn't have eaten that peanut butter. You're getting fatter!"*
CLIENT: "I only had one bite of peanut butter on my apple!"
DISORDER: *"You think you can get away with that? I thought you didn't want to get fat."*
CLIENT: "I don't want to! But it wasn't even a teaspoonful!"
DISORDER: *"And every teaspoonful counts! You're thighs are getting bigger as you sit here!"*
CLIENT: "Okay. Maybe you're right. I'll have to run an extra mile."
DISORDER: *"That's right. You've got to really watch it or your thighs will just get bigger!"*
CLIENT: "I know, I know. I'll do better next time."

The client gives in, defeated; she couldn't out-argue her eating disorder. But now the therapist moves to the side of her chair and speaks for her, as the client continues to alternate between chairs and speaks for her eating disorder:

THERAPIST AS CLIENT: "Whoa! On second thought, I'm not giving in so easily. I think I need that peanut butter for protein and energy, and it will make me feel stronger."

DISORDER: *"At the cost of getting fat!"*

T AS C: "Not so! My doctor said I need to eat more, that I'm too thin to get fat. And he knows better!"

DISORDER: *"Since when did you start listening to your doctor. Who made him the god of fat?"*

T AS C: "He knows more than I do! He knows more than you do! For now, I'm going to listen to him."

DISORDER: *"You're going to get fat!"*

T AS C: "I'm going to get strong!

This two-chair exercise provides a concrete, experiential, yet oblique way for the anorexic to communicate to her therapist about her inner struggle. When her therapist speaks for her, the client can experience her therapist's support more concretely than through direct dialogue. Psychodramatic enactments such as this can be a useful adjunct in working with anorexics because they can feel like safer ways of communicating than direct dialogue.

In psychodrama, the internal reality of the client is enacted externally and the client's perceptions become larger than life. For example, when the client role-plays *both* people in an interaction, she develops a more complex understanding of the interchange than if she were simply to talk about it. Psychodrama and Gestalt use similar techniques in integrating psychotherapy and action to increase awareness on a physical level; for simplicity I use the term "psychodrama" to refer to them both. The psychodramatic therapist uses action-oriented interventions to help the client develop both a physical and a mental experience of an event. The goal of psychodrama is "action insight," and it works on the assumption that experimentation with new behaviors creates an experiential body awareness which involves avenues beyond cognitive understanding. Furthermore, psychodrama increases body consciousness and fosters reliance on body sensations; these can help the anorexic develop an experiential sense of Self (Hudgins, 1989, pp.236–237).

Psychodramatist Kate Hudgins proposes a three-stage sequential approach to using psychodrama to treat anorexic clients. Each stage builds on the previous one. The first is focused on developing a therapeutic alliance, the second on discriminating between false Self and true Self, and the third on developing autonomy.

In using psychodrama to build a therapeutic alliance, the therapist can use the technique of "doubling," described in the two-chair example above. In doubling, the therapist (or, if this is done in a group, another member of the group) sits next to the client, adopts the client's posture, and speaks as though she is part of the client's internal world. In this way, the therapist can verbalize hypotheses about the client's internal state without confrontation or direct questioning, both of which would likely be met with resistance. The therapist can also make a suggestion about a change in posture as a way to feel differently. For example, if the client is slumped as if she is carrying the weight of the world on her shoulders while she is attempting to confront her eating disorder voice, the therapist might have her experiment with sitting up straighter (Hudgins, 1989, p.239). This approach is a very gentle process of figurative handholding as the client begins to notice any internal sensation, thought or image (Hudgins, 1989, pp.238–242).

Hudgins' second stage uses the two-chair technique to discriminate among internal parts of the individual and create dialogue between them (Hudgins, 1989, p.242). In this exercise, when the client is trying to make a decision or resolve a situation that is causing her internal conflict, the therapist directs her to sit in one chair, facing the second, empty chair. In the first chair, the client role-plays one part of herself, and speaks to the empty chair, which is a different part. The client then moves to the second chair and replies to the first part. The client goes back and forth between the two chairs, guided by the therapist in how to speak with her other part. The two-chair dialogue continues until the client is able to achieve some resolution about the issue. This technique can help teach the client about handling internal and external conflict.

In another two-chair technique focused on role reversal, the client learns more about interpersonal boundaries. By playing herself in one chair and a family member in the other, she also learns to stand up for herself (Hudgins, 1989, pp.244–246). Role reversal can help an anorexic with the threat of separation-individuation; it gives a chance to clarify her wants and needs relative to another person, thus strengthening her sense of Self. In acting as another person, she can develop a "felt sense" of what is going on with the other person, which in turn can help her develop empathy for others, and in time, for herself. As she switches back to being herself, she learns she can tolerate another person's demands, which further strengthens her sense of Self.

Focusing, the central technique used in stage three, facilitates the anorexic's capacity for introspection, which will further strengthen her sense of Self. Introspection also helps her differentiate her authentic feelings (true Self) from those stemming from pleasing behaviors (false Self) and facilitate her becoming more autonomous. In this stage, she learns to translate the awareness gleaned from introspection into a cognitive understanding of the experience (Hudgins, 1989, pp.246–249). In other words, the anorexic integrates her internal sense of a feeling with talking about the feeling. Thus she has moved from an initial place of not knowing what she was feeling, to learning to experience her feelings and adopt new behaviors, to talking about her feelings from a physical and emotional experience of them. Psychodrama builds from the internal awareness to the verbalization of the physical in cognitive terms. This process enables the anorexic to gradually develop a more solid internal self-structure in a way that may be more palatable to her than pure talk, and at the same *to* talk about her internal world. In these ways, psychodrama and gestalt techniques can complement psychotherapy.

Psychodramatic techniques such as the two-chair exercise are sometimes used by psychotherapists who aren't necessarily specialists in psychodrama, as a part of a comprehensive therapy to help an anorexic work with her "eating disorder voice," or the internal critic driving her perfectionism, body hatred, and self-destructive behaviors. The two-chair method can also be used to help an anorexic with both decision-making and handling conflict, two areas which are particularly challenging for her. In addition, anorexics may find it helpful to work with a certified psychodrama practitioner. These practitioners often lead groups which can give the anorexic an opportunity to "try on" different roles. In a psychodrama group, generally a situation pertaining to one group member is enacted by the members of the group under the direction of the practitioner. After the enactment, individuals talk about what it was like to play a certain role. For example, a group may enact a family scene in which the anorexic acts as a wife and mother who is at odds with her husband. The anorexic would act out the mother's role in the conflict and the mother's interactions with other family members, giving her a sense of how a person in that situation might feel and act. The anorexic can also observe others, and learn more about the feelings and thoughts they demonstrate and talk about. She can experiment with expressing herself in new ways in a setting that is non-judgmental and therapeutic. In addition, by playing a role, she is making a contribution to the psychodrama, which can give her a sense of effectiveness. Plus, while psychodrama is therapy, it can also be fun — which is important for the anorexic to experience in recovery!

Therapeutic Bodywork

The anorexic generally holds her body in a rigid, tight manner. She carries herself with her head down, her shoulders slumped and her rib cage collapsed. Her breathing is shallow; even if she is a heavy exerciser, her breathing is not deep. She appears to carry the weight of the world on her shoulders and, indeed, she toils under the conviction that this is her lot: to try to be perfect, but invariably, to fail; to please others, no matter what; to shrink into invisibility for the sake of safety — these are the burdens she bears. Her despair and discouragement are visible in her posture before she even speaks. And of course, her emaciation tells still another part of her story, that of her fight for self-preservation, which almost robbed her of life itself. For the anorexic in recovery — when she has the physical strength — bodywork can help dismantle the physical correlates to her psychological stance. When she ceases feeling called to prop up the world, bodywork, massage and other hands-on body therapies can help restructure the posture she adopted to meet that challenge. When she finds she no longer needs to fend off humanity or use starvation as defense, bodywork can help disassemble the impenetrable walls she had erected against intruders.

While the body is genetically programmed, with aspects of physical character and body type determined long before birth, the body also is molded throughout life by both physical and emotional circumstances. The body constructs armor in the form of muscular tension, or holding patterns, in response to life events. But sometimes that armor outlives its usefulness; sometimes protection that was necessary as a young child is no longer useful to the adolescent or adult. When old patterns embedded in the body are no longer constructive, they can rob the individual of energy and cause illness and emotional distress. The goal of therapeutic bodywork is to help release and realign neuromuscular patterns and postural configuration to free up the energy that has held the old patterns in place. Lessening defensive body tension enhances the person's well-being, aliveness and vitality.

Therapeutic bodywork is body-based but also psychological in content. As old body defenses are released, the psychological wounds they protected can emerge. Body and mind are intricately intertwined and events that affect one affect the other. The psyche accumulates a person's history, encoding it in memory — a physical entity — as well as in the structure of the body. The body remembers and houses the residue of the individual's experiences, physical and emotional. While psychotherapy is the healing medium for the psyche and body therapy for the body, each modality affects both mind and body. Healing the body can help heal the mind, although it is generally not the most direct approach; similarly, psychotherapy can help alleviate body tensions, though bodywork can do it more directly. For the anorexic, whose physical armoring is pronounced and whose psychological issues are complex, bodywork can augment the work of psychotherapy.

The use of massage and bodywork for healing has a long history. The therapeutic use of touch has been depicted on cave paintings in the Pyrenees dating to 15,000 B.C. Ancient Chinese civilization wrote about manipulated pressure points, and an Egyptian papyrus from 1700 B.C. described adjusting the spinal column through use of massage. The modern Western practice of massage was systemized in the early 19th century (Claire, 1995, p.10).

There are dozens of different kinds of bodywork, including various types of massage and numerous forms of therapeutic bodywork. Each kind of bodywork is distinguished by its philosophy, focus and techniques. All healing practices that work with the body are designed to improve well-being, although some are uncomfortable in the moment. This cursory discussion is in no way meant to cover the broad range of bodywork types available or the therapeutic benefit of each.

In general, bodywork can produce some level of change relatively quickly. However, just as happens with psychological issues, body issues surface in an unpredictable manner. They are multi-layered and complex, and old patterns that are exposed and explored don't disappear immediately. As with psychological issues, body patterns can be tenacious. Bodywork is often conducted in a series of sessions to effect and sustain change, and attention must be given to the psychological issues that arise from these treatments. Every person, anorexic or not, possesses a measure of body-based defenses, some of which are valuable and healthy, and all of which warrant respect. However, those individuals suffering from serious psychological disturbances or who have suffered prolonged or recurrent trauma are likely to harbor a correspondingly significant amount of body armor. Bodywork with these individuals generally is protracted and best done in conjunction with psychotherapy.

Bodywork has particular value in recovery from anorexia because of the anorexic's extreme distortion in body perception and body use. The anorexic has generally used her body as a machine, exercising obsessively and ignoring exhaustion. Her body is an automaton that she wills to keep going. She feels a heightened sense of the physical sensations of fatigue and cold. She has stifled emotional sensations, and interred pleasure with her pain. Fluid movement and physical pleasure are foreign concepts. The anorexic holds a lot of tension in her defensive posture and patterns of movement.

Forms of bodywork differ both in philosophy and methodology. Some use a lot of hands-on manipulation, while others use light touch or, paradoxically, no touch at all. Some integrate psychological work into the process, others are truly body-centered. Some focus on holding patterns, others address patterns of movement. Most types of bodywork ultimately promote greater body awareness in a way that leads to more pleasure, freedom of movement, relaxation and broader range of sensation, all of which can benefit the anorexic in developing a more healthful body awareness. Here I discuss but a few of the many types of bodywork that either have been or potentially could be used in the treatment of anorexia.

Massage manipulates the soft tissue of the body, using stroking, kneading and pressure, and can be soothing, nurturing and relaxing. It can provide an increased sense of body awareness and well-being. The anorexic has little real sense of her body and mostly thinks of it as a foreign object that she is trying to starve into submission. Becoming conscious of her body in a new way is an important step in recovery. Massage can also feel pleasurable and help the anorexic develop a sense of body-pleasure. Massage can further help relieve the chronic tension that the anorexic often holds in her muscles and soft tissues.

Rolfing and the remaining techniques in this section are forms of therapeutic bodywork. Rolfing uses deep muscle and connective tissue manipulation to restructure the body's counterproductive holding patterns. According to Ida Rolf, developer of this approach, gravity affects organization and physical movement; when a person is affected by emotional events, such as defeat or disappointment, the body responds. That response is affected by gravity, which tends to shorten soft tissue and cause corresponding psychological changes (Claire, 1995, pp.59–60). The physical intensity of this approach makes it appropriate only with an anorexic who has made significant physical recovery.

Other techniques derived from Rolfing do not do such deep work. These include *Aston Patterning*, which combines Rolfing with movement education, and *Hellerwork*, which combines hands-on work that is less invasive than Rolfing with movement evaluation and interactive dialogue between practitioner and client. Hellerwork is a highly structured approach consisting of eleven sessions. It is developmental in perspective, moving through body holding patterns, starting with those presumed to be formed in infancy and going forward through childhood, adolescence and maturity. This developmental progression makes Hellerwork of particular benefit in working with psychological issues. The initial sessions focus on more superficial tissues of the body and on the developmental phases of infancy and early childhood. In the next four sessions, the practitioner works with deeper tissue layers and their psychological corre-lates, issues of adolescence. The final four sessions are integrative and focus on maturity (Claire, 1995, p.74). Because Hellerwork work focuses developmentally on holding patterns that have become fixed in the body, this work can be useful for the anorexic who may have experienced deficits in touch as a baby.

Another therapeutic bodywork approach that can be useful in addressing the body's hold-ing patterns is the *Rosen Method*, which Marion Rosen developed by combining physical ther-apy with verbalization of psychological content that emerged during the work. A Rosen practitioner uses gentle touch and light massage to relax a client and help release holding in some parts of the body. In this state, unconscious psychological material, forgotten emotions and memories can surface. Rosen work relies on the breath as a signal of change; that is, as the client's breathing patterns change during the session, they signal the practitioner that uncon-scious material is becoming conscious (Claire, 1995, p.170). The Rosen worker then gently encourages the client to speak about the experience that is surfacing; in doing so, the client both releases the holding and constriction in the body and becomes more cognitively aware of the source of the tension. In the process of letting go of suppressed emotions, clients can expe-rience improvement in both emotional and physical well-being. Because the anorexic client experiences chronic and severe body tension, she may benefit from the release of chronic mus-cular tightness and the gradual emergence of psychological material that Rosen work elicits.

The *Alexander Technique* works with movement integration to reeducate the body to pro-mote more ease of movement and better postural alignment. Using gentle manual guidance accompanied by verbal instruction, the practitioner assists the individual to notice, then change, movement patterns. An Australian actor, F. Matthias Alexander, who was plagued by losing his voice midway through theatrical productions, originated this method. As he discovered body patterns associated with the vocal change, he worked to modify the body alignments, and even-tually not only regained his voice but improved his physical and emotional functioning as well. Alexander summarized the goal of this work as "developing a better use of the self" (Claire, 1995, p.79). As developing more optimal ways of using the body, and the Self, is central to recov-ery in anorexia, Alexander work can be a helpful modality for the recovering anorexic.

Moshe Feldenkrais, an engineer and neurophysicist, synthesized knowledge from physics, biomechanics and physiology to help himself recover from a debilitating knee injury, and in the process developed the *Feldenkrais Method* (Claire, 1995, p.101). This practice, like the Alexan-der Technique, uses gentle movements to improve movement integration. According to Feldenkrais practitioners, movement patterns become established and fixed at a young age. By reeducating the body to move differently, we can open to wider freedom of movement and pleasure in movement. The Feldenkrais method seeks to make unconscious movement con-scious, and to then provide the individual with other options in how she moves and behaves. This work does for the body what psychotherapy does for the mind: it makes the unconscious conscious, and thus allows choice (Claire, 1995, p.103). The practitioner verbally guides the client to make very small, precisely defined movements. As the client becomes aware of which movements are easier and smoother and which are difficult, she can repeat and reinforce the preferred movement. For example, she may notice that one way of moving from sitting to stand-ing strains a back muscle while another feels fine. An anorexic may be hyperactive and exhibit a great deal of movement, but her rhythms of movement are often very rigid and tense. The awareness of freedom of movement that Feldenkrais encourages can address the very driven, unconscious nature of movement of the anorexic, offering her a choice in how she moves.

Integrative Body Psychotherapy (IBP) is predicated on the belief that everyone has an "essen-tial Self," and that "this Self comes from the soul, the universal energy embodied in the indi-vidual and made unique by its presence in that body" (Rosenberg et al., 1991, p.12). IBP combines bodywork with psychotherapy. The practitioner uses a focus on the breath and hands-on massage to help the client release energy blocks that impede the experience of a full and vital Self. A trusting relationship between therapist and client is key as it is through the therapeutic process, the interaction between client and therapist, that the Self is healed. IBP practitioners work from a developmental perspective, exploring the impact of the person's childhood on the body. They guide the individual through reliving problematic developmental stages, with adult ego, perspective, intellect and language present, in order to break the spell of the past. Because of the particular formulation and integrative foundation of IBP, it seems particularly suited to the treatment of anorexia (Rosenberg et al., 1991, pp.30–31).

Somatic Experiencing (SE) is a form of bodywork developed by Peter Levine specifically to help heal trauma (Levine and Frederick, 1997, p.152). Levine's work grew out of his observation that in the wild, when an animal gets traumatized by an attacker and then escapes, it immediately goes through a flurry of movements that help release the trauma from its body; hence polar bears that shake off their trauma do not develop post-traumatic stress disorder. Human beings, however, largely out of cultural learning, tend to freeze in the aftermath of fear or trauma, and so they harbor the trauma and its residue in the body. Traumas vary significantly in degree, as does the intensity of a body's tension or holding patterns. In Levine's view "posttraumatic symptoms are incomplete physiological responses suspended in fear" (Levine and Frederick, 1997, p.35). So long as the responses remain incomplete, the symptoms will remain.

The SE practitioner sits several feet in front of the client and observes the client's body. The practitioner has a keenly developed capacity to notice minute holding patterns in the client's body — perhaps the client tilts her head ever so slightly to the right. The practitioner then guides the client to make small movements or shifts in body posture to "complete" the trauma or response, thereby releasing the tension. For example, the practitioner might ask the client whose head is tilted to slowly move her head further to the right, and then to very gradually lift her head. The practitioner will then talk with the client about what change she noticed from the movements. In this way, the SE practitioner can help the client to discover what movement she needs to make in order to complete the movement and release the tension.

Finding the right kind of bodywork as well as the right bodyworker is important. Bodywork is generally conducted by certified practitioners, and each modality requires particular qualifications. About two-thirds of the states recognize the certification which is overseen by the National Certification Board of Therapeutic Massage and Bodywork. Some states have city or county licensing requirements. Specific training and certification in specialized bodywork approaches is required to practice in those modalities. In order to become a certified Rolfer, an individual must attend an eighteen-month or longer training at the Rolfing Institute. Alexander Technique, Feldenkrais Method and Somatic Experiencing practitioners are required to attend a three- or four-year training in the particular discipline to obtain certification. Rosen Method bodyworkers attend a two-year study program followed by a two-year internship. (See "Bodywork Certifications" in the Bibliography's list of Internet references for links to more information.)

In addition to finding someone who is certified and experienced, it is essential for the anorexic to find a practitioner she can trust, and for both practitioner and client to understand that building trust can take time. Therefore, bodywork needs to be undertaken gradually, gently and at the pace the anorexic finds useful. An anorexic may be slow to accept the idea of bodywork; after all, her body is her identity, her *raison d'être*, and her sole protection. Relaxing those defenses in the presence of a stranger is a daunting prospect. Non-invasive massage is often the most useful introduction to bodywork for the anorexic. She may discover that massage improves her mood and alleviates her depression. As the anorexic feels more aliveness and well-being in her body, this vitality can promote her work in psychotherapy or other modalities. In time the anorexic may find it helpful to experiment beyond massage to other forms of bodywork.

I have had the opportunity to experience several forms of bodywork and massage, and found each helpful in its way. Massage has helped me to appreciate my body's capacity for relaxation and pleasure. Massages provide healing in two ways: in the actual release of physical tension in my body and in receiving nurturing touch from the expert practitioner. Also, as noted earlier, I experienced a couple of sessions of bodywork while at Cathexis. However, in the years after I left Cathexis, I was quite aware that my body still felt rigid and disconnected; I didn't know if it would ever feel otherwise. Since then, I have had the opportunity to experience a few different kinds of bodywork which have changed not only how my body feels, but also how I feel about my body.

About six years after leaving Cathexis, I started to see a Rosen Method bodyworker. The psychotherapist with whom I was working at the time thought bodywork might help my progress in therapy. To my amazement, week after week, the Rosen practitioner found an area of tension in my body that I had assumed was a permanent part of my body structure. She encouraged me to pay attention to any feelings or pictures that emerged as she gently massaged the areas to unlock the tightness. I held the most tension in my neck, shoulders and upper back. There were many times during bodywork sessions that I would simply cry and cry, feeling profound sadness without ever knowing its source or meaning. Often, I left the Rosen worker's office feeling emotionally exhausted from releasing the powerful feelings that had emerged during my session. And gradually, my body started to feel more pliable and more real. Once in a while some of the tightness would return, and the Rosen practitioner would do another round of work which always seemed to afford a more sustained release in the area. Occasionally the muscular release was companied by forgotten memories—or what I assumed were memories; they may have been constructs of my mind, but they certainly fit what I knew of my childhood and growing up. I explored the memories both with my Rosen practitioner and with my therapist. I was especially grateful for the softening of overall body rigidity that I experienced from Rosen work.

A few years later, I undertook a course of Hellerwork with an experienced practitioner. As a result of these sessions, I was able to experience breathing from my diaphragm — something I thought I had been doing for years! I had not realized how constricted my breathing had actually been. The practitioner massaged my diaphragm while instructing me to take extra deep inhalations and exhalations. My rib cage seemed to expand as a result of the work, as if my lungs had actually grown larger. The Hellerworker also had me experiment with walking with a different rhythm — I hadn't known how stiff my posture really was, or how narrow the range of motion of my gait. I learned to move my foot through the complete sequence of putting my heel on the ground, moving from heel to ball of foot and lifting my foot in a way that made my connection with the earth feel solid. When I first saw the Hellerwork practitioner, I had simply been aware that certain areas in my torso seemed somewhat stiff and inflexible; eleven sessions later, I was breathing deeper, standing straighter, and walking more fluidly and solidly — bonuses I had never anticipated.

A series of sessions in Somatic Experiencing also helped me in ways that I had never thought possible. Many months after my mother passed away, I was cycling through unabating periods of grief and depression. At the suggestion of a naturopath, I went to see an SE practitioner, who had me sit, relaxed and at ease, in a chair about eight feet in front of where he sat. The practitioner casually looked at me and pointed out an area of holding in one shoulder that I hadn't even been aware of. We talked a bit about what I thought the shoulder tightness might mean. Then, at his suggestion, I consciously released and tightened the spot in my shoulder. He next suggested I move my shoulder just a little forward and to the side. It felt weird, but I followed his instructions as he guided me through several more small movements, and then asked me to follow my shoulder's lead and let my shoulder complete the movement. Though I had no clue what he meant by this suggestion, my shoulder did seem like it was suspended in mid-movement. As I let my shoulder shift a little more, I had the sense of how else it needed to shift to complete the movement — slowly moving my shoulder back and down. Each movement was tiny and probably would have been imperceptible to anyone else watching the scene. But for the SE practitioner, this little exercise was cause for celebration! My shoulder had completed a movement; in essence, it had moved through and resolved a trauma pattern.

Each SE session after this seemed to release one more little piece of stuckness in my body, usually a piece that I wasn't fully aware existed. In one session, I felt grief for my mother in my throat, and despite all the tears I had already shed, seemed able to let go of my sadness a little more and a little differently than I'd done with all my crying. In other sessions, I became aware of body-holding related to other people or events. In each session, the SE practitioner simply had me work with whatever tightness he or I noticed was present. Eventually I came to realize that my pattern in the face of fear or shock was to freeze; what I didn't know was that these miniature ice cubes remained in my body. I also didn't know that the little blocks could thaw and leave me feeling more whole and connected inside. This work bestowed unimaginable gifts. For decades I'd been aware of having little numb places in my chest that my breath couldn't access. My breath somehow navigated around these obstacles, and I had assumed they were a permanent part of my interior structure, like my liver and heart. I was amazed to find out that I was now able to breathe into my whole chest and torso; that my insides felt like one open space without jagged edges or obstacles. It felt as if my parts inside were actually interconnected and forming a whole, and I was finally able to glimpse on a physical level the inner cohesiveness and sense of continuity that psychologist Rosenberg and his co-authors describe as essential to a healthy Self (Rosenberg et al., 1991, p.20).

Psychopharmacology

Drug treatment in anorexia is difficult because the anorexic is already in a physiologically compromised state and the side effects of drugs can have more dramatic consequences than in someone who is physically stable. Though the world of psychopharmacology has expanded dramatically in the last several decades, psychotropic medication in anorexia has been used more successfully to alleviate symptoms of the disorders that *occur with anorexia*, especially depression and obsessive-compulsive symptoms, than to treat actual symptoms *of anorexia*. However, improving mood with medication can help the anorexic's overall functioning to a degree. In some cases, psychotropic medication has been used to encourage eating behavior in severely undernourished patients. To date, there has been little success in identifying an agent which counteracts the core problems of anorexia, body image disturbance and intense fear of gaining weight. This field of research is hampered by the fact that relatively few controlled medication trials with anorexia have been conducted. It seems that the value of medication in treatment of anorexia is best determined on a case-by-case basis.

In the 1960s and 1970s, drug treatment of anorexia was largely conducted in inpatient settings with patients suffering from acute or chronic cases. In inpatient settings, psychological and physiological reactions to medication could be monitored closely and treated when necessary. Nowadays, medication can be used in outpatient as well as inpatient settings, but for the most part, medication has been used as part of a treatment protocol which also includes psychotherapy or behavior modification.

The earlier medication trials focused on use of tri-cyclic anti-depressants (TCAs) or the anti-psychotic drug chlorpromazine, sometimes in conjunction with insulin. The TCAs seemed neither to help weight gain nor to address other symptoms of anorexia, and had the drawback of potentially causing cardiac arrhythmias, although they did help the depression symptoms. Administration of chlorpromazine yielded some positive results in treating depression, and some of the earlier protocols are still in use. More recently, medication trials have focused on inpatient and outpatient administration of antipsychotic medication, olanzapine and of selective serotonin reuptake inhibitors (SSRIs)—a class of antidepressant medications that can improve mood by increasing the available neurotransmitter serotonin. SSRIs have not yielded generally positive results, perhaps in part because anorexic patients have insufficient serotonin to begin with. A few trials of olanzapine are reported to have produced somewhat promising results, but there are concerns about side effects, and the drug is not approved for treatment of depression.

To get a sense of both older and newer medications used to treat anorexia, let's look at some specific studies. In 1965, British psychiatrist Arthur Crisp reported that chlorpromazine appeared to have a significant effect on eating behavior in anorexia both experimentally and clinically (Crisp, 1965, p.75). Chlorpromazine is an anti-psychotic medication that can help reduce anxiety. Crisp monitored 21 hospitalized patients ranging in age from 17 to 55 who had been ill for from under one to over ten years. The patients were also treated psychotherapeutically, with a focus on the causes of their illness. It is unclear how long the study lasted, but follow-up data were available for an average of one and a half years after the treatment was completed. Of the original 21 patients, 19 were of normal weight at follow-up while two had died. Eleven had normal eating behavior. In three patients, weight gain was followed by the emergence of a severe depressive illness (Crisp, 1965, p.75). Given the variation in patients treated and the lack of information presented about the immediate results of the course of treatment, it is difficult to evaluate Crisp's results, although Crisp himself considered the outcome positive.

In the same era, two other British psychiatrists, Peter Dally and William Sargant, employed a combination of chlorpromazine and insulin to treat a group of 20 hospitalized anorexics ranging in age from 11 to 33 who had been ill for from nine months to ten years prior to hospitalization. Each patient was administered a daily dosage of chlorpromazine, which was gradually increased. Insulin administration was begun the first morning. Meals were small at first and gradually increased in size. The clinicians treated the patients empathetically and gave them reassurance, but no attempt was made to deal with psychological problems until the patients had gained weight (Dally and Sargant, 1960, p.1771). The patients remained on this regimen approximately one month, gaining about four pounds each week. After a follow-up period of undisclosed length, eleven were seen to have made a good recovery, in terms of regaining normal weight and reestablishing menstruation, while three maintained a stable although subnormal weight and three had recurrent relapses. For the remaining three, no follow-up data were available.

Dally and Sargant compared their results with those from an undescribed treatment regimen applied to 24 anorexics treated at another hospital. They noted that in the other group, patients gained weight less rapidly and were hospitalized for longer periods, and concluded that their treatment method was more effective than any other form of treatment used previously (Dally and Sargant, 1960, p.1772). It appears that it is the *combination* of chlorpromazine and insulin which was effective, for neither drug given alone produced such effective results. Furthermore, if treatment with either drug was stopped before the weight gain was achieved, relapse occurred.

However, there were several downsides to the chlorpromazine-insulin regimen. Both drugs have potentially dangerous side effects. Hypotension may result from administration of large dosages of chlorpromazine, giving rise to symptoms of restlessness and shakiness; ingestion of insulin can cause hypoglycemia. In a later study, Dally and Sargant further discovered that bulimia can develop in anorexics treated with this drug regimen. They suggested that the occurrence of bulimia might be related to the mechanism of action of chlorpromazine, which affects the appetite-regulating centers in the hypothalamus (Dally and Sargant, 1960, p.795). While bulimia is an undesirable consequence, its incidence appeared to be largely transitory in those who developed it.

One further disadvantage of the chlorpromazine-insulin regimen is that the drugs appear to delay the return of menstruation. This is problematic because without menstrual cycles and the hormonal fluctuations that accompany them, bone formation is compromised. A great many anorexics suffer from osteopenia or osteoporosis, and this is rarely fully reversible. In chlorpromazine-insulin treated clients, menses reappeared an average of fourteen months later than in the drug-free or insulin-only treated clients. However, Dally and Sargant concluded that in the longterm view of anorexia and recovery, fourteen months can be considered temporary and not of overall significance.

According to Dally and Sargant, one advantage of the chlorpromazine-insulin regimen over other treatment methods is that in *chronic anorexics*— defined as those in whom the symptoms persist for more than five years and in whom weight restoration has never been achieved — treatment with chlorpromazine and insulin together was sometimes effective in inducing weight gain where all previous treatments (chlorpromazine or insulin alone, antidepressant drugs, electric shock, intensive psychotherapy) had failed. Thus the main advantage of the chlorpromazine-insulin treatment appears to be in its *initial stimulation of the appetite regulation center of the brain*, resulting in a change of eating behavior and consequently a gain in weight. Considering the potential hypotensive and hypoglycemic effects of the chlorpromazine-insulin treatment and the possibility that the treatment regimen may induce bulimia during the recovery phase, it seems that the chlorpromazine-insulin regimen should be limited to individuals who are resistant to other forms of therapy. To be effective, treatment must be tailored to the needs of the patient, and what works for one may not work for another.

With the advent of SSRIs, and the fact that depression is quite common in anorexia, it has seemed reasonable that SSRIs might play a role in the treatment of anorexia. Also, SSRIs have helped reduce appearance-related obsessions and compulsions in some clients with body dysmorphic disorder, further suggesting they might be able to work similarly in anorexia (Allen and Hollander, 2004, p.932). However, the significance of SSRI medication in the treatment of anorexia remains unclear. In 2002, American psychiatrists M.B. Tamburrino and R.A. McGinnis reported that the most promising finding in medication treatment of anorexia suggests that fluoxetine, or Prozac, may help prevent relapse in the weight-restored anorexic (Tamburrino and McGinnis, 2002, pp.301–311). Researchers Andrea Allen and Eric Hollander at Mt. Sinai School of Medicine note that preventing relapse in anorexia is significant as weight gain is easier to obtain than weight maintenance in this disorder, and the majority of patients relapse within one year (Allen and Hollander, 2004, p.932). In 2008, researchers Reinblatt, Redgrave and Guarda at Johns Hopkins University concluded after a review of the literature that for anorexia "there are no pharmacotherapies of proven efficacy in either adults or youths" (Reinblatt et al., 2008, pp.183–188). However, they noted that some clients may benefit from the thoughtful use of psychotropic medication on an individualized basis when it is part of a multimodal treatment plan.

On the other hand, two French researchers who have investigated hyperactivity and self-starvation have noted that hyperactivity can lead to self-starvation and create a self-maintained cycle. Based on animal studies, they have noted that self-starvation aggravated by hyperactivity generates an opioid and also causes an increased hypothalamic serotonin metabolism. They have hypothesized that SSRIs or an opioid antagonist (a medication that prevents the opioid response) might be effective in the treatment of anorexics exhibiting hyperactivity, who comprise a large subset of anorexics (Kohl and Guelfi, 2004, pp.482–489).

A class of drugs known as atypical antipsychotic agents has been used more recently in treating anorexia; these medications, which include olanzapine, quetiapine, clozapine, ziprasidone, atriprazole and risperidone, have fewer neurological side effects than some other antipsychotic medications, and they have been reported to reduce anxiety and dampen obsessions. In addition, dramatic weight gain has been noted as a side effect of olanzapine, leading researchers to consider its use for anorexics. Approved by the FDA in 1996 for treatment of schizophrenia, olanzapine has been used "off label" for anorexia in both inpatient and outpatient settings. In 1999, British psychiatrist L. Hansen used olanzapine with a group of hospitalized anorexics and reported weight increase, decreased fear of fatness, reduced agitation and less resistance to treatment in the patients (Hansen, 1999, p.592). In 2001, a group of German clinicians noted that with five hospitalized adolescents with anorexia, olanzapine helped to lessen their fear of gaining weight and their rigid thinking, although it had no apparent impact on weight gain (Mehler et al., 2001, pp.151–157). There have been a couple of reports of single-case use of olanzapine. In 2003, a group of clinicians in Turkey reported marked improvement both in weight and psychological adjustment when they used olanzapine with a hospitalized 15-year-old girl suffering from severe anorexia (Ercan et al., 2003, pp.401–403). Psychiatrists in Taiwan combined treatment of olanzapine with a non–SSRI anti-depressant, mirtzapine, in treating a 27-year-old seriously depressed anorexic. These researchers reported success both in relieving the woman's depression symptoms and in helping to restore her weight (Wang et al., 2006, pp.306–309). In 2008, a study in Ontario, Canada, used a larger sample size and treated adult women who had both obsessive symptoms and anorexia. Seventeen of the women were treated with olanzapine and 17 were given a placebo. The researchers reported that compared with the placebo, olanzapine resulted in a greater rate of increase in weight, earlier achievement of target body mass index and a greater rate of decrease of obsessive symptoms. Furthermore, no differences in adverse effects were noted between the two groups. However, the researchers recommended that additional trials with larger sample size be undertaken (Bissada et al., 2008, pp.1281–1288). And the potential for side effects with olanzapine remains problematic.

One drawback in using olanzapine is that most anorexics do not *want* to gain weight, and the rapid, dramatic weight gain that has been reported as a side effect of olanzapine is likely to seriously distress an anorexic. Also, some disturbances in metabolism such as insulin resistance may develop, and the drug may have an alarming impact on blood sugar and cholesterol levels. Furthermore, olanzapine and similar drugs have a sedating quality; this quality is part of their usefulness in counteracting anxiety, but calming to the point of sleepiness is not a well-liked effect. As with other medications, or indeed, all treatment protocols, of course it is essential to tailor the treatment to the individual in a case-by-case basis.

Personal Note

I was twenty years old when my older brother committed suicide. I'd been anorexic for almost ten years at that point. With my brother's death, I became very depressed and had little desire to eat or sleep. After several weeks, I went to see a psychiatrist who prescribed the tricyclic antidepressant Elavil. This was before the advent of SSRIs. Within a couple of months, I began to see a psychiatrist regularly for psychotherapy. During the time I was taking Elavil and in therapy, I became less depressed than I had been initially, but I continued to be somewhat depressed. My eating habits returned to where they had been before my brother's death: minimalist, restricting and rigid. To the extent that my mood did improve, I have no way of knowing whether it was the effect of time, of medication, of psychotherapy, or of some combination of the different factors. After about a year, I stopped taking Elavil.

Several years later I experienced another bout of severe depression. I was no longer in therapy and I was a graduate student in biology. I had completed all of my work towards a Ph.D. except researching and writing a thesis. The prospect of spending two years in a lab collecting data by doing invasive procedures on small creatures— probably horseshoe crabs— was unappealing. And I was questioning whether I was really suited to a career as a biologist or biology professor.

I decided to try antidepressants again, but I couldn't really afford to see a psychiatrist. Instead, feeling dread and fear that I'd be turned away, I went to a walk-in psychiatric clinic at Bellevue Hospital in New York City. The psychiatrist on staff was actually very kind. He was amenable to prescribing Elavil for me again, since I had taken it before and thought it had helped.

For about three weeks, I struggled with side effects of the drug. I was so sleepy at times during the day that I felt like I dozed off standing up. Fortunately, the drowsiness eventually subsided, and I also started to feel less depressed.

I saw the clinic doctor each week. He monitored my drug dosage and we talked about the drug's effects, but we never discussed my life or any emotional problems. I don't know if I was helped as much by the medication as by my decision to leave graduate school, but my mood did improve, and I stopped taking the Elavil after about six months.

What I refused to acknowledge at the time, however, was that I was anorexic and underweight, which doubtless had an impact on my mood. I did not want to eat for fear of gaining weight, and medication did not help my anorexic mindset. However, medication somewhat improved my general sense of well-being. When I experienced more anxiety and depression in subsequent years, I could at least remember times I had felt *less* bad, which helped motivate me to seek assistance so I could again feel better.

I suspect I have been somewhat depressed during much of my life but have not wanted to admit it. Saying I was depressed seemed tantamount to advertising a character flaw. In hindsight, I also realize my mother was depressed when I was a child, and that I hated it, and her, when she was moody and would withdraw. For a long time, I didn't know that depression was really a disease. To a degree, I excused my brother's depression, which led to his suicide, because his depression seemed so horribly severe, and I wasn't dependent on him like I had been on my mother when I'd been younger. As an adult, I had experienced bouts of deep, dark moods, but I resisted labeling these as "depression," or at least as depression serious enough to warrant medication. However, when in quick succession a long-term relationship ended, a close friend died and another friend moved away, I felt like I had fallen into a big, black hole. I kept telling myself I could handle this on my own; after all, I was in therapy, these were situational events, it was normal to feel down under the circumstances, and my mood would pass. Finally, I realized it wasn't passing, and I reluctantly went to see a psychiatrist.

By that time SSRIs were in common use for depression, and some older anti-depressants were still being prescribed as well. The psychiatrist I saw thought I would be best helped by the SSRIs. It took considerable trial and error. Prozac put me to sleep; Zoloft made me sick to my stomach; on Celexa, I dozed off in the middle of the afternoon any time I sat down; and Lexapro also made me too sleepy to function well. Having been through four SSRIs, I then tried Wellbutrin, which is in a different class of antidepressants. Fortunately, Wellbutrin helped ease my depression without giving me intolerable side effects. As my mood began to improve, I was very grateful for the help of medication.

I don't know whether there is a link between my susceptibility to depression and my developing anorexia. Either one, I'm sure, could have exacerbated the other. In anorexia, despite the fact that no medication seems to address the core issue of body image distortion, relieving coexisting mood problems can at least improve the individual's overall functioning. My view of psychotropic medication today is that for those whom it helps, it can be a blessing. It may not be clear how medication helps; there may be a large placebo component, or it may really be doing something to neurotransmitters that we can only hypothesize about at this point. For those fortunate ones that are helped by medication, however, whatever difference it makes is worth celebrating. If unnecessary pain can be alleviated and quality of life improved, then perhaps other healing can commence as well.

9

Therapy for Families and Family Members

Anorexia nervosa is a disorder not only of an individual, but also of the individual in context. The culture plays a role — including the media, the community and the peer group — as does the family milieu, particularly when the anorexic is an adolescent or young adult living at home. Whatever may have contributed to the origin of the disorder, once it starts, it is sustained within the family system. And the family system consists not just of the current family members, but also of the family culture, both biological and social, inherited from previous generations and reenacted in present time. In some ways, anorexia can be seen as a symptom of something gone awry in the family system. Family systems therapy, more simply called family therapy, can be critical in helping restructure the family dynamics which are contributing to the persistence of the disorder.

Family Therapy

Family therapy addresses the structural organization of the family, or the bonds which tie some family members more closely than others; the family life cycle, which is the family's developmental process as a unit; and the patterns of interaction among family members. There are a number of different approaches to family therapy, and I will summarize only a few types below.

Whatever the theoretical orientation of the family therapist, however, some basic considerations seem clear. First, family therapy is but one component of treatment for anorexia. In addition to family therapy, the anorexic needs the forum and support of individual therapy in dealing with emotional and developmental issues; she needs to be medically monitored throughout the course of treatment, although frequency is generally at the discretion of the physician, and to work with a qualified nutritionist. Second, it is essential for the family therapist to connect with and understand the inner world of *every* family member, and to not make assumptions about, for example, an over-involved mother or a distant father. Third, a family therapist needs to maintain a positive, supportive and empathic attitude to offset the guilt and self-blame which is often significant both for the parents and the anorexic. And finally, while a family therapist should have a conceptual framework, each family is unique, and the therapist's responses in the moment must be tailored to the specific family in that particular moment.

Family Systems Theory

Psychiatrist Murray Bowen developed Family Systems Theory in the 1960s, and family therapy owes a great deal to his conceptualizations. Bowen views the family as an emotional unit and describes the interactions among family members using systems theory. Emotionally, members of a family are highly interconnected — although the degree of interconnectedness varies between families — and if one person in the family changes, it has an impact on how each other person in the family functions.

One of Bowen's key concepts is differentiation of self: the more differentiated the self, the less the person depends on approval from others and the greater his tolerance for difference and conflict. Differentiation of self is determined in large part by interpersonal relationships within the family during childhood and adolescence. Differentiation is largely an unconscious process: no one "chooses" his or her level of differentiation. At times of higher anxiety in the family, there tends to be more fusion between some family members than others. Often one child carries more of the family anxiety, and is less differentiated than other children in the family. Birth order can also play a role in degree of differentiation — generally, first-born children tend to be more differentiated than last-born (Gilbert, 2006, pp. 85–100).

Another central precept in Bowen's work is multigenerational transmission: The capacity for differentiation is transmitted through the family culture from one generation to the next. This means that the degree to which a mother has differentiated in her family of origin will affect the degree to which she is able to encourage differentiation of her offspring. The concept of differentiation is critical in anorexia, since it is this process which is thwarted at adolescence when the anorexic regresses emotionally and physiologically. Bowen described other patterns within the family that are helpful in understanding family relationships, including the existence of sub-units or triangles of family members. Although Bowen did not apply his theory specifically to anorexia, his work is foundational in understanding how families operate.

Two German therapists, Helm Stierlin and Gunthard Weber, did apply family systems theory to the treatment of anorexia. They describe families with an anorexic child as characteristically exhibiting a high degree of binding, or fusion, both inter-generationally and in the immediate nuclear family, which leads to a blurring of boundaries and a "seismographic sensitivity towards the mental and emotional processes of the others" (Stierlin and Weber, 1989, p.31). In other words, family members are very tightly bonded and hypervigilant, and there is a lot of concern about what is going on with other family members. Also, loyalty, cohesion and self-sacrifice are idealized in these families (Stierlin and Weber, 1989, p.34). These characteristics contribute to the anorexic's difficulty in developing an identity and a life of her own. A major focus of family therapy is to activate each individual in the family to develop initiative and to accept responsibility for his or her own actions. At the same time, it is necessary to address the forces in the family that may thwart individual motivation. The work of family therapy is thus to promote differentiation of each family member, including the anorexic. The authors conclude that in such systems, it is not only the anorexic, but all family members who can benefit from family therapy (Stierlin and Weber, 1989, p.254).

Structural Family Therapy

In the late 1970s, the clinician Salvador Minuchin and his colleagues at the Philadelphia Child Guidance Center developed a Structural Family Therapy approach for working with what they termed "psychosomatic families." Minuchin and his colleagues believed that in these families, each of which had a child suffering either from anorexia or diabetes, family dynamics were contributing to the persistence of the medical disorder. Among the dynamics they identified were indirect communication, blurred boundaries and avoidance of conflict. The focus of their work was to change interactional patterns of family members, thereby strengthening some family bonds (such as those between the parents) and weakening others (such as those between mother and anorexic daughter) and promoting the anorexic's autonomy (Minuchin et al., 1978, pp. 59–99).

Minuchin and his co-workers asserted that "anorexogenic families," families in which a child develops anorexia, exhibit four major characteristics. First, these families are highly enmeshed, with poor interpersonal boundaries, and the roles of parents and siblings not well differentiated. Second, the families tend toward conflict avoidance, which can cause suppression of significant problems. Third, parents in these families are overly protective towards their children, causing their children to have more difficulty becoming independent and autonomous. Fourth, these families exhibit a limited range of problem-solving skills and are somewhat rigid in the solutions they will accept from outsiders. Their organization is such that "loyalty and protection take precedence over autonomy and self-realization" (Minuchin et al., 1978, p.59). A child in this kind of family environment is very protected emotionally and physically. If she develops symptoms, the family unites in their concern for the anorexic child, which in turn reinforces her dependency and lack of autonomy.

While all four of the traits may not be present in every family with an anorexic child, Minuchin's family therapy can still be a useful approach in conceptualizing therapy for many families. In this approach, the task of a family therapist is to join the family system, then to challenge the family dynamics and restructure the family organization. Initially, the therapist enters the family system by supporting the family's strengths and respecting the family hierarchy. But eventually the therapist assumes leadership in establishing the rules of the system and controlling family interactions, particularly around the eating disturbance. In Minuchin's view, the family of an anorexic tends to be courteous and cooperative and creates a semblance of willingness to change, but in reality is quite resistant to change. Therefore, says Minuchin, relatively dramatic maneuvers are required to facilitate change. To this end, Minuchin developed his unusual "family meal": He joins the family for lunch, and uses the meal as an opportunity to either under- or over-focus on food in order to modify the family's interactions around the girl's anorexia. Later family sessions are focused on reframing the problem from the girl's eating to intra-familial communications.

Once Minuchin met for lunch with a fifteen-year-old anorexic girl and her parents. He engaged the parents in lively, detailed discussion about everything *except* their daughter and her eating, refocusing the conversation and the parents' attention anytime either began to look at her. To prevent the mother from overseeing her daughter's eating, which evidently was a common occurrence in the family, Minuchin deftly built a wall of milk cartons between the daughter's plate and her mother's gaze. Minuchin repeated several times that eating was not a problem, and pointed out that normal people eat lunch, and that was in fact was what their daughter was doing. He also encouraged the daughter to assert herself when he asked for her permission to let her parents talk about her. At one point, Minuchin asked the girl if he could eat a piece of her celery, indicating that she was in charge of her own food. In this situation, Minuchin disrupted and redirected a number of the family's usual dynamics: he encouraged the parent-child separation and the daughter's autonomy; he reinforced adult-to-adult connection by carrying on a conversation with the parents while their daughter was eating; he refocused the family onto non-food topics; he disrupted the mother-daughter alliance, reducing the mother's capacity to oversee and direct her daughter's eating; and he encouraged the daughter to take control of eating in a healthy way, and to be assertive on her own behalf, thus lessening her dependence.

Minuchin and his coauthors report that their results were dramatically successful. They evaluated their outcome both medically, based on the degree of remission of anorexic symptoms — including resumption of normal eating patterns and stabilization of body weight within normal limits — and clinically, using psychosocial criteria such as adjustment to the family situation, involvement with peers, and participation in academic and extracurricular activities (Minuchin et al., 1978, pp. 132–138). Judging the patients' condition both at the end of therapy and after a period of from eighteen months to seven years after treatment ended, 86 percent of the 53 cases they treated recovered from both the medical and psychosocial components of the disorder (Minuchin et al., 1978, p.133).

Probably few clinicians possess Minuchin's charisma and chutzpah, which may have played a role in his success. However, Minuchin's principles, with less radical tactics, can be used effectively in working with families of anorexics. It is important for the family therapist to reframe and relabel the presenting problem. Usually the family believes that the problem is the disturbance in their daughter's eating and that they are helpless in remedying the situation. The family therapist challenges this view and declares that the problem is actually the way the family members interact with each other, specifying where in the family these interactions are problematic. Essentially, the therapist challenges whatever in the family structure might be contributing to curtailing the anorexic's autonomy and growth. By insisting that all family members speak for themselves and not be allowed to say how another person thinks or feels, the therapist encourages each person to claim his or her own space. The therapist also blocks any intrusion by a third person into an interaction between two others. Furthermore, by supporting the individual strengths of each family member and, in particular, the ability of the anorexic to do things for herself, the therapist undermines any overprotectiveness which may have precluded the anorexic's self-assertiveness and expression of independence. In addition, if there are dysfunctional family dyads, or two-person coalitions— perhaps between the mother and daughter — the family therapist structures alliances that serve the health of the family, and thus the health of the anorexic child. Essentially, Minuchin's Structural Family Therapy method defines structural deficits in the family —communication patterns, coalitions and inappropriate roles— and then modifies those structures to promote the child's growth and individuation.

Family Developmental Model

Another school of clinicians used a Family Developmental Model in working with families of anorexics. These therapists suggested that both the anorexic and her family members were developmentally arrested at the separation-individuation stage of the family life cycle. In other words, at the point when the anorexic and other family members should be moving towards separation, with the anorexic developing more autonomy, instead intra-familial ties impeded this transition (Stern et al., 1981, pp. 396–98). What is important about this model is that it recognizes that not just the anorexic's life cycle, but the *family life cycle* has been arrested developmentally in the process of separation.

The Family Developmental Model proposes a five-stage process in which basic parenting functions are provided initially for *both* the anorexic and her family by a therapeutic team. During the initial "holding" stage, the therapists provide protective, empathic environments for both the anorexic and the other family members *separately*, similar to what an infant requires early on for healthy maturation. It is assumed that the parenting received by the parents of the anorexic, as well as the parenting they were in turn equipped to provide for their daughter, was deficient in the reliable and dependable responsiveness and support of initiative that encourages an infant to differentiate and later to develop autonomy. Therefore, parents and offspring alike can benefit from receiving this kind of support (Stern et al., 1981, p.398).

Subsequent stages are instructive because they demonstrate the process of healthy family development that therapists hope to foster in any recovering family. In the second stage, termed the "battle for structure," the therapists exert effective leadership of the family and establish therapeutic guidelines for the anorexic and for family members. Then, in the "battle for initiative," the therapeutic team encourages the family to take responsibility for its own functioning. While the family of an anorexic may be adept at displacing responsibility and initiative onto others, and particularly the therapist, the therapist continually shifts the responsibility back to the family. In the next stage, labeled "availability," the therapist refrains from being directive and encourages family members to resolve their issues with minimal therapeutic input. The final stage is "separation." At this point, the family leaves treatment; this is tantamount to the developmental phase in which an adolescent matures and becomes autonomous, and parents and offspring go through an appropriate process of separation and individuation (Stern et al., pp.396–398). The Family Developmental Model demonstrates the significance of the family developmental process both in the origin and the resolution of anorexia.

Strategic Family Therapy

A few schools of clinicians developed variants of Strategic Family Therapy. The most noted of these groups include the practitioners affiliated with Jay Haley in Philadelphia and those working with Mara Selvini Palazzoli in Milan. Strategic Family Therapy views anorexia as a symptom that strongly influences the family. The therapist's goal is to disconnect the symptom from its role in directing family interactions through prescribing specific behaviors for family members. As family members change their behaviors, the symptom fades from its central role in the family, the family organization shifts, and the anorexic and other individuals in the family develop more appropriate ways of functioning (Palazzoli, 1981, pp.193–230).

Feminist Family Therapy

Feminist Family Therapy provides another viewpoint. In the feminist perspective, anorexia develops within a social and familial context that views women as nurturers and places emphasis on their conforming to culturally defined norms of physical attraction. It is not the family that is dysfunctional in this conceptualization; societal expectations are at the root of the problem.

Feminist Family Therapy practitioners explore the way cultural values get expressed in the family, and their approach is much less directive than that of some other schools: the practitioner tends to ask questions, listen and explore rather than giving specific instructions to family members (Perlick and Silverstein, 1994, pp.77–93). The contributions of Feminist Family Therapy include the therapeutic attitude of equality, an opposition to any use of male power against women, and "a special respect for the emerging individuality and feminity of an anorexic woman" (Dare and Eisler, 1997, p.316). Whatever the therapeutic approach of the practitioner, feminist therapy reminds us that anorexia in adolescent girls emerges as a reaction to individuation and intimations of womanhood — and to the cultural expectations that womanhood implies.

Maudsley Method

An approach to family therapy which is increasing in popularity, especially with treating younger adolescents, is the Maudsley Method, named after the hospital in London where the approach was developed in the 1980s. The method has continued to evolve, through collaborative work of British clinicians Christopher Dare, Ivan Eisler, Daniel LeGrange and W. Stewart Agras; James Lock, psychiatrist at Stanford University in California; and the Eating Disorders Commission, a group of psychiatrists and psychologists funded by a grant to prepare a comprehensive manual of mental health treatment for adolescents (Grilo, 2006, pp.82–83). Maudsley practitioners look at anorexia as the result of multiple factors. Anorexic symptoms influence both the individual and the family; conversely, both the individual and the family also influence anorexic symptoms. Once a child has developed the disorder, interactional patterns within the family serve to maintain the problem.

The Maudsley Method is an outpatient, family-based therapy which takes place in three stages. In the first stage, the parents are engaged in re-feeding their anorexic adolescent. The family therapist unites the family in developing a consistent eating plan for the anorexic. The therapist also provides considerable education about anorexia, as well as structure and support, and helps the family deal with their frustrations about the situation. When the anorexic has siblings, the therapist engages them to support their anorexic sister.

The second phase begins when steady weight gain has been achieved and the family has some sense of control over the anorexia. Family therapy at this stage focuses not only on the anorexic's behaviors and beliefs, but also on stressors the family is facing regarding the anorexic, such as how to handle eating if she goes to a social event. When the anorexic has achieved a stable and appropriate weight, therapy enters the third stage, which focuses on developmental issues, boundaries, autonomy for the anorexic, the ways the symptoms affect the anorexic and her developmental process, and the effect of her disorder on the relationship between the anorexic and her family (Lock and le Grange, 2007, pp.155–161).

Research suggests that this method has been very helpful in working with young adolescents with a relatively short duration of anorexia, and that length of treatment required and outcome is determined by severity and duration of the disorder as well as by the functioning of the family (Dare and Eisler, 1997, p.319). Other approaches to family therapy are more appropriate with older adolescents and adults with anorexia, because family organization tends to be different when the child is older and sometimes no longer living at home, and also because the anorexia at that stage is likely to be more chronic.

In sum, the goal of all family therapy in anorexia is to promote overall family health as well as a healing environment for the anorexic. Just as individual psychotherapists working with anorexia may draw from several psychotherapeutic approaches, so too may family therapists adopt concepts from more than one orientation. Murray Bowen's work provides a framework for understanding how families function; Minuchin added specific insight about dynamics in families of anorexics. Other theorists have shed additional light on the developmental rupture that happens with anorexia. The Maudsley Method differs in its initial phases from other approaches to anorexia in that it initially gives the parents responsibility for managing all aspects of their daughter's food. However, later family work addresses the issues central to other family therapies for anorexia: promoting individuation of each family member, clarifying roles and boundaries, encouraging direct communication, handling conflict, and developing more intimacy. The gift of effective family therapy in the treatment of anorexia is not just healing for the anorexic, but family recovery.

Therapy for Individual Family Members

I believe individual family members of an anorexic deserve help. When a loved one is suffering from anorexia, it can stir up tremendous emotional pain and confusion for those who are close to her, and they may not have a helpful forum for handling their distress.

In my work as a psychotherapist specializing in eating disorders, I have devoted special attention to mothers whose daughters are suffering from anorexia. (I include information about this work in the following section.) I also work with fathers, spouses and other family members. Their pain is no less significant; it simply manifests differently because they have a different relationship with the anorexic than the mother does.

Depending on the orientation of the therapist and on the situation, the anorexic's therapist may choose not to work with individual members of her family but to refer them to another eating disorder specialist. Sometimes an anorexic benefits from having her own therapist whom she does not have to share with her family; this can help her feel safer and trust that her concerns are being held in confidence.

When the anorexic is an adolescent or young adult, couples therapy for the parents may be helpful. Difficulties between the parents can contribute to the anorexic's unwillingness to get better, although she may not necessarily be conscious of her behavior. The anorexic may believe it is her role to keep her parents together or to act as a buffer between them. Certainly having an anorexic in the household will divert attention from any issues between the parents to their mutual concern for their daughter.

In the case of an older anorexic who is married or in a significant relationship, couples therapy can be valuable for her and her partner. Partners of anorexics are generally scared, angry, overwhelmed and at a loss for how to support their anorexic loved one. Having a forum both to share their feelings and to learn specific ways to communicate can help the relationship as well as support the anorexic's recovery.

Groups for parents of eating-disordered daughters, which may include step-parents as well, provide the adults an opportunity to learn together how to better support their daughters—and each other—in managing this difficult situation. These groups can help ease the burden on each individual parent. Like couples therapy, they can open up communication between parents and allow them to express difficult feelings regarding their situation that they may not have talked about before. Ultimately, help for the parents benefits the child.

Therapy for Mothers

"She is so smart, and she used to be so pretty. Now she's just skin and bones, and her eyes are hollow and dark." "She used to care how she looked and now she just dresses in baggy sweatshirts and never even combs her hair." "It's terrible seeing her like this. What did I do wrong?"

These are the plaintive cries of mothers whose daughters are in the throes of anorexia, mothers who have only wanted the best for their daughters, mothers who have worked and sacrificed so their daughters would grow up happy and healthy, mothers who now are witnessing a tragic drama unfolding before their eyes. There are few things more painful to a mother than watching the child that she has nurtured and protected from infancy abuse herself and threaten her own life.

When I think about what my own mother experienced during the years I was anorexic, I grieve that she had no support beyond my father's presence. My father, too, was distressed, but he seemed better able to cope, and less burdened by self-blame. During my twenties, when I was unrelenting in my weight restriction and never allowed the scale to register 80 pounds, my mother suffered terribly. She already had lost one child to suicide, and she was terrified of losing another. And her fear was aggravated by substantial guilt: she believed that in some way she was responsible for my illness and that it was also her responsibility to make me well. I tried to reassure her, both that I was not going to die, and that my anorexia was neither her fault nor her responsibility. But my attempts were fruitless, just as were her pleas for me to get help. Eventually, when I did decide to enter treatment, she was relieved. But, sadly, she never received help for the pain she suffered over my anorexia.

Family therapy has long been a component of treatment of anorexia, but special support for mothers of anorexic daughters has not been sufficiently recognized for its potential benefit both to mothers themselves and to their daughters' recovery. Family members have myriad uncomfortable feelings about the person in their midst who has developed anorexia, and they walk on eggshells lest they do anything to make a bad situation worse. But mothers are in a particularly vulnerable position. Mothers of anorexic daughters generally feel scared, frustrated, guilty and helpless. Their self-esteem as mothers is compromised: they are terrified that they have done something to *cause* their daughters' illness, and yet they are helpless to *save* their daughters. They feel ashamed that their efforts to be good mothers have failed. And they may feel horribly alone. They find that their friends can't relate to their experience, and that their spouses have a different perspective on the situation as well.

Even if a mother has the good fortune to be sharing the emotional burden of her child's anorexia with a supportive partner, she may not feel understood by her mate because generally men and women think differently about emotional problems and their solutions. And men, for biological and psychosocial reasons, tend to relate differently to weight and body size and shape than do women. A father can have difficulty comprehending his daughter's pain or her body hatred, much less her choice to starve. Fathers' most common refrain is "*Why doesn't she just eat?*"

However, a mother also has a lot of trouble understanding what is going on with her daughter. Time after time I hear the fearful and frustrated complaint from a mother: "But my daughter is so bright, talented and attractive. Why is she doing this?" And so mothers of anorexic daughters need information support, guidance and an opportunity to voice their fears and frustrations. Without a venue for handling her feelings, a mother tends to move toward her suffering daughter in a protective and caretaking way at the very time the daughter is seeking a voice of her own. The mother senses her daughter's ambivalence, even if she comprehends neither its origin nor its intensity. The mother can be aware that her daughter wants to make her own choices, but also that her daughter shrinks from that responsibility; similarly, a mother may sense that her daughter is frustrated and angry, but that she is unable to express these feelings.

The anorexic's mother often feels compelled to rescue her daughter from silence and indecision, to speak for her daughter, and to absolve her child of the need to choose by making choices for her. But when the mother usurps her daughter's self-expression, she unwittingly robs the girl of mastering the very challenges that would support her daughter's development and maturity.

The course of healthy child development is fraught with minor and major parent-child clashes, setting of limits, testing the limits, defiance, consequences, agreements, compromises, harmony restored and disturbed with regularity, and new rules established. It is through this endless dance that children learn appropriate behaviors which promote their healthy functioning and protect their safety. This back-and-forth dialogue teaches kids about boundaries: what a child is and is not in charge of, where her province ends and another's begins. It is in part through having her thoughts and feelings heard and understood — not that she gets to use them to run the family — that a girl comes to value herself and to develop a consistent sense of who she is. This healthy boundary-setting is the foundation of forming a separate, differentiated self.

The development of anorexia derails this normal process of differentiation. Mother and daughter become more merged and their differences are stifled. Differentiation can't occur when mother and daughter are engaged in an endless cycle of daughter-pleasing-mother by refraining from voicing contrary feelings, mother-speaking-for-daughter and choosing either what she thinks her daughter wants or what she wants for her daughter. As anorexia progresses and the mother becomes more terrified, she tries to predict her daughter's needs and satisfy them before they even surface. Her daughter complies with this behavior, preserving peace while risking her life; she diverts her feelings into the tormented world of body hatred and food restriction. She is beleaguered between food eaten and not eaten, and self-recrimination for both.

A mother is often terrified that she will say the wrong thing and provoke her daughter to eat even less. She vacillates between biting her tongue and directing her daughter. Out of fear, she may try to coax her daughter to eat, and then get scared she is making a mistake. The mother may try to put herself in her daughter's shoes, then give up in despair because she simply cannot comprehend her daughter's self-destructive actions.

When a scared and desperate mother comes to me, she wants me to tell her what to do, a reenactment of her role with her daughter: just as she would like to make her daughter's suffering disappear, she would like me to make hers evaporate. She may fervently wish — as I often do myself — that I could wave a magic wand and make her daughter's illness vanish. However, the therapist is neither guru nor magician and I am unable to perform this vanishing act. What I *can* do is encourage the mother to talk about her own experience, to express her fears and concerns (although inevitably she drifts almost imperceptibly into a catalogue of her daughter's food choices and restricting behaviors).

I work with mothers both individually and in groups. Each venue has its benefits. When working with an individual mother, I have the opportunity to explore with her the nuances of her feelings, concerns and fantasies about herself and her daughter. In elaborating both the course of her daughter's illness and her own experience, the mother gradually begins to feel less alone in her plight. A fuller picture slowly emerges of who she is as a person, woman, mother, daughter, wife, caregiver, worker and friend. As she reveals the intricate details of her many roles and relationships, as much to herself as to me, she better understands herself, and through this knowing she is able to more clearly delineate herself both as an individual and as a mother of an anorexic daughter.

Mothers are desperate to "fix" their daughters, but just as fervently, they want to understand them. I usually ask a mother to talk about her specific concerns, and our ensuing discussion focuses on what she needs. Just like her daughter, a mother requires her own venue to differentiate from her daughter and to focus on her personal needs and her own recovery. When a mother works with me, we explore her own experience as an adolescent and how she accomplished the task of separation from her family. We ponder the impact her own history may be having on her response to her daughter's behavior, and postulate what her daughter might be trying to communicate through food restriction that she can't say through words. We talk about how the mother can voice her concerns to her daughter while leaving her daughter to her own emotional space. Finally we develop a plan for the mother to take care of herself, physically, emotionally and spiritually.

We also address her concerns about the impact of her daughter's illness on other members of the family and how she can best handle those. So often, when the anorexic daughter has required substantial and focused attention, other children have been neglected and feel resentful. When there are younger female siblings, we talk about how they do and don't resemble their anorexic sister and what precautions may reduce the risk of their becoming anorexic.

With this foundation, we can also orchestrate in more detail the mother's role in contributing to her daughter's recovery. Very often, the most painful part for the mother is learning how to step back and let go of some of the tasks — internal and external — that she has taken over for her daughter. Her attempts to rescue or control her daughter actually impede her daughter's recovery and produce more frustration for the mother at the same time. A mother's helplessness in the face of her daughter's life-threatening illness is excruciating. Most mothers would do almost anything — including trading places with their daughter — to rid their daughter of this disorder. It is heartwrenching for a mother instead to be standing on the sidelines, watching a situation that she feels powerless to change.

But there are tasks that the mother can perform to assist her daughter's recovery. First of all, she can arrange appropriate professional treatment for her daughter. The daughter should be evaluated medically by her physician and see a psychotherapist specializing in treating eating disorders. From there, the psychotherapist will generally guide the treatment, including specifying the need for other adjunctive therapies for the daughter and for the family. Nutritional counseling and psychiatric consultation for the daughter and family therapy may be recommended as part of her daughter's treatment. A mother's role is thus to ensure that her daughter gets appropriate help and to participate in any recommended therapy for the family or for herself. She needs to be a nurturing, loving parent and to treat her daughter as a responsible individual, not as a sick child. It is important for her to relate to her daughter as a maturing adolescent who is responsible for her own choices.

And the mother needs to grieve. Her daughter has been changed by her anorexia and will continue to change throughout the process of recovery. The girl will not return to being the docile, all-smiling, always helpful, pleasing and almost-perfect child. Neither will she continue to be the depressed, withdrawn, moody, controlling and supersensitive waif she has become. The mother may fear that she has lost her daughter — the innocent, happy little girl she remembers. In fact, she has. Some of her daughter's apparent good-naturedness masked pain and other feelings that the girl could not reveal or express. Her daughter will change and grow throughout treatment, and as her daughter recovers, the young woman will emerge as a real, multidimensional being. More facets of her daughter's character will manifest, and some of them will not be as shiny or bright as they may have seemed in the past.

One mother I worked with lamented that her daughter, currently in therapy, dressed in sloppy, over-sized garments, rarely washed her hair and left her room a mess. The mother was disappointed and chagrined that her formerly appearance-conscious daughter was now oblivious to how she and her surroundings looked. However, as I explained, neither the perfectly coiffed and immaculately groomed princess of the past nor the sloppy anti-appearance maven of the present was likely to characterize her daughter's eventual personification. To the mother, unaware of her daughter's anguish, her little girl had been happy. For her daughter, however, her former dress and demeanor hid her inner turmoil and pain, and she was now feeling relieved of an unwanted burden. The mother's challenge was to accept her daughter's current wardrobe choices and hygiene standards, as well as the other anomalies of attitude and behavior that her daughter exhibited. She needed to give her daughter room to grow into her own person.

Mothers in a group therapy situation grapple with the same painful feelings and difficult tasks as they do in individual therapy. However, the opportunity to be with other mothers facing similar struggles offers a unique kind of support. A mother's connection to her peers can help ease her loneliness and isolation. Women recognize themselves and their own struggles in other mothers' stories. Hearing other loving and well-intentioned mothers voice their fear that they may have contributed to their daughters' illness helps assuage their own guilt and self-blame. While each mother has her unique situation and concerns, the fear and grief each experiences in facing a daughter's life-threatening illness forges a bond that is both comforting and empowering. A group is more than the sum of its parts, and offers each mother a stronghold in facing her own challenges.

My groups include from six to eight mothers — a size small enough to preserve a sense of safety and to permit each mother to receive individual attention, but large enough to represent a range of experience. The mothers yearn for information and advice; they want to understand and help their daughters; and they want to feel understood, connected, and relieved of a smidgen of the crushing burden of responsibility they feel. They are often reassured to find that it is typical for mothers in this situation to feel such a broad range of emotions. Mothers in these groups are also generally relieved to voice their anger and frustration, as well as their fear and sadness. Many of the mothers have shored up their reserves to appear strong, in control, responsive and nurturing. They have believed it is wrong to feel annoyed, irritated and angry at their daughters who are suffering and at risk. But as they hear other mothers expressing their difficult feelings, they feel permission to voice their own. It comes as a comfort and a gift to them when the other mothers in the room nod their heads in recognition and acknowledgment.

Mothers in groups are also visibly calmed to learn about the complex origins of anorexia, the genetic and physiological components, the impact of external triggering events and the cycle of addiction. No longer do they point their fingers unwaveringly at themselves. They begin to understand that many factors coalesce in the origin of anorexia, and recognize that even if their mothering has been imperfect, they are not "the cause" of their daughters' illness. Blame and fault are concepts I help them dispel — no one factor, no one person, can be held responsible. The culprit is neither the mother, nor the daughter, nor the diet industry, nor the spouse's insistence on sterling grades, nor their mother-in-law's obsession with clothing size, nor the cousin's constant refrain to the kids of "how much you've grown." Looking for cause deflects the mothers' pain and mires them in guilt. If we do uncover any particular transgressions, they can take responsibility for these, and follow through with whatever action, if any, is called for — perhaps acknowledging their error to their daughter, or apologizing, or simply grieving and letting go.

Usually, the biggest task for mothers is learning to forgive themselves for their perceived transgressions. They need to focus on the present and to take care of themselves and their daughters. Self-care is often the last item on their long lists of things to do; taking care of their husbands and children tends to be a much higher priority. However, they learn they can feel less stressed and be more present to others' needs by taking time out for themselves. It can be useful for a mother to create a list of activities she finds fun or nurturing, even if she needs to be nudged to do them.

I work with individual mothers in person and by phone, and lead in-person groups for mothers. For mothers who are outside of my geographical area and who have no groups near them, I offer a free monthly teleclass for mothers with eating disordered daughters; this is a conference call open to mothers in any geographical location. Information about the conference call is available on my Website for mothers, www.HelpYourDaughter.com, or by calling me at 415-924-2100. What mothers learn through getting help for themselves often has much more to do with themselves than with their daughters. They do find out how to support their daughters, but also, how to have a more authentic relationship with their daughters — and with other family members — with less tension, confusion and vagueness and more direct communication, clarity and intimacy. They learn they are not alone and they can look outside themselves for support. They find out how to focus on their needs, and allow others to focus on theirs. They learn to listen and not to offer help when their own reservoirs are dry. They learn acceptance and forgiveness; they learn who they are and how to create more fulfilling lives for themselves and their families. Recovery is not just about their daughters; it is about them — recovering their own lives, and building lives that are more solid, fulfilling, interconnected and fun.

When mothers of anorexics get help for themselves, however, it can also assist their daughters' recovery. As a mother begins to clarify her role with respect to her daughter's illness, and to draw clearer boundaries for herself, defining how she can and cannot help her daughter, it helps her daughter understand her own role in her recovery. When a mother lets go of responsibilities she has usurped from her daughter, such as making choices and decisions, it allows her daughter the space to wrestle with these herself — which the daughter must do, because deciding what she wants is part of differentiating and becoming her own person. Plus, her daughter gains self-esteem through addressing these life challenges. As a mother discovers that anorexia is a complex disorder with many causes contributing to its onset, and that other equally well-meaning mothers also suffer from doubt and self-recrimination, she can begin to let go of her guilt and forgive herself; also, when she has a deeper understanding of anorexia and is not burdened by her own guilt, she can have more patience with her daughter's plight and empathy for her daughter's pain. Furthermore, as a mother expresses her grief and pain, she can let go of the past, focus on the present and future, and relate to her daughter as she is, rather than to how she remembers her or wishes she were. The mother then becomes available for a more authentic relationship with her daughter. In addition, in seeking help for herself, the mother models the value of self-care and of using outside resources, which can ease the shame an anorexic often feels about needing help.

In sum, mother and daughter grow together. As a mother focuses on herself and identifies and communicates her feelings, needs and wants, she begins to differentiate from her daughter; conversely, as her daughter grapples with defining and expressing herself and facing the challenges of being her own person, she differentiates from her mother. As this separation occurs, mother and daughter can relate to each other as two distinct individuals, capable of mutual empathy and understanding, of intimacy and of sharing, but each on her own life course. These changes happen in the context of the family, and other family members can also progress with their lives. Thus, the family developmental process that has been arrested can resume, and the daughter's healing from anorexia can proceed.

10

12-Step Programs

12-Step programs for eating problems can be a powerful adjunct to therapy for an anorexic. Such programs are not considered therapy, but they do offer a supportive community and many resources to help individuals cope with destructive, compulsive and addictive behaviors. All 12-Step programs are based on the format, principles and steps of Alcoholics Anonymous (AA), which was founded in Akron, Ohio, in 1935. There are four 12-Step programs which support people with food and eating issues: Overeaters Anonymous (OA), Food Addicts Anonymous (FAA), Eating Disorders Anonymous (EDA), and Anorexics and Bulimics Anonymous (ABA). The four programs have some similarities in principles and structure, as well as some differences in philosophy, format, methodology and tools.

The twelve steps of AA are the foundation of all of these support groups. Those famous twelve steps, adapted for recovery from food problems, are:

1. We admitted we were powerless over alcohol — that our lives had become unmanageable.

2. Came to believe that a Power greater than ourselves could restore us to sanity.

3. Made a decision to turn our will and our lives over to the care of God *as we understood Him.*

4. Made a searching and fearless moral inventory of ourselves.

5. Admitted to God, to ourselves and to another human being the exact nature of our wrongs.

6. Were entirely ready to have God remove all these defects of character.

7. Humbly asked Him to remove our shortcomings.

8. Made a list of all persons we had harmed and became willing to make amends to them all.

9. Made direct amends to such people wherever possible, except when to do so would injure them or others.

10. Continued to take personal inventory and when we were wrong, promptly admitted it.

11. Sought through prayer and meditation to improve our conscious contact with God *as we understood Him*, praying only for knowledge of His will for us and the power to carry that out.

12. Having had a spiritual awakening as the result of these Steps, we tried to carry this message to alcoholics, and to practice these principles in all our affairs.

[Copyright A.A. World Services, Inc., www.aa.org].

Each program changes the wording in the first part of step one to name the particular addiction, but the remaining eleven steps are identical in all programs. For example, OA literature says, "We admitted we were powerless over food, and that our lives had become unmanageable." EDA says "powerless over our food behaviors," FAA says "powerless over our food addictions," and ABA says "powerless over our eating disorders."

Admitting powerlessness can be a difficult concept both to understand and to acknowledge, but it is fundamental to the 12-Step philosophy and speaks to the nature of addiction. Addictions and compulsions have a genetic component which renders people susceptible to developing these problems, just as some people are susceptible to developing diabetes or heart disease: in those individuals who are biologically vulnerable, certain circumstances will trigger expression of the disease. In the Big Book of Alcoholics Anonymous—which was first published in 1939, long before any of the research showing that specific irregularities in brain chemistry contribute to vulnerability to certain disorders—alcoholism is described as an "allergy," hence as a biological vulnerability which drives the compulsion to drink (*Alcoholics Anonymous, 2004*, p.xxviii). Research into the origins of anorexia and other eating disorders now indicates that they, too, have a biological basis. In these contexts, being "powerless" over a substance or behavior does not mean giving up doing anything about the problem. It means acknowledging that the problem is more powerful than the person. Being powerless means being out of control, and being victim to the very behaviors and thinking patterns that one has tried to control; being powerless means owning that the eating disorder symptoms are the result of a brain disease and accepting that you can't recover by using willpower. In fact, a supporter of OA's founder suggested thinking of "powerlessness" as "willpowerlessness" (*Overeaters Anonymous*, 2001, p.17).

The companion principle to admitting powerlessness is acknowledging that recovery cannot be done alone: relying on "a power greater than ourselves" is essential. This means that the brain, which is skewed by the disorder, cannot think itself out of the mess it got itself into and needs help. This help can be the power of the group — the people in the meetings and the experience and hope they share that support the person in changing her behavior. This resource is labeled "higher power." It is a power with a higher good — the healthier person — as goal. For some, higher power means a spiritual entity; for others, it can mean the caring and compassion of others in the program. Relying on a "power greater than ourselves" entails letting go of the belief that one can do it oneself. Most people with food issues are convinced that if they just try harder, or maybe do one thing differently, it will fix them — they just have to figure out what that one thing is. Step Two reminds them that they can share their burden.

Belief in something larger, more powerful, or more meaningful than oneself can provide a healing perspective and a welcome relief. The knowledge that "I am not alone and I don't have to do it all my own," for someone who has been convinced that "the only way to do life is entirely on my own" is refreshing and encouraging. Differentiating what one can and can't do—rather than believing one can and should be able to do it all — helps reduce unrealistic expectations. Whether supported by a belief in God, a universal goodness, a higher power, a healthier inner voice, or the members at the meeting, accepting the reality that our bodies look, act and operate in certain ways liberates us from a war we cannot win. The 12-Step programs rely heavily on the words attributed to Reinhold Niebuhr, "God, grant me the serenity to accept the things I cannot change, the courage to change the things I can, and the wisdom to know the difference" (*www.aa.org*). That there are things we are not in charge of and cannot change may be a major disappointment, but it is also a relief: it is a gift to know we no longer have to keep pushing water uphill and contorting our bodies in opposition to genetics and biology.

What 12-Step programs offer is a structure, a philosophy and a community — in sum, a kind of support not available anywhere outside of a residential treatment program. Outpatient therapy groups do not offer the frequency of meetings, number of members, or consistent structure of the 12-Step community. The 12-Step programs offer structure: the meetings have a format and a routine; the steps provide a solid foundation; a sponsor serves as a mentor; other program members recount the messages of reason, hope and serenity. The philosophy is simple: do what others in the program do, and you, too, will be on a path of recovery. And the community is worldwide, with phone-based meetings available for those who are not able to get to a meeting of OA, FAA, EDA or ABA. Through meetings and phone calls, the anorexic has unlimited access to caring individuals committed to finding their way through the labyrinth of life without resuming self-harming behaviors. The only condition for membership is the desire to stop the food-related self-destructive behaviors.

The 12-Step philosophy extends beyond offering the anorexic tools to handle impulses, symptoms and behavior. It provides guidance to move beyond the me-centered focus of an eating disorder. It provides a recipe for handling life: for being a responsible person, discerning where one's boundaries end and the other person's begin, being accountable, being kind to others, helping others, making amends for transgressions. The community provides a means to be accountable — to commit to a service position at a meeting, and to follow through and do what you have committed to do. This accountability is one way self-esteem is built. The steps provide a way to live in the world — to notice when one has behaved in an offending way, and to "make amends" — to take responsibility for one's behavior, apologize for mistakes, act differently in the future. This practice builds integrity. It also allows the person to let go of mistakes and move on, rather than to add to her burden of shame.

In addition, there are particular issues in anorexia that 12-Step programs address. The anorexic suffers from developmental deficits and lacks a sense of self; 12-Step programs provide tools for growth and for learning self-responsibility, developing boundaries, and turning to people in place of restricting food or obsessing about weight. The anorexic suffers from self-hatred; 12-Step programs foster self-acceptance and self-forgiveness, and caring individuals can reflect back a picture that is more realistic than the anorexic's skewed self-perceptions. The anorexic has difficulty self-soothing; 12-Step programs encourage meditation and prayer, which are sources of solace and self-comfort. Anorexia is a disease of isolation; 12-Step programs offer opportunities for connection.

12-Step programs are not a replacement for therapy, but they can augment therapy and enhance its effectiveness. Recovery from anorexia is multimodal and complex. There is room and reason to build new growth from many resources. It takes a village — and 12-Step programs provide, if not a village, at least a hamlet of humane and caring individuals who want the same thing: recovery.

The four 12-Step programs that address food-related behaviors have similar principles, with some differences in philosophy, format, and tools. Overeaters Anonymous was the first 12-Step program designed for those with food issues, and the program welcomes anorexics and bulimics, as well as compulsive eaters. The philosophy of OA is that "the only requirement for membership is the desire to stop compulsive eating." For some anorexics, this concept is difficult to relate to; for many, however, their food restricting has been punctuated by occasional, and frightening, episodes of bingeing, and their greatest fear is of not being able to stop eating once they start. The phrase "compulsive undereating" or "disordered eating" can replace "compulsive overeating" and the remaining precepts of OA fit quite well for the anorexic.

Developed in 1960, OA adapted the principles and structure of AA fairly literally. The founder of OA, Rozanne, was actually inspired to apply12-Step principles to overeating after attending a meeting of Gamblers Anonymous, and recognizing the similarity of her behaviors with food to those of a gambler with money (*Overeaters Anonymous*, 2001, p.11). OA believes that compulsive eating has physical, emotional and spiritual roots. The physical problem of overeating (or other disordered eating behavior) leads to the emotional distress of feeling out of control and experiencing self-disgust and self-hatred, as well as the added physical problems resulting from the overeating. As despair and self-hatred continue, the inner emptiness and loneliness (which may have contributed to the food abuse in the first place) continue to grow. The person has no love or respect for herself. One aspect of what OA offers is the warmth and caring from recovering members. "Love is a spiritual quality," says the Rev. Rollo Boas, one of OA's earliest supporters (Boas, 2001, p.243). OA members often say, "They love us until we can love ourselves." The members of OA provide community, as well as support in handling emotions and changing behaviors, which fosters recovery for the undereater or overeater physically, emotionally and spiritually, one day at a time.

In addition to the steps, 12-Step programs offer specific tools to help with behavior change. At times in its history, OA has suggested members follow a very specific food plan. More recently, the guidelines have suggested that a member follow a food plan, but one that she creates — often with the assistance of a nutritionist or a sponsor — that addresses her own nutritional and physiological needs. A food plan is a therapeutic tool that most anorexics need in some form in order to help change their eating behavior, and all four of the eating behavior-related 12-Step programs incorporate some type of food plan. Other OA tools include making phone calls, doing service and working with a sponsor, someone who has sufficient recovery in OA to act as a program mentor.

Some anorexics and bulimics have found they relate better to the program of Food Addicts Anonymous than to Overeaters Anonymous. Founded in 1987, FAA views food addiction as a biochemical disease, and requires that participants follow a rigorous food plan, including abstinence from eating white flour and sugar. These particular substances can trigger addictive behaviors for some people, and are viewed the way alcohol is in AA. FAA is considerably more rigid in structure than OA, with specific guidelines for quantity and type of food allowed, schedule for support phone calls, and number of days of abstinence required before participating in meetings. The additional structure and support of FAA are helpful for some anorexics, while others find the requirements too rigid.

In 1992, Anorexic and Bulimics Anonymous was developed to meet the needs of anorexics and bulimics. One focus of the program is to educate its members about the physiological bases of eating disorders. The philosophy of ABA is that "the only requirement for membership is a desire to stop unhealthy eating practices." ABA considers a range of eating practices — restricting food, bingeing on food, purging through vomiting, laxatives or compulsive exercise — as "true addictions over which we were powerless, just as surely as an alcoholic is powerless over drinking."

The most recent 12-Step program developed for recovery from eating problems is Eating Disorders Anonymous. Founded in 2000, EDA states that their "primary purpose is to recover from eating disorders." The concept of balance, not abstinence, is central to recovery in the EDA program, meaning that neither living with the extremes of behavior characteristic of eating disorders nor living by rigid recovery rules is the answer. Rather, the goal is to learn to manage the emotions that lead to disordered eating behaviors. EDA does not require any specific food plan but, much like OA, suggests than each individual determine — with a professional, if desired — an appropriate food plan for herself.

Some find fault with 12-Step program language. One complaint is that defining oneself as an anorexic in meetings reaffirms the very identity that treatment is seeking to dispel. A related complaint is that there is no way within the 12-Step structure to graduate: once in recovery, always in recovery. However, "labeling" oneself as an anorexic does not mean one never improves; it reflects the idea that recovery from using destructive behaviors is a process. It does not mean that anorexia is the same as alcoholism; one missed meal is unlikely to send someone headlong down the skid row of starvation. But reaffirming that one is an anorexic, or a recovering anorexic, can be viewed simply as acknowledging, "My biochemistry is vulnerable. When I give in to my impulses, I am susceptible to resuming self-harming behaviors."

Another complaint with 12-Step language is the use of the term "abstinence." One cannot abstain from food in the same way as from drugs or alcohol. Food is a necessity of life, alcohol is not, and the anorexic already is abstemious with respect to food. "Abstinence," however, does not mean abstaining from food (although for some individuals, and in FAA, it may entail abstaining from specific, *triggering* foods). Abstinence means refraining from impulse-driven self-harming eating behaviors.

Individuals may initially find not only the language but the format of 12-Step meetings off-putting and unfamiliar. However, anything new is unfamiliar. By going to a number and variety of meetings, and trying out OA, FAA, EDA and ABA, and even some AA or other 12-Step meetings, attending meetings can become more comfortable. Also, every meeting is different and has its own atmosphere, and finding one that feels like a good fit is important. Going with someone to a meeting can be good a way to try it out. Arriving early at meetings and staying afterwards to have one-on-one conversations can help. The 12-Step practice of "no-crosstalk"— that when talking in the meeting, no one is to comment on what another person says—can also strike some people as strange, especially if someone has attended interactive therapy groups. This practice, however, actually provides safety and respect for the person who has shared. Someone is likely to be less inhibited about speaking up if she knows that what she says will not be judged or criticized.

While the anorexic may find aspects of 12-Step programs foreign at first, it can be worth tolerating the early discomfort to discover whether she can find any potential benefit. There is probably no one for whom the meetings are contraindicated, but some people may have more difficulty than others in facing the unfamiliarity of the environment. One way to adapt to the program and the meetings is to do exactly as one 12-Step motto recommends: Take what you like and leave the rest.

Personal Note

My father was an active alcoholic when I was growing up. When I was 18, his alcoholism cost him his job. AA was a godsend; he remained active in the program until he died over 25 years later. Eventually, I had skirmishes with alcohol, but mostly I didn't like how I felt when I drank a lot. But though I knew about alcohol addiction and AA, and although I had a very compulsive relationship to exercise, not-eating, and self-criticism, I never thought of my anorexia as an addiction.

In 1997, it had been over fifteen years since I'd entered treatment for anorexia. My weight was healthy but my nutrition was not. I was working with a financial consultant and regularly shared with her the details about how I spent money. It was clear that the majority of my food budget was actually financing a sugar habit: I was spending more on café mochas, brownies and chocolate each week than on groceries or meals. I resisted calling myself a "sugar addict" (her words), but the reality was evident. The consultant may have told me 30 or 100 times about Overeaters Anonymous, but one day it clicked—I realized I *was* addicted to sugar, or at least I was using it compulsively and self-destructively.

Initially, I didn't like the meetings or the program and had lots of complaints. The meetings were too big; my compulsive use of sugar wasn't terrible; I wasn't in as bad shape as the other people; the terminology was cultish. But I kept going back, and ultimately, I received gifts from the program that I had never anticipated. I already had some close friends, but none who had had food issues like mine. Suddenly in these groups, I felt understood in a new way. Also, the process helped me learn the difference between the things I could and couldn't change— and along with this understanding, I learned acceptance, a concept that at least half a dozen therapists had tried to help me grasp. I also learned about gratitude — not that the concept was new to me, but the *practice* of acknowledging my gratitude was new. In sum, I learned valuable tools to help get me through the rough times.

And, most importantly, I found a spiritual center and an antidote to the emptiness I had long felt inside. For years I had envied the apparent contentment that some of my friends found in their religious or spiritual practices. Even when I tried doing what they did, it didn't resonate for me and I still felt empty and hollow. I'd pretty much decided that this was one of those birth things— that maybe there was a gene for "ability to develop spirituality," and since apparently I hadn't been born with it, I was unlikely to get it later in life. I wasn't actually looking for a spiritual practice when I arrived in OA; I just wanted to stop destroying myself with sugar. But in fact I did find a path towards building a spiritual practice of my own. It wasn't any one aspect of the program that made the difference for me, and it certainly wasn't an epiphany; building a spiritual connection was a gradual process that happened almost without my realizing it. I went to meetings, read AA and OA literature, spent time with program people, found a sponsor, worked the steps, recited the serenity prayer and wrote gratitude lists. I stopped subsisting on mochas and brownies. And slowly, over the course of months, then years, I noticed something was different. I could actually feel serene not trying to control every outcome. I could believe that some force greater than myself could help me handle the stuff I couldn't deal with on my own. I had faith that I could get through hard times without falling apart like the empty shell of Humpty Dumpty. I was feeling more real and whole. I had a sense of something solid and foundational inside called "me." This is the "me" that I lacked as an anorexic and couldn't even imagine in early recovery, the "me" that felt like a safe place, the "me" that was my home.

11

Intervention

Sometimes anorexics who are clearly in dire need of treatment refuse to seek help. When that anorexic is a minor, it is the responsibility of the parents or guardians to seek and provide treatment for her. If the anorexic who is a minor is in a hospital and still refuses treatment, then the parents in coordination with the staff have to choose the best route to assure the child's safety. However, an adult generally does not fall under the legal jurisdiction of her parents or anyone else, and the anorexic adult is entitled by law to refuse treatment. But there are situations in which the anorexic is undoubtably psychologically and cognitively compromised and may be incapable of making a well-reasoned decision. She may appear quite lucid in all areas, except in evaluating her own condition, and she may be able to convince family and friends of her well-being despite her appearance. Family and friends may then assume her condition is not severe enough to warrant intervening, while in fact the anorexic's competence to choose or not choose treatment is impaired.

How to proceed in these cases poses a quandary. Below I discuss briefly some of these legal and ethical considerations encountered with treatment refusal and suggest a format for family intervention — a very loving, caring, and non-confrontational approach to encourage an anorexic to accept help. I also include some considerations for the clinician in working with an adult anorexic who is either refusing treatment or refusing a higher level of care.

Determination of the right to refuse treatment in anorexia generally hinges on four elements: the anorexic's physical state and the potential risks of her condition; the likely benefit of treatment; the likely harm of treatment; and the competence of the anorexic to make the choice of treatment refusal (Goldner et al., 1997, p.452).

In evaluating *potential risks* of the anorexic's condition, it is important to realize that premature death is a very real possibility in anorexia. When the anorexic shows signs of severe emaciation and physical deterioration, it is the medical practitioner, if the anorexic is being seen by one, who must decide whether hospitalization is required, even against the patient's will. Joel Yager, an eating disorder psychiatrist and professor, recommends refraining from considering legal means of treatment imposition — involuntary hospitalization — unless treatment refusal is judged to constitute a serious risk (Yager, 2007, p.430). The potential for death is certainly a risk serious enough to warrant consideration of involuntary hospitalization. However, premature death in anorexia generally results from cardiac failure which cannot usually be predicted. It is also estimated that from one-third to one-half of premature deaths in anorexia are due to suicide (Goldner et al., 1997, p.452).

Potential benefit or harm as a result of treatment also needs to be considered. While generally treatment of anorexia results in improvement, these results are debatable for sufferers of extreme, chronic anorexia. How humane is it to intervene with someone whose physical deterioration will prevent her from ever returning to normal life? Chronic anorexia leads to loneliness, isolation, and stunted development emotionally, physically, socially and vocationally. It has been noted that the anorexic's "rigid control of all aspects of life tends to kill life as other people know it, and indeed as the patient herself has known it" (Nielsen and Bará-Carril, 2003, p.192). To what degree is this reversible? Or can we assume that there is always at least the possibility that quality of life will improve, even if only marginally so? There are cases where long-term sufferers of anorexia have made remarkable recovery, generally where starvation has not caused serious damage to vital organs or systems. Also, there certainly are situations where some kind of forced nutrition has resulted in the anorexic's later improvement; but in others this has not been true. There are also cases in which chronic anorexics have been, perhaps mistakenly, labeled "incurable." In Great Britain, treatment of a 24-year-old anorexic was deemed "futile" and her condition "incurable." The young woman was admitted into a terminal care facility where she received morphine injections and died after eight days. The anorexic's records were reviewed after her death by a special interest group at the Royal College of Psychiatrists, and the psychiatrists concluded that the patient in fact had likely *not been* incurable (Goldner et al., 1997, p.453). Ethical concerns such as those raised by these cases must be considered in choosing how to proceed.

In the case of chronic anorexia, however, sometimes the pain of continuing life is more than the anorexic can bear; the prospect of any significant recovery is grim and the ordeal of struggling to continue a miserable existence is overwhelming. Often the anorexic who reaches this stage has experienced several hospitalizations or may even currently be in the hospital and refusing treatment. If legal authorization has been obtained, medical staff can tube feed a hospitalized anorexic, but anorexics have been known to tear out the tubes. Treatment can actually be potentially damaging if aggressive or intrusive feeding measures are used. Yager notes that when the willing cooperation of the anorexic is absent, treatments based on invasive feeding are usually short-lived and likely to fail (Yager and Powers, 2007, p. 431). There is also the issue of what constitutes quality of life: if increasingly aggressive measures are required to prolong an anorexic's life, her physical and psychological capacities certainly will deteriorate. In addition, few facilities can treat these patients indefinitely, and families can rarely pay for prolonged care. In these instances, Yager poses the question: "How long can or should such drawn-out suicides or dying processes continue?" (Yager, 2007, pp.430–431). The most humane stance for the clinician at this point may be to help the family develop compassion and understanding for the anorexic's perspective and to prepare everyone involved for the possibility or even likelihood of a fatal outcome (Yager, 2007, p.431).

There are other situations where treatment can create more harm than good. In a hospital or outpatient setting where staff members do not understand the plight of the severely ill anorexic or do not know how to work with her, staff may become angry about the way she is manipulative or not trying to get better (Goldner et al., 1997, pp.453–454). An anorexic who feels blamed for her condition is likely to experience further psychological distress, which can make her more resistant to making use of the available help. Even an experienced clinician can become discouraged at a client's lack of progress or apparently oppositional behavior, and may withdraw or disengage from the anorexic (Yager, 2007, p. 432). Working successfully with an anorexic whose illness is either severe or long-standing requires considerable patience, compassion, empathy and fortitude.

The question of an *anorexic's competence to make choices* about her own health care is complicated. The anorexic doubtless chose to lose weight initially. However, starvation leads to psychological and biological consequences over which the anorexic has no control. Her mental distortion may preclude her from comprehending the extent of her medical danger. Also, she probably is more afraid of treatment than of continuing to live as she has been living — marginally, starving, weak, but still under the impression that somehow she is in control. Her eating disorder is her trusted safety net; the specter of treatment is tantamount to prison.

Criteria that indicate that the anorexic is *not* competent to make decisions on her own behalf include a distinct inability to communicate choices, to understand relevant information, and to appreciate the severity of her situation and its consequences (Goldner et al., 1997, p. 454). This assessment mostly rests on the anorexic's capacity to take rational steps to preserve her health and life. While the anorexic may be lucid in respect to other aspects of life, anorexia can disable her capacity to make a free and rational decision about the condition itself. An anorexic can sincerely declare her *intention* to resume eating, but when actually faced with food, she may be fraught with anxiety stemming from the thought disturbances of anorexia (Goldner et al., 1997, p.455). Research clinicians Tiller, Schmidt and Treasure note that "the desire, when emaciated, to avoid treatment leading to weight gain is not comparable to a decision to refuse medical intervention; rather it is a psychiatric symptom" (Tiller et al., 1993, p.679).

In situations where family members of an anorexic are concerned that their loved one either is not seeking treatment or is not progressing in treatment, family members can seek the help of a trained interventionist who is also an eating disorder specialist. An intervention is a transformative process in which the goal is to help *both* the anorexic and her loved ones get appropriate support and help. The problem with treatment refusal may not rest solely with the anorexic but also with friends or members of her family who unwittingly enable the anorexic's continuing demise. Both because family members may be distraught and unclear how to be of help, and because the anorexic may not be psychologically able to comprehend the severity of her illness, it is essential that an empathic, compassionate, but firm eating disorder interventionist with experience, knowledge and expertise guide the intervention process. Sometimes, in the interest of trying to "help" or to "not rock the boat," family members have held back from voicing important thoughts and feelings, or have communicated them only indirectly. They may have attempted to be encouraging, but have been counterproductive instead. For example, a worried mother may refrain from voicing to her adult anorexic daughter her fear that her daughter is not getting help, because she is afraid her daughter will eat even less. Instead, when the daughter comes to visit, her mother may leave in plain view books about anorexia or pamphlets from treatment centers. But the anorexic cannot know the content and depth of her mother's concerns if they are not spoken. A dynamic can develop where well-meaning friends and family tiptoe around the anorexic; they may feel helpless, scared and distressed, and can develop symptoms of stress such as anxiety, moodiness, sleep disorders and difficulty concentrating. Also, family members often struggle with feelings of guilt and self-blame which get in the way of their knowing what to say or do. An intervention can help everyone involved better understand the complex causes of anorexia as well as the potential consequences of the disorder.

There are two types of interventions, traditional and systemic. In the traditional model, family members come up with a strategy to confront the individual about her illness. She is generally given a choice between intensive treatment, which has been pre-arranged, and a consequence, which may involve the family members' withdrawing support or moving towards implementing involuntary treatment. Sometimes as a result of this kind of intervention, the anorexic may choose to go into treatment, but she may not actually *engage* in treatment. Alternatively, the anorexic may enter treatment and improve, but then return to family dynamics which are unchanged and can undermine her recovery.

In the more recently developed systemic family model, the anorexic's illness is viewed as a part of a family process. In this model, it is assumed that not only is the anorexic in pain, but others in the family are suffering as well. Not only does the anorexic need help to heal; so, too, do her family members, and family recovery can be essential to the anorexic's recovery. A systemic intervention can be a compassionate and respectful way for everyone involved to communicate care and concern for the anorexic in a loving way. Through this process it is not unusual for the dynamics and outcome to be altered sufficiently that the anorexic embraces treatment. In addition, the intervention process can provide guidance and relief for suffering family members.

A systemic family intervention begins when a concerned family member calls a systemic eating disorder interventionist to talk about the situation and his or her concerns. The systemic family interventionist then sets up an initial meeting that includes the caller, immediate family members, friends, or anyone else who is close to the anorexic. What follows is a process choreographed in a way that changes the focus from the anorexic to the family system. The interventionist's goals are to look at the family as a whole, to view the problem as systemic (perhaps multigenerational), to assess the family dynamics and to gather information about the concerns of each person present, whether family member or friend. Is enabling happening — that is, are any family members unknowingly fostering the anorexic's disease? The dynamics of the family often create an environment that actually supports the development of anorexia, and the goal of the interventionist is to alter this course.

The next step of the systemic family intervention is setting up a family workshop or meeting conducted by the interventionist and tailored to the specific needs of the family, perhaps including friends or others close to the anorexic. The anorexic is asked to join the process that was set in motion by the initial meeting. She is invited to participate with the concerned others in the family workshop which resembles a protracted family therapy session. In the family workshop, each family member or friend is invited to speak about his own pain, not just about his desire for the anorexic loved one to get help. The interventionist will uncover problems and offer support, guidance and specific recommendations for each family member as well as for the anorexic. If there is enabling, for instance, the family member may be referred to Al-Anon, the program of support for family members of alcoholics and addicts. (No comparable program exists specifically for loved ones of anorexics.) If someone in the family is having mood or sleep problems, individual therapy may be recommended. If treatment, or a change in treatment, is recommended for the anorexic, the interventionist will work closely with the anorexic to establish what she is and is not willing to do.

No intervention can guarantee any particular outcome. However, when an experienced interventionist who is leading the systemic intervention guides the family in an open and supportive discussion, making room for each person to have a voice, family members can develop new ways of interacting with each other as well as with their anorexic loved one, and family dynamics begun to shift. Family members may choose to enter treatment for their own issues, including codependency. Often the family has spiraled down with the problems of the anorexic in their midst, and conducting a systemic intervention can reverse the fortunes of the family members as well as create an environment that can encourage the anorexic's recovery. In this way, an intervention can initiate a process of recovery for the family as well as for the anorexic.

Interventions with an anorexic should be conducted by a certified interventionist with eating disorder intervention expertise. Board Registered Interventionists are certified by the Illinois Alcohol and Other Drug Abuse Professional Certification Association or IAODAPCA (*http://iaodapca.org/index.cfm*). BR I interventionists specialize in drugs and alcohol while BR II interventionists have other specializations. Some BR II interventionists specialize in eating disorders. The newly-formed Network of Independent Interventionists (NII) (*independentinter ventionists.org*) will be a referral source for certified interventionists.

There are some important guidelines to heed in understanding and working with an anorexic, whether for the interventionist working with an anorexic and her family, or for a therapist meeting with an anorexic either whose treatment is not progressing or who is refusing a higher level of care. First, it is essential that the interventionist or therapist develop a heartfelt connection with the anorexic; otherwise, the anorexic is likely to perceive any suggestions as coercive and controlling. Also, the interventionist or therapist should seek to fully understand an anorexic's reasons for treatment refusal. Sometimes she is refusing certain treatment *methods* rather than actually refusing treatment. The interventionist or therapist needs to be prepared for the possibility of negotiation: an anorexic may be willing to go along with some parts of a treatment plan, but not with others. Conducting a thorough review with the anorexic and going over the psychological, medical and psychopharmacological aspects of her previous therapy can be invaluable. With the anorexic's permission, the interventionist or therapist can explore the client's treatment history with her prior practitioners, if there are any. Developing a solid understanding of what did and did not help, and the likely reasons for success and failure, can offer insight into the anorexic's current situation. In addition, the interventionist or therapist can assess the anorexic's beliefs about future treatments that might or might not work, and plan, if reasonable, to implement those she believes can help. Taking into account the client's suggestions and wishes is important in her maintaining autonomy. Also, a change in strategy, or in therapy modality — perhaps some experiential therapy — can provide a new beginning (Yager, 2007, pp.432–436).

It is also important that the interventionist or therapist offer neither false optimism nor harsh pessimism. Pessimism can be a practitioner's defense against frustration, discouragement, and the pain of potential loss, but it is not useful to the client. Many anorexics can exist for a very long time on meager amounts of food, and no one can predict an anorexic's life expectancy. A stance that offers the *possibility of change* is of most service; none of us can foresee what will happen in the future. Sometimes chronic anorexics eventually do make changes; other times not. The best approach is usually to include a reality-based explanation of risks and benefits of any treatment suggestions given to the anorexic.

One option an interventionist or therapist can offer when an anorexic refuses more structured treatment is to encourage the anorexic to meet with a therapist to develop and follow a plan that will address life-preserving medical and nutritional needs. If the client has the capacity and willingness to take small steps to change any aspect of her life, a therapist can help her develop a plan of very basic, low-stress actions. It is essential in these situations to coordinate parameters with the anorexic's physician to establish basic limits regarding medical severity beyond which hospitalization for medical stabilization will be necessary. If the anorexic does not have a physician, her first step, and the prerequisite for any further planning, must be to see one. However, when a client has adamantly refused inpatient treatment, it is essential that it be understood that hospitalization, if required, is for stabilization *only* (Yager, 2007, p.421). If hospitalization is extended longer than is medically required, or as a means of convincing the anorexic to move into residential treatment, the client understandably will feel resentful and betrayed. This betrayal will damage the clinician's credibility and erode the client's trust in the clinician, the physician and the therapeutic process.

In cases where an anorexic is refusing help or where her condition remains marginal and her physical condition compromised despite the treatment she has received, ongoing contact with a caring and involved clinician can convey meaning and hope. The client still may receive psychological benefit even if she is not making cognitive or behavioral changes. A clinician can listen compassionately and be a thoughtful, caring witness to her pain. The clinician can provide reassuring companionship for the anorexic. Acceptance and refusal of treatment are evolutionary processes; an individual who initially refuses help may alter her response over time, particularly with the investment of supportive individuals. It is important to never underestimate an individual's potential for change, or the value of compassionate human interaction.

Personal and Professional Note

In working as a psychotherapist, I've encountered many of the dilemmas that arise in seeing severely anorexic clients. For instance, I once met with a fifty-year-old anorexic woman.

She was quite thin; her body was stooped, her hair was thinning, her skin was pallid, her legs were swollen, and her eyes bulged. She had a child-like, sickly presence but when she smiled, she beamed. She had been anorexic to some degree since the age of twelve. The woman had multiple physical problems—a non-functioning thyroid, severe edema, osteoporosis, leg and back pain—in addition to being able to consume only minimal amounts of food each day. She had been hospitalized involuntarily on two occasions and each time left against medical advice. She was adamant about not returning to the hospital. Her physician and I talked, and referred her to a psychiatrist. The psychiatrist, physician and I discussed her situation at length, and consulted with other practitioners as well. We concluded that another involuntary hospitalization was counterproductive.

Although the woman was unable to change her eating habits, she wanted to meet with me. I was in a quandary. She was quite debilitated; shouldn't she be in the hospital? Was it ethical of me to see her rather than to have her involuntarily placed in the hospital again? What value could I be to her, given her compromised condition, both physically and psychologically? How would it be for me to sit with a client who was gaunt and cadaverous?

I struggled to figure out the "right" thing to do—right for her, right for me. I consulted with the client's physician who was monitoring the woman twice weekly. In the end, I chose to see her, to at least find out if there was any value for her in our meeting. It was painful to see her so ill, and clearly she was quite depressed. Yet a certain indescribable brightness shone through her; and besides, she welcomed our meetings. In her words, she "treasured" the sessions and was grateful she could talk with me because "no one else could understand her." Probably no one else actually *listened* to her; the family members she had contact with alternately fawned over her, told her what to do, or yelled at her. I met with the woman every week for several months, until she moved out of the area to live with a relative. In our meetings, I offered her a service—a human presence and a connection, a listening ear, and an opportunity for her to speak out loud what was in her heart. In return, I received *her* presence, and the gifts of her trust and appreciation. Even when visible change does not occur and behaviors are unmodified, human beings cannot know the impact they have on one another.

Epilogue

As of this writing it is estimated that 30 percent of American children and 25 percent of American adults are obese, and that 98 percent of diets fail. These numbers, along with the prevalence of anorexia, suggest that our culture's values regarding food, body image and health are seriously askew. Advances in medical research and prescriptions for anti-depressants and anti-anxiety aids will not eradicate anorexia. These may help, but the underlying issue is not the genetic foundation of the disorder or the largely unavoidable environmental stressors and human hurdles that pose enormous challenges. The big problem is the psychological undercurrent that makes so many young men and women prone to focus on what is wrong with their bodies. If healthy attitudes about weight and body image were more prevalent, fewer females would use thinness as the measure of self-worth or engage in weight manipulation as the solution to life's ills.

To combat anorexia, we need change of a huge magnitude, essentially a cultural overhaul. This would mean stepping off the speed train, arresting the addictive elements that permeate our society, investing in personal growth, differentiating what we can and cannot change, accepting what we can't, and acting with compassion and grace as we change what we can. And it would entail dismantling the multi-billion dollar weight loss industry, diminishing dollars spent on defense, and investing instead in a national movement to implement life-affirming behaviors.

But we don't have to renovate the entire culture in order to begin to address eating disorders. We can start with a change in consciousness, and then disseminate that through available avenues. Healthy attitudes about food and weight need to be promulgated in the media as well as in schools and homes. It's not so much about preventing young people from having "fat days" but about how to help them deal with "feeling fat" when they have those days.

We now recognize the severity of the problem of anorexia nervosa. The challenge from here is the hard work of reeducating a population that has been saturated with images of perfect bodies and inundated with misinformation, confusion and bias about food and body image. But healing can happen — one step at a time.

Appendix A.
Treatment Centers for Eating Disorders
(Alphabetically by State)

Key: ip — inpatient; op — outpatient; php — partial hospitalization;
f —female; m — male; adol — adolescent

Alabama

Magnolia Creek Treatment Center for Eating Disorders
Columbiana, AL
Phone: 205-678-4373; 888-762-46654
Fax: 205-678-4632
Email: info@magnolia-creek.com
Website: *www.magnolia-creek.com*
ip, f, 18+

Arizona

Mirasol
7650 E. Broadway, Suite 303
Tucson, AZ 85710
Phone: 888-520-1700
Fax: 520-546-3200
Email:jrust@mirasol.net
Website: *www.mirasol.net*
ip, f, adol+

Remuda Ranch West
One East Apache St.
Wickenburg, AZ
Phone: 1-800-445-1900
Fax: 928-684-4801
Email: info@remudaranch.com
Website: *www.remudaranch.com*
ip, php, f/m, 8+, Christian

Rosewood Ranch
36075 S. Rincon Road
Wickenburg, AZ 85390
Phone: 928-684-9594
Fax: 928-684-9562

Email: cindy.mealpin@rosewoodranch.com
Website: *www.rosewoodranch.com*
ip, op, php, f/m, 18+

Sierra Tucson
39580 South Lago del Oro Parkway
Tucson, AZ 85739
Phone: 800-842-4487
Fax: 520-818-5869
Email: via website
Website: *www.sierratuscon.com*
ip, f/m, adult

California

Alta Bates Summit Medical Center, Behavioral Health
Herrick Campus
2001 Dwight Way
Berkeley, CA 94704
Phone: 510-204-4405 inpatient; 510-204-4569 partial hospitalization
Fax: 51-0-204-4046
Email: via website
Website: *www.altabatessummit.org*
ip, php, f/m, 12+

Alta Mira Recovery
125 Bulkley Ave.
Sausalito, CA 94965
Phone: 415-332-1350
Fax: 415-332-3793
Email: via website
Website: *www.altamirarecovery.com*
ip, php, f/m, 18+

Ananda Institute
401 South A Street
Santa Rosa, CA 95401
Phone: 707-544-4441, ext. 304
Fax: 707-544-4492
Email: dr.ireneives@prodigy.net
Website: *www.ananda-institute.com*
op, f/m, child+

Casa Palmera Treatment Center for Eating Disorders
14750 El Camino Real
Del Mar, CA 92014
Phone: 888-481-4481
Fax: 858-350-1378
Email: via website
Website: *www.casapalmera.com*
ip, f/m, 17+

Casa Serena Intensive Outpatient Program
1868 Clayton Road, Suite 123
Concord, CA 94520
Phone: 925-682-8252
Fax: 925-682-8313
Email: info@casaserenaedp.com
Website: *www.casaserenaedp.com*
op, f, 15+

Center for Discovery and Adolescent Change
4281 Katella Avenue
Los Alamedas, CA 90720*
Phone: 866-833-9969
Fax: 714-828-1870
Email: via website
Website: *www.centerfordiscovery.com*
ip, f/m, 10–19
*Also centers in La Habra, Lakewood, Long Beach, Menlo Park and Whittier

Del Amo Hospital
23700 Camino del Sol
Torrance, CA 90505
Phone: 800-533-5266
Email: via website
Website: *www.delamotreatment.com*
ip, php, f (adol+) m (adult)

La Ventana Eating Disorder Programs
Malibu, CA
Phone: 888 528 3682
Fax: 818-712-9447
Email: info@laventanaeatingdisorder.com
Website: *www.laventanaeatingdisorder.com*
op, m/f, 13+

Lucille Packard Children's Hospital at Stanford
Outpatient:
Psychiatry and Behavioral Science Building

401 Quarry Road
Palo Alto, CA 94304
Adolescent Medicine
1174 Castro Street, Suite 250A
Mountain View, CA 94040

Inpatient:
El Camino Hospital
2500 Grant Road
Mountain View, CA94040
Phone: 650-498-4468
Fax: 650-694-0610
Email: via website
Website: *www.lpch.org*
ip, op, php, f/m, child+

Monte Nido Treatment Center
27162 Sea Vista Drive
Malibu, CA 90265
Phone: 310-457-9958
Fax: 310-457-8442
Email: mntc@montenido.com
Website: *www.montenido.com*
ip, php, f, adol+, not a twelve-step program

Montecatini
2524 Lacosta Avenue
Carlsbad, CA 92009
Phone: 760-436-8930
Fax: 7604368143
Email: via website
Website: *www.montecatinieatingdisorder.com*
ip, php, f, 12+

New Dawn Eating Disorders Recovery Centers
Outpatient:
2320 Marinship Way, Suite 240
Sausalito, CA 94965

Inpatient:
San Francisco, CA
Phone: 415-331-1383
Fax: 415-331-1392
Email: erin@newdawnrecovery.com
Website: *www.newdawnrecovery.com*
ip, op, php, f, 18+

Rader Programs
2130 North Ventura Road
Oxnard, CA 93036
Phone: 800-841-1515
Fax: 818-880-3750
Email: rader@raderprograms.com
Website: *www.raderprograms.com*
ip, f/m, 18+

Rebecca's House
23861 El Toro Road
Lake Forest, CA 92630
Phone: 800-711-2062

Fax: 949-900-8268
Email: rebecca@rebeccashouse.org
Website: *www.rebeccashouse.org*
op, f/m, adol+

Summit Eating Disorders and Outreach
Program
601 University Avenue, #225
Sacramento, CA 95825
Phone: 916-920-5276
Fax: 916-920-5221
Email: via website
Website: *www.sedop.org*
op, php, adol+

UCSD Eating Disorder Treatment Center
Department of Psychiatry
La Jolla Village Professional Center
8950 Villa La Jolla Drive, Suite C-207
La Jolla, CA 92037
Phone: 858-534-8019
Fax: 858-534-6727
Email: via website
Website: *www.health.ucsd.edu/specialties/psych/*
    eatingdisorders/
op, f/m, adol+

Colorado

Eating Disorder Center of Denver
950 South Cherry Street, Suite 1010
Denver, CO 80246
Phone: 866-771-0861; 303-771-0861
Fax: 720-889-4258
Email: via website
Website: *www.edcdenver.com*
op, php, f/m, 16+

District of Columbia

Children's Hospital
Inpatient Program:
111 Michigan Avenue NW
Washington, DC 20010
Phone: 202-476-4085
Children's Outpatient Center in Spring Valley
4900 Massachusetts Avenue, NW, Washington,
    DC 20016
Phone: 202-476-2164
Website: *www.dcchildrens.com*
ip, op, php, f/m, 10–21

Florida

Fairwinds Treatment Center
1569 S. Fort Harrison Ave.
Clearwater, FL 33756
Phone: 800-226-0301

Fax: 727-467-0438
Email: fairwinds@fairwindstreatment.com
Website: *www.fairwindstreatment.com*
ip, php, f/m, adol+

The Renfrew Center of Florida
7700 Renfrew Lane
Coconut Creek, FL 33073
Phone: 800-736-3739
Fax: 954-698-9007
Email: via website
Website: *www.renfrewcenter.org*
ip, op, f, 14+

Illinois

Evanston Northwestern Healthcare
    at Highland Park Hospital
777 Park Avenue West
Highland Park, IL 60035
Phone: 847-480-2617
Fax: 847-480-2647
Website: *www.northshore.org*
op, php, f/m, 13+

Timberline Knolls
40 Timberline Drive
Lemont, IL 60439
Phone: 877-257-9611
Fax: 630-257-9708
Email: via website
Website: *www.timberlineknolls.com*
ip, php, f, 12+

Indiana

Charis Center for Eating Disorders
Clarian Health — Riley/Methodist Indiana Uni-
    versity Hospital
6640 Intech Boulevard, Suite 195
Indianapolis, IN 46278
Phone: 317-295-0608
Fax: 317-295-0622
Email: chariscenter@clarian.org
Website: *www.clarian.org/charis*
op, php, f/m, child+

Iowa

University of Iowa Hospitals and Clinics
Highland Park Hospital
Dept. of Psychiatry
200 Hawkins Drive, 2800 JPP
Iowa City, IA 52242
Phone: 319-356-2263
Website: *uihealthcare.com*
ip, op, php, f/m, adol+

Louisiana

**The Eating Disorders Treatment Center
  at River Oaks Hospital**
1525 River Oaks Road
New Orleans, LA 70123
Phone: 800-366-1740
Fax: 504-733-7020
Email: via website
Website: *www.riveroakshospital.com*
ip, php, f/m, adol+

Maryland

**The Center for Eating Disorders at Sheppard
  Pratt**
Physicians Pavilion North
6535 North Charles Street, Suite 300
Baltimore, MD 21204
Phone: 410-938-5252
Fax: 410-938-5250
Email: eatingdisorderinfo@shepardpratt.org
Website: *www.eatingdisorder.org*
ip, op, php, f/m, 10+

**The Johns Hopkins Eating Disorders
  Program**
The John Hopkins Hospital
600 North Wolfe Street
Baltimore, MD 21287
Phone: 410-938-5252 (outpatient); 410-502-
  5467 (inpatient)
Fax: 410-955-6155
Email: aguarda@jhmi.edu
Website: *www.hopkinsmedicine.org*
php, f/m, adol+

Massachusetts

Cambridge Eating Disorder Center
3 Bow Street
Cambridge, MA 02138
Phone: 617-547-2255
Fax: 617-547-0003
Email: seda@cedcmail.com
Website: *www.eatingdisordercenter.org*
ip, op, php, f/m, adol+

**The Klarman Eating Disorders Center at
  McLean Hospital**
115 Mill Street
Belmont, MA 02478
Phone: 617-855-3412
Fax: 617-855-3409
Email: Klarmancenter@mclean.harvard.edu
Website: *www.mclean.harvard.edu*
ip, php, f, 13–23

Minnesota

Emily Program
2265 Como Avenue, Suite 1002550
St. Paul, MN 55108
Other treatment centers in Stillwater, St. Louis
  Park, Burnsville, Chaska and Duluth
Phone: 651-645-5323
Fax: 651-647-5135
Email: info@emilyprogram.com
Website: *www.emilyprogram.com*
ip, op, f/m, child+

Mississippi

**Pine Grove Women's Center of Forrest
  General Hospital**
2255 Broadway Drive
Hattiesburg, MS 39404
Phone: 888-574-4673
Email: info@pinegrovetreatment.com
Website: *www.pinegrovetreatment.com*
ip, op, f, 18+

Missouri

Castlewood Treatment Center
800 Holland Road
St. Louis, MO 63021
Phone: 888-822-8938
Fax: 636-386-6622
Email: via website
Website: *www.castlewoodtc.com*
ip, op, f/m, 16+

McCallum Place
231 West Lockwood Avenue, Suite 201
St. Louis, MO 63199
Phone: 800-828-8158; 314-968-1900
Fax: 314-968-1901
Email: info@mccallumplace.com
Website: *www.mccallumplace.com*
ip, op, php, f/m, adol+

Nevada

Center for Hope of the Sierras
1453 Pass Drive
Reno, NV 89509
Phone: 866-690-7242
Fax: 775-322-4556
Email: via website
Website: *www.centerforhopeofthesierras.com*
ip, f, 16+

New Jersey

Somerset Medical Center
110 Rehill Avenue

Somerville, NJ 08876
Phone: 800-914-9444
Fax: 908-685-2458
Email: via website
Website: *www.somersetmedicalcenter.com*
ip, op, php, f/m, 10+

University Medical Center at Princeton
253 Witherspoon Street
Princeton, NJ 08540
Phone: 877-932-8935; 609-497-4490
Fax: 609-497-4412
Email: via website
Website: *www.princetonhcs.org*
ip, php, f/m, 8+

New Mexico

The Life Healing Center
PO Box 6758
Santa Fe, NM 87502
Phone: 866.806.7214
Fax: 505-820-8161
Email: via website
Website: *www.life-healing.com*
ip, f/m, adol+

New York

**Eating Disorders Center at Schneider
    Children's Hospital**
410 Lakeville Road, Suite 108
New Hyde Park, NY 11040
Phone: 516-465-3270
Fax: 516-465-5299
Email: via website
Website: *www.schneiderchildrenshospital.org*
ip, op, php, f/m, adol/young adult

Mount Sinai Medical Center
Eating and Weight Disorders Program
One Gustave L. Levy Place
Box 1230
New York, NY 10029
Phone: 212-659-8724
Fax: 212-849-2561
Email: Lauren.alfano@mssm.edu
Website: *www.mountsinai.org*/eatingdisorders
op, m/f, child+

The Renfrew Center of New York
11 East 36th Street, 2nd Floor
New York, NY 10016
Phone: 800-736-3739
Fax: 212-686-1865
Email: via website
Website: *www.renfrewcenter.com*
op, f, 14+

North Carolina

The Renfrew Center of Charlotte
6633 Fairview Rd
Charlotte, NC 28210
Phone: 800-736-3739
Email: via website
Website: *www.renfrewcenter.com*
op, f, 14+

North Dakota

Eating Disorder Institute
Merit Care South University
1720 University Drive South
Fargo, ND 58103
Phone: 800-437-4010; 701-461-5300
Fax: 701-461-5373
Email: via website
Website: *www.meritcare.com*
ip, php, f/m, adol+

Oklahoma

Laureate Psychiatric Clinic and Hospital
6655 South Yale Avenue
Tulsa, OK 74136
Phone: 800-322-5173
Fax: 918-491-3765
Email: via website
Website: *www.eatingdisorders.laureate.com*
ip, op, f, adol+

Oregon

**Kartini Clinic for Disordered Eating—
    Intensive Outpatient for Children
    and Adolescents**
2800 North Vancouver, Suite 118
Portland, OR 97227
Phone: 503-249-8851
Fax: 503-282-3409
Email: help@kartiniclinic.com
Website: *www.kartiniclinic.com*
op, php, f/m, 6–21

Pennsylvania

**Center for Overcoming Problem Eating
    (COPE)**
Western Psychiatric Institute and Clinic
University of Pittsburgh Medical Center
3811 O'Hara Street
Pittsburgh, PA 15213
Phone: 412-246-5117
Fax: 412-246-6370
Website: *www.wpic.pitt.edu*
ip, op, php, f/m, child

The Penn State Eating Disorder Program at
    Milton S. Hershey Medical Center
Briarcrest Office Building
905 W. Governor Road, Suite 250
Hershey, PA 17033
Phone: 800-243-1455; 717-531-2099
Fax: 717-531-0067
Email: via website
Website: *www.hmc.psu.edu*
op, php, f/m, 8+

The Renfrew Center of Philadelphia
475 Spring Lane
Philadelphia, PA 19128
Phone: 800-736-3739
Fax: 215-482-7390
Email: via website
Website: *www.renfrewcenter.com*
ip, f, 14+

The Renfrew Center of Radnor
320 King of Prussia Road
Radnor, PA 19087
Phone: 800-736-3739
Email: via website
Website: *www.renfrewcenter.com*
op, f, 14+

Tennessee

The Renfrew Center of Nashville
1624 Westgate Circle
Brentwood, TN 37027
Phone: 800-736-3739
Email: via website
Website: *www.renfrewcenter.com*
op, f, 14+

Texas

The Menninger Clinic Eating Disorders
    Program
2801 Gessner Drive
Houston, TX 77080
Phone: 800-351-9058
Fax: 713-275-5107
Email: via website
Website: *www.menningerclinic.com*
ip, f/m, 18+

Santé Center for Healing
914 Country Club Road
Argyle, TX 76226
Phone: 800-258-4250
Fax: 940-464-0323
Email: intake@santecenter.com
Website: *www.santecenter.com*
ip, op, f/m, adult

Shades of Hope
P.O. Box 639
Buffalo Gap, TX 79508
Phone: 800.588.4673
Email: via website
Website: *www.shadesofhope.com*
ip, op, f/m, adol+

Stepping Stones Intensive Outpatient
Medical City Dallas
7777 Forest Lane, Suite B-142
Dallas, TX 75230
Phone: 972-566-8514
Fax: 972-566-8497
Email: via web
Website: *www.steppingstonesdallas.com*
op, m (11–20), f (adol+)

The Walker Wellness Clinic
100 Highland Park Village, Suite 320
Dallas, TX 95205
Phone: 214-521-8969
Fax: 214-522-1150
Website: *www.walkerwellness.com*
op, f (adol+), m (adult)

Utah

Avalon Hills
Adolescent facility:
7852 West 600 North
Petersboro, UT 84325
Phone: 435-753-3760
Fax 435-753-3760

Adult treatment facility:
8530 South 500 West
Paradise, UT 84328
Phone: 800-330-0490; 435-245-4537
Fax: 435-245-4537
Email: via website
Website: *www.avalonhills.org*
ip, f, adol+

Center for Change
1790 North State Street
Orem, UT 84057
Phone: 888-224-8250; 801-224-8255
Email: via website
Website: *www.centerforchange.com*
ip, f, 16+

Virginia

Remuda Ranch East
2500 Remuda Lane
Milford, VA 22154
Phone: 800-445-1900
Fax: 928-684-4801

Email: info@remudaranch.com
Website: *www.remudaranch.com*
ip, php, f/m, 9+, Christian

Washington

The Center
547 Dayton Street
Edmonds, WA 98020
Phone: 888-771-5166
Fax: 425-670-2807
Website: *www.aplaceofhope.org*
ip, op, f/m, child+

Eating Disorders Program
Seattle Children's Hospital
Department of Child and Psychiatry and Behavioral Health
PO Box 5371/W3636
4800 Sand Point Way NE
Seattle, WA 98105
Phone: 206-987-3560
Fax: 206-987-2246

Website: *www.seattlechildrens.org*
ip, op, f/m, 13+

Wisconsin

Aurora Psychiatric Hospital
1220 Dewey Avenue
Wauwatosa, WI 53213
Phone: 414-454-6694
Fax: 414-773-4330
Email: sandra.blaies@aurora.org
Website: *www.aurorahealthcare.org*
ip, op, php, f/m, 13+

Rogers Memorial Hospital — Oconomowoc
34700 Valley Road
Oconomowoc, WI 53066
Phone: 800-767-4411
Fax: 414-327-6045
Email: via website
Website: *www.rogershospital.org*
ip, php, f/m, child+

Appendix B.
Resources for Information and Referral

Organizations

Academy for Eating Disorders
111 Deer Lake Road, Suite 100
Deerfield, IL 60015 USA
http://www.aedweb.org/
Phone: 847-498-4274
Fax: 847-480-9282
Email: *info@aedweb.org*
Website: *www.aedweb.org*

Association for Professionals Treating Eating Disorders — San Francisco
3195 California Street
San Francisco, California 94115
Phone: 415-771-3068
Email: *AptedSF@aol.com*
Website: *www.aptedsf.com*

Duke University Eating Disorders Program
Box 3842
Duke University Medical Center
Department of Psychology
Durham, NC 27710
Phone: 919-668-7301
Fax: 919-681-7347
Website: *www.eatingdisorders.mc.duke.edu*

Eating Disorders Coalition for Research, Policy and Action
720 7th Street NW, Suite 300
Washington, DC 20001
Phone: 202-543-9570
Email: *manager@eatingdisordercoalition.org*
Website: *www.eatingdisorderscoalition.org*

Harris Center for Education and Advocacy in Eating Disorders at Massachusetts General Hospital (Formerly Harvard Eating Disorders Center)
2 Longfellow Place, Suite 200
Boston, MA 02114
Phone: 617-726-8470
Fax: 617-726-1595
Email: *infohedc@comcast.net*
Website: *www.harriscentermgh.org*

International Association of Eating Disorder Professionals
PO Box 1295
Pekin, IL 61555
Phone: 800-800-8126
Fax: 800-800-8126
Email: *iaedpmembers@earthlink.net*
Website: *www.iaedp.com*

National Association of Anorexia Nervosa and Associated Disorders
PO Box 7
Highland Park, IL 60035
Phone: 847-831-3438
Fax: 847-433-4632
Email hotline: anadhelp@anad.org
Support Groups: *Anadgroup@aol.com*
Advocacy: *Anadadvocacy@aol.com*
Website: *www.anad.org*

National Eating Disorder Association
603 Stewart Street, Suite 803
Seattle, WA 98101
Phone: 206-382-3587
Information and Referral Helpline: 800-931-2237
Fax: 206-829-8501
Email: *info@NationalEatingDisorders.org*
Website: *www.nationaleatingdisorders.org*

National Eating Disorder Information Centre
ES 7-421, 200 Elizabeth Street
Toronto, Ontario M5G 2C4

Phone: 866-633-4220; 416-340-4156
Fax 416-340-4736
Email: *nedic@uhn.on.ca*
Website: *www.nedic.ca*

12-Step Programs

Anorexics and Bulimics Anonymous
Main P.O. Box 125
Edmonton, AB T5J 2G9
Edmonton Central Information Line: 780-443-6077
Email: *aba@shawbiz.ca*
Website: *www.anorexicsandbulimicsanonymous aba.com*

Eating Disorders Anonymous
Email: *info@eatingdisordersanonymous.org*
Website: *www.eatingdisordersanonymous.org*

Food Addicts Anonymous
World Service Office Phone: 561-967-3871
Website: *www.foodaddictsanonymous.org*

Overeaters Anonymous
World Service Office
PO Box 44020
Rio Rancho, NM 87174
Phone: 505-891-2664
Fax: 505-891-4320
Email: *info@oa.org*
Website: *www.oa.org*

Other Helpful Internet Resources

Addictions.Net
www.addictions.net

After the Diet (info on medical complications)
www.afterthediet.com

Anorexia Nervosa & Related Eating Disorders
www.anred.com

Body Icon
http://nm-server.jrn.columbia.edu/projects/ masters/bodyimage/food/

Body Image Coalition of Peel
www.bodyimagecoalition.org

The Body Positive, Inc.
www.bodypositive.com

Caring Online
www.caringonline.com

Dads and Daughters
www.dadsanddaughters.org

The Eating Disorder Foundation
www.eatingdisorderfoundation.org

Eating Disorder Services
www.eatingdisorderservices.net

EDReferral.Com (resource locator)
www.edreferral.com

Focus Adolescent Services
www.focusas.com/EatingDisorders.html

Gürze Books
www.bulimia.com

Help Your Daughter
www.helpyourdaughter.com

Interventions
www.interventions.net

Medline Plus
www.nlm.nih.gov/medlineplus/eatingdisorders. html

Mirror-Mirror
www.mirror-mirror.org

Pale Reflections
www.pale-reflections.com

The Recovery Group (online meetings & more)
www.therecoverygroup.org

Something Fishy
www.something-fishy.org

Bibliography

Adams, Eileen, Marian Eberly, Kevin Wandler, and Yong Lee. "Body Dysmorphic Disorder and Eating Disorders." *The Remuda Review: The Christian Journal of Eating Disorders*, 2007, 6(3): 26–33.

Agras, W. Stewart, David Barlow, Harvey Chapin, Gene Abel, and Harold Leitenberg. "Behavior Modification of Anorexia Nervosa." *Archives of General Psychiatry*, 1974, 30(3): 279–286.

Ainsworth, M.D.S., and J. Bowlby. "An Ethological Approach to Personality Development." *American Psychologist*, 1991, 46: 331–341.

Alcoholics Anonymous: The Story of How Many Thousands of Men and Women Have Recovered from Alcoholism. 4th ed. New York: Alcoholics Anonymous World Services, 2001. 575pp.

Allen, Andrea, and Eric Hollander. "Similarities and Differences Between Body Dysmorphic Disorder and Other Disorders." *American Psychiatric Annals*, December 2004, 34(12): 927–933.

Andersen, Arnold E. *Practical Comprehensive Treatment of Anorexia Nervosa and Bulimia.* Baltimore, Maryland: The Johns Hopkins University Press, 1987. 207pp.

Bachrach, Arthur J., William J. Erwin, and Jay P. Mohr. "The Control of Eating Behavior in an Anorexic by Operant Conditioning Techniques." In Ullmann, Leonard P., and Leonard Krasner, eds., *Case Studies in Behavior Modification.* New York: Holt, Rinehart and Winston, 1965, pp.153–163.

Bailer, U.F., G.K. Frank, S.E. Henry, C.C. Melzer, L. Weisfield, C.A. Mathis, W.C. Drevets, A. Wagner, J. Hoge, S.K. Zilka, C.W. McConaha, and W.H. Kaye. "Altered Brain Serotonin 5-HT1A Receptor Binding after Recovery from Anorexia Nervosa Measured by Positron Emission Tomography and [Carbonyl11C]WAY-100635." *Archives of General Psychiatry*, September 2005, 62(9): 1032–1041.

Bailer, U.F., G.K. Frank, S.E. Henry, J.C. Price, C.C. Meltzer, C.A. Mathis, A. Wagner, L. Thornton, J. Hoge, S.K. Zilko, C.R. Becker, C.W. McConaha, and W.H. Kaye. "Exaggerated 5-HT1A but Normal 5-HT2A Receptor Activity in Individuals Ill with Anorexia Nervosa." *Biological Psychiatry*, May 1, 2007, 61(9): 1090–1099.

Bailer, U.F., and W.H. Kaye. "Review of Neuropeptide and Neuroendocrine Dysregulation in Anorexia and Bulimia Nervosa." *Current Drug Targets CNS Neural Disorders*, February 2003, 2(1): 53–59.

Barabasz, M. "Efficacy of Hypnotherapy in the Treatment of Eating Disorders." *International Journal of Clinical and Experimental Hypnosis*, July 2007, 55(3): 318–335.

Bardone-Cone, A.M., and K.M. Cass. "What Does Viewing a Pro-Anorexia Website Do? An Experimental Examination of Website Exposure and Moderating Effects." *International Journal of Eating Disorders*, September 2007, 40(6): 537–548.

Bemis, Kelly. "The Present Status of Operant Conditioning for the Treatment of Anorexia Nervosa." *Behavior Modification*, 1987, 11: 432–463.

Betts, Donna J. "Art Therapy Approaches to Working with People Who Have Eating Disorders." In Brooke, Stephanie, ed., *The Creative Therapies and Eating Disorders.* Springfield, Illinois: Charles C. Thomas, 2008, pp.12–27.

Bissada, Hany, Giorgio Tasca, Ann Marie Barber, and Jacque Bradwejn. "Olanzapine in the Treatment of Low Body Weight and Obsessive Thinking in Women with Anorexia Nervosa: A Randomized, Double-Blind, Placebo-Controlled Trial." *The American Journal of Psychiatry*, June 16, 2008, 165: 1281–1288.

Boas, Rollo. "A Disease of the Spirit." In *Overeaters Anonymous.* 2d ed. Rio Rancho, New Mexico: Overeaters Anonymous, Inc., 2001, pp.242–247.

Bobilin, Marah. "Music Therapy in the Treatment of Eating Disorders." In Brooke, Stephanie, ed., *The Creative Therapies and Eating Disorders.* Springfield, Illinois: Charles C. Thomas, 2008, pp.142–158.

Boodman, Sandra G. "*Thin* and Eating Disorders." *Charlotte Observer*, November 14, 2006, p.3E.

Bowers, W.A., and L.S. Ansher. "The Effectiveness of Cognitive Behavioral Therapy on Changing Eating Disorder Symptoms and Psychopathology of 32 Anorexia Nervosa Patients at Hospital Discharge and One Year Follow-Up." *Annals of Clinical Psychiatry,* April-June 2008, *20*(2): 79–86.

Boyd, Harry S., and Vernon V. Sisney. "Immediate Self-image Confrontation and Changes in Self-Concept." *Journal of Consulting Psychology,* 1967, *31*(3): 291–294.

Brady, J.P., and W. Rieger. "Behavioral Treatment of Anorexia Nervosa." In Brady, J.P., and H.K.H. Brodie, eds., *Controversy in Psychiatry.* Philadelphia, Pennsylvania: W.B. Saunders, 1978.

Bremner, Charles, and Marie Tourres. "French Anorexia Law Targets Websites." *The Australian,* April 10, 2008. http://www.theaustralian.news.com.au/story/0,,23515919-26040,00.html

Brisman, Judith. "Psychodynamic Psychotherapy and Action-Oriented Technique." In Werne, Joellen, ed., *Treating Eating Disorders.* San Francisco, California: Jossey-Bass, 1996, pp.31–70.

Brody, Sylvia. *The Hunger Artists: The Development of Anorexia Nervosa.* Rev. ed. Madison, Connecticut: International Universities Press, 2007. 277pp.

Brooke, Stephanie, ed. *The Creative Therapies and Eating Disorders.* Springfield, Illinois: Charles C. Thomas, 2008. 291pp.

Brotsky, S.R., and D. Giles. "Inside the Pro-Ana Community: A Covert Online Participant Observation." *Eating Disorders,* March-April 2007, *15*(2): 93–109.

Brown, Stephanie. *A Place Called Self: Women, Sobriety, and Radical Transformation.* Center City, Minnesota: Hazelden, 2004. 182pp.

Bruch, Hilde. *Eating Disorders: Obesity, Anorexia Nervosa, and the Person Within.* New York: Basic Books, 1973. 396pp.

_____. "Perils of Behavior Modification in Treatment of Anorexia Nervosa."
Journal of the American Medical Association, December 9, 1974, *230*(10): 1419–1422.

_____. "Psychotherapy in Primary Anorexia Nervosa." *The Journal of Nervous and Mental Disease,* 1970, *150*(1): 51–67.

Cash, Thomas. *The Body Image Workbook: An Eight-Step Program for Learning to Like Your Looks.* 2d ed. Oakland, California: New Harbinger, 2008. 216pp.

Cash, Thomas, and Thomas Pruzinsky, eds. *Body Image: A Handbook of Theory, Research and Clinical Practice.* New York: Guilford, 2004. 530pp.

Chernin, Kim. *The Hungry Self: Women, Eating and Identity.* New York: HarperPerennial, 1985. 240pp.

_____. *The Obsession: Reflections on the Tyranny of Slenderness.* New York: Harper & Row, 1981. 240 pp.

Claire, Thomas. *Body Work: What Type of Massage to Get and How to Make the Most of It.* New York: William Morrow, 1995. 440pp.

Cortright, Brant. *Psychotherapy and Spirit: Theory and Practice in Transpersonal Psychotherapy.* Al-

bany: State University of New York Press, 1997. 257pp.

Costin, Carolyn. *The Eating Disorder Sourcebook: A Comprehensive Guide to the Causes, Treatment and Prevention of Eating Disorders.* 3d ed. New York: McGraw Hill, 2007a. 334pp.

_____. *100 Questions and Answers about Eating Disorders.* Sudbury, Massachusetts: Jones and Bartlett, 2007b. 221pp.

Crisp, A.H. "Clinical and Therapeutic Aspects of Anorexia Nervosa: A Study of 30 Cases." *Journal of Psychosomatic Research,* 1965, *9:* 67–78.

Crisp, Arthur H. "Anorexia Nervosa as Flight from Growth: Assessment and Treatment Based on the Model." In Garner, David M., and Paul E. Garfinkel, eds., *Handbook of Treatment for Eating Disorders.* 2d ed. New York: Guilford, 1997, pp.248–277.

Crowther, Janis, and Nancy Sherwood. "Assessment." In Garner, David M., and Paul Garfinkel, eds., *Handbook of Treatment of Eating Disorders.* 2d ed. New York: Guilford, 1997, pp.34–49.

Cuzzolaro, M., G. Vetrone, G. Marano, and P.E. Garfinkel. "The Body Uneasiness Test (BUT): Development and Validation of a New Body Image Assessment Scale." *Eating and Weight Disorders,* March 2006, *11*(1): 1–13.

Dally, Peter J., and William Sargant. "A New Treatment of Anorexia Nervosa." *British Medical Journal,* June 1960, *2*(5187): 1770–1773.

Daniels, Lucy. *With a Woman's Voice: A Writer's Struggle for Emotional Freedom.* Lanham, Maryland: Madison, 2001. 320pp.

Dare, Christopher, and Ivan Eisler. "Family Therapy for Anorexia Nervosa." In Garner, David M., and Paul Garfinkel, eds., *Handbook for Treatment of Eating Disorders.* 2d ed. New York: Guilford, 1997, pp.307–324.

Dennis, A.B., and R. Sansone. "Treatment of Patients with Personality Disorders." In Garner, David M., and Paul Garfinkel, eds., *Handbook of Treatment of Eating Disorders.* 2d ed. New York: Guilford, 1997, pp.437–449.

Deter, H.C., W. Herzog, and R. Manz. "Do Patients with Anorexia Return to Psychological Health?" *Z Psychosomatik Medizinische Psychoanalysis,* 1994, *40*(2): 155–173.

Diagnostic and Statistical Manual of Mental Disorders, Text Revision: DSM-IV-TR. Washington, D.C.: American Psychiatric Association, 2000. 943pp.

Eisler, Ivan, Daniel Le Grange, and Eia Asen. "Family Interventions." In Treasure, Janet, et al., eds., *Handbook of Eating Disorders.* 2d ed. Chichester, West Sussex, England: John Wiley, 2003, pp.291–310.

Ercan, Eyüp Sabri, Hakan Copkunol, Sibel Çÿkööl, and Azmi Varan. "Olanzapine Treatment of an Adolescent Girl with Anorexia Nervosa." *Human*

Psychopharmacology: Clinical and Experimental, July 7, 2003, *18*(5): 401–403.

Fairburn, C.G., Z. Cooper and R. Shafran. "Cognitive Behaviour Therapy for Eating Disorders: A "Transdiagnostic" Theory and Treatment." *Behaviour Research and Therapy,* 2003, 41(5): 509–528.

Fallon, Patricia, and Stephen Wonderlich. "Sexual Abuse and Other Forms of Trauma." In Garner, David M., and Paul Garfinkel, eds., *Handbook of Treatment of Eating Disorders.* 2d ed. New York: Guilford, 1997, pp.394–414.

Fleming, Mari. "Art Therapy with Anorexia: Experiencing the Authentic Self." In Hornyak, Lynne, and Ellen Baker, eds., *Experiential Therapies for Eating Disorders.* New York: Guilford, 1989, pp. 279–304.

Fox, N., K. Ward, and A. O'Rourke. "Pro-Anorexia, Weight-Loss Drugs and the Internet: An "Anti-Recovery" Explanatory Model of Anorexia." *Sociology of Health and Illness,* November 2005, *27*(7): 944–971.

Fraiberg, Selma H. *The Magic Years: Understanding and Handling the Problems of Early Childhood.* New York: Scribner's, 1959. 305pp.

Garfinkel, Paul E., Stephen A. Kline, and Harvey C. Stancer. "Treatment of Anorexia Nervosa Using Operant Conditioning Techniques." *The Journal of Nervous and Mental Diseases,* 1973, *157*(6): 428–433.

Garner, David M., "Psychoeducational Principles in Treatment." In Garner, David M., and Paul Garfinkel, eds., *Handbook of Treatment of Eating Disorders.* 2d ed. New York: Guilford, 1997, pp.145–177.

Garner, David M., and Paul Garfinkel, eds., *Handbook of Treatment of Eating Disorders.* 2d ed. New York: Guilford, 1997. 528pp.

Garner, David, Kelly Vitousek, and Kathleen Pike. "Cognitive-Behavioral Therapy for Anorexia Nervosa." In Garner, David M., and Paul Garfinkel, eds., *Handbook of Treatment of Eating Disorders.* 2d ed. New York: Guilford, 1997, pp.94–144.

Gilbert, Roberta M. *The Eight Concepts of Bowen Theory: A New Way of Thinking about the Individual and the Group.* Falls Church, Virginia: Leading Systems, 2006. 127pp.

Gilligan, Carol. *In a Different Voice: Psychological Theory and Women's Development.* Boston, Massachusetts: Harvard University Press, 1993.

Goldner, Elliot M., C. Laird Birmingham, and Victoria Smye. "Addressing Treatment Refusal in Anorexia Nervosa: Clinical, Ethical and Legal Considerations." In Garner, David M., and Paul Garfinkel, eds., *Handbook of Treatment of Eating Disorders.* 2d ed. New York: Guilford, 1997, pp. 450–461.

Gottheil, Edward, Clifford E. Backup, and Floyd S. Cornelison. "Denial and Self-image Confronta-tion in a Case of Anorexia Nervosa." *The Journal of Nervous and Mental Disease,* 1969, *448*(3): 238–250.

Greenfield, Lauren, filmmaker. *Thin.* HBO Documentary, November 2006.

Grice, D.E., K.A. Halmi, M.M. Fichter, M. Strober, D.B. Woodside, J.T. Treasure, A.S. Kaplan, P.J. Magistretti, D. Goldman, C.M. Bulik, W.H. Kaye, and W.H. Berrettini. "Evidence for a Susceptibility Gene for Anorexia Nervosa on Chromosome 1." *American Journal of Human Genetics,* March 2002, *70*: 787.

Grilo, Carlos. *Eating and Weight Disorders.* New York: Psychology Press, 2006. 246pp.

Gross, Meir. "Anorexia Nervosa." *Medical Hypnoanalysis,* August 1981, *2*(3): 95–l0l.

Hall, Lindsey. *Anorexia Nervosa: A Guide to Recovery.* Carlsbad, California: Gurze, 1998. 192pp.

Hallsten, Edwin A., Jr. "Adolescent Anorexia Nervosa Treated by Desensitization." *Behaviour Research and Therapy,* 1965, *3*(2): 87–91.

Halmi, K.A., P. Powers, and S. Cunningham. "Treatment of Anorexia Nervosa with Behavior Modification." *Archives of General Psychiatry,* January 1975, *32*(1): 93–96.

Hansen, L. "Olanzapine in the Treatment of Anorexia Nervosa." *British Journal of Psychiatry,* 1999, *175*: 592.

Head, Jacqueline, "Seeking 'Thinspiration.'" *BBC News/UK/Magazine,* August 8, 2007. http://news vote.bbc.co.uk/mpapps/pagetools/print/news. bbc.co.uk/2hi/uk_news/magazine/6935768.stm.

Heischman, Nancy. "A Paper about Anorexia Nervosa." *Redwoods,* 1981, *1*(1): 10–25.

Herzog, David, and Kamryn Eddy. "Diagnosis, Epidemiology and Clinical Course of Eating Disorders." In Yager, Joel, and Pauline Powers, eds., *Clinical Manual of Eating Disorders,* Washington, D.C.: American Psychiatric Publishing, 2007, pp.1–30.

Hinshaw, Stephen, and Rachel Kranz. *The Triple Bind: Saving Our Teenage Girls from Today's Pressures.* New York: Ballantine Books, 2009, 256pp.

Hobbes, Thomas. *Leviathan: Parts One and Two.* (1651). Indianapolis, Indiana: Bobbs-Merrill, 1977. 432pp.

Hornyak, Lynne M., and Ellen K. Baker. *Experiential Therapies for Eating Disorders.* New York: Guilford, 1989. 338pp.

Hudgins, M. Katherine. "Experiencing the Self through Psychodrama and Gestalt Therapy in Anorexia Nervosa." In Hornyak, Lynne, and Ellen Baker, eds., *Experiential Therapies for Eating Disorders.* New York: Guilford, 1989, pp.234–251.

Hudson, J.I., E. Hiripi, H.G. Pope, Jr., and R.C. Kessler. "The Prevalence and Correlates of Eating Disorders in the National Comorbidity Survey Replication." *Biological Psychiatry,* 2007, 61(3): 348–358.

Huebner, Hans F. *Endorphins, Eating Disorders and Other Addictive Behaviors.* New York: W.W. Norton, 1993. 272pp.

Hutchinson, Marcia Germaine. "Imagining Ourselves Whole: A Feminist Approach to Treating Eating Disorders." In Fallon, Patricia, Melanie Katzman, and Susan Wooley, eds., *Feminist Perspectives on Eating Disorders.* New York: Guilford, 1994, pp.152–168.

Hutchinson-Phillips, Susan, Graham Jamieson, and Kathryn Gow. "Differing Roles of Imagination and Hypnosis in Self-Regulation of Eating Behaviour." *Contemporary Hypnosis,* February 2006, *22*(4): 171–183.

Hutchinson-Phillips Susan, Kathryn Gow, and Graham Jamieson. "Hypnotizability, Eating Behaviors, Attitudes, and Concerns: A Literature Survey." *International Journal of Clinical and Experimental Hypnosis,* January 2007, *55*(1): 84–113.

Johnson, Craig, ed. *Psychodynamic Treatment of Anorexia Nervosa and Bulimia.* New York: Guilford, 1991. 404pp.

Kabat-Zinn, Jon. *Full Catastrophe Living.* McHenry, Illinois: Delta, 1990. 512pp.

_____. "Mindfulness-Based Interventions in Context: Past, Present and Future." *Clinical Psychology: Science and Practice,* 2003, *10*(2): 144–156.

Kaplan, Allan, and Sarah Noble. "Management of Anorexia Nervosa in an Ambulatory Setting." In Yager, Joel, and Pauline Powers, eds., *Clinical Manual of Eating Disorders.* Washington, D.C.: American Psychiatric Publishing, 2007, pp.127–147.

Kaplan, Allan, and Marion Olmsted. "Partial Hospitalization." In Garner, David, and Paul Garfinkel, eds., *Handbook of Treatment of Eating Disorders.* 2d ed. New York: Guilford, 1997, pp.354–360.

Kaye, W.H., U.F. Bailer, G.K. Frank, A. Wagner, and S.E. Henry. "Brain Imaging of Serotonin after Recovery from Anorexia and Bulimia Nervosa." *Physiology and Behavior,* September 15, 2005, *86*(1–2): 15–17.

Kearney-Cooke, Ann. "Reclaiming the Body: Using Guided Imagery in the Treatment of Body Image Disturbances among Bulimic Women." In Hornyak, Lynne M., and Ellen K. Baker, eds., *Experiential Therapies for Eating Disorders.* New York: Guilford, 1989, pp.11–33.

Kearney-Cooke, Ann, and Ruth Striegel-Moore. "The Etiology and Treatment of Body Image Disturbance." In Garner, David M., and Paul Garfinkel, eds., *Handbook of Treatment of Eating Disorders.* 2d ed. New York: Guilford, 1997, pp.295–306.

Kohl, M., C. Foulon, and J.D. Guelfi. "Hyperactivity and Anorexia Nervosa: Behavioural and Biological Perspective." *Encephale,* September-October 2004, *30*(5): 492–9.

Kroger, William, and William D. Fezler. *Hypnosis and Behavior Modification: Imagery Conditioning.* Philadelphia, Pennsylvania: J.B. Lippincott, 1976. 426pp.

Lavin, Cheryl. "So Thin She May Disappear." *The State Magazine,* Columbia, South Carolina, October 4, 1981, *90*(277): 5–6.

Lessem, Peter A. *Self Psychology: An Introduction.* New York: Jason Aronson, 2005. 262pp.

Levine, Peter A., and Ann Frederick. *Waking the Tiger: Healing Trauma.* Berkeley, California: North Atlantic, 1997. 274pp.

Lilenfeld, L.R., W.H. Kaye, C.G. Greeno, K.R. Merikangas, K. Plotnicov, C. Pollice, R. Rao, M. Stroeber, C.M. Bulik, and L. Nagy. "A Controlled Family Study of Anorexia Nervosa and Bulimia Nervosa: Psychiatric Disorders in First-Degree Relatives and Effects of Proband Comorbidity." *Archives of General Psychiatry,* July 1998, *55*(7): 603–610.

Linehan, Marsha. *Cognitive-Behavioral Treatment of Borderline Personality Disorder.* New York: Guilford, 1993. 558pp.

Liu, Aimee. *Gaining: The Truth about Life after Eating Disorders.* Boston, Massachusetts: Wellness Central, 2008. 336pp.

_____. *Solitaire.* New York: Harper & Row, 1979. 215pp.

Lock, James, and Daniel le Grange. "Family Treatment of Eating Disorders." In Yager, Joel, and Pauline Powers, eds., *Clinical Manual of Eating Disorders.* Washington, D.C.: American Psychiatric Publishing, 2007, pp.149–170.

_____, and _____. *Help Your Teenager Beat an Eating Disorder.* New York: Guilford, 2005.

Lock, James, Daniel le Grange, W. Stuart Agras, and Christopher Dare. *Treatment Manual for Anorexia Nervosa: A Family-Based Approach.* New York: Guilford, 2002. 270pp.

Lucas, Alexander R., Jane Duncan, and Violet Piens. "The Treatment of Anorexia Nervosa." *American Journal of Psychiatry,* September 1976, *133*(9): 1034–1038.

Luepnitz, Deborah Anna. *Schopenhauer's Porcupines: Intimacy and Its Dilemmas.* New York: Basic Books, 2002. 288pp.

McAll, Robert K., and Frances M. McAll. "Ritual Mourning in Anorexia Nervosa." *Lancet,* August 16, 1980, *2*(8190): 368.

McIntosh, V.V., J. Jordan, F.A. Carter, S.E. Luty, J.M. McKenzie, C.M. Bulik, C.M. Frampton, and P.R. Joyce. "Three Psychotherapies for Anorexia Nervosa: A Randomized, Controlled Trial." *American Journal of Psychiatry,* April 2005, *162*(4):741–747.

McKay, Matthew, Jeffrey Wood, and Jeffrey Brantley. *The Dialectical Behavior Therapy Skills Workbook.* Oakland, California: New Harbinger, 2007. 232pp.

McNear, Suzanne. "The Curse of Perfectionism." *Cosmopolitan*, October 1981, *191*(4): 294–297, 319.

Maine, Margo. *Father Hunger: Fathers, Daughters and the Pursuit of Thinness*. Carlsbad, California: Gurze, 2004. 288pp.

Maine, Margo, William N. Davis and Jane Shure, eds. *Effective Clinical Practices in the Treatment of Eating Disorders: The Heart of the Matter*. New York: Routledge, Taylor & Francis, 2009. 262pp.

Marnilli, A., A. Pinto, A.S. Guarda, L.J. Heinberg, and C.C. Dialemente. "Self-Report of Self-Efficacy to Recover from an Eating Disorder." *International Journal of Eating Disorders*, July 2006, *39*(5): 376–84.

Martin, Courtney E. *Perfect Girls, Starving Daughters: The Frightening New Normalcy of Hating Your Body*, New York: Free Press, 2007. 330pp.

Mehler, C., C. Wewetzer, U. Schulze, A. Warnke, F. Theisen, and R.W. Dittman. "Olanzapine in Children and Adolescents with Chronic Anorexia Nervosa. A Study of Five Cases." *European Child and Adolescent Psychiatry*, June 2001, *10*(2): 151–157.

Minuchin, Salvador, Bernice L. Rosman, and Lester Baker. *Psychosomatic Families: Anorexia Nervosa in Context*. Cambridge, Massachusetts: Harvard University Press, 1978. 351pp.

Mitchell, James, Claire Pomeroy, and David Adson. "Managing Medical Complications." In Garner, David M., and Paul Garfinkel, eds., *Handbook of Treatment of Eating Disorders*. 2d ed. New York: Guilford, 1997, pp.383–393.

Montagu, Ashley. *Touching: The Human Significance of the Skin*. New York: Harper & Row, 1978. 384pp.

Morenoff, Andrea, and Barbara Sobol. "Art Therapy in the Long-Term Psychodynamic Treatment of Bulimic Women." In Hornyak, Lynne, and Ellen Baker, eds., *Experiential Therapies for Eating Disorders*. New York: Guilford, 1989, pp.144–166.

Munoz, Sara Schaeffer. "When a Child Is Afraid to Eat: Coping with Allergy Anxieties." *The Wall Street Journal*, October 2, 2007, p.B11.

Nielsen, Soren, and Nuria Bará-Carril. "Family, Burden of Care and Social Consequences." In Garner, David M., and Paul Garfinkel, eds., *Handbook of Treatment of Eating Disorders*. 2d ed. New York: Guilford, 1997, pp.191–206.

Overeaters Anonymous. 2d ed. Rio Rancho, New Mexico: Overeaters Anonymous, 2001. 252pp.

Palazzoli, Mara Selvini. *Self-Starvation: From Individual to Family Therapy in the Treatment of Anorexia Nervosa*. Northvale, New Jersey: Jason Aronson, 1985. 296 pp.

Parente, Alice Ball. "Music as a Therapeutic Tool in Treating Anorexia Nervosa." In Hornyak, Lynne, and Ellen Baker, eds., *Experiential Therapies for Eating Disorders*. New York: Guilford, 1989, pp.305–328.

Pecarvé, Reuben. *The Hypnosis Book: How to Use Modern Hypnotic Techniques to Improve Physical and Mental Health*. Montreal, Canada: Optimum, 2002. 276pp.

Perlick, Deborah, and Brett Silverstein. "Faces of Female Discontent: Depression, Disordered Eating, and Changing Gender Roles." In Fallon, Patricia, Melanie Katzman, and Susan Wooley, eds., *Feminist Perspectives on Eating Disorders*. New York: Guilford, 1994, pp.77–93.

Pinto, A., L.J. Heinberg, J.W. Coughlin, J.W. Fava, and A.S. Guarda "The Eating Disorder Recovery Self-Efficacy Questionnaire (EDRSQ): Change with Treatment and Prediction of Outcome." *Eating Disorder Behavior*, April 2008, *9*(2): 143–153.

Rayner, Claire. *Where Do I Come From?* Ottawa, Ontario: Arlington, 1974. 128pp.

Reaves, Jessica. "Anorexia Goes High Tech." *Time.com*, July 31, 2001. http://www.time.com/health/article/0,8599,169660,00.html.

Reinblatt, S.P., G.W. Redgrave, and A.S. Guarda. "Medication Management of Pediatric Eating Disorders." *International Review of Psychiatry*, April 2008, *20*(2): 183–188.

Rice, Julia B., Marylee Hardenbergh, and Lynne M. Hornyak. "Disturbed Body Image in Anorexia Nervosa: Dance/Movement Therapy Interventions." In Hornyak, Lynne, and Ellen Baker, eds., *Experiential Therapies for Eating Disorders*. New York: Guilford, 1989, pp.252–278.

Rodin, Judith. *Body Traps: Breaking the Binds that Keep You from Feeling Good About Your Body*. New York: William Morrow, 1992. 299pp.

Rollins, N., and A. Blackwell. "The Treatment of Anorexia Nervosa in Children and Adolescents: Stage I." *Journal of Child Psychology and Psychiatry*, 1968, *9*: 81–91.

Rosenberg, Jack Lee, Marjorie L. Rand, and Diane Asay. *Body, Self and Soul: Sustaining Integration*. Atlanta, Georgia: Humanics, 1991. 339 pp.

Ryan, Joan. "The Internet Is Where 'Anas' Meet." *San Francisco Chronicle*, February 16, 2003, pp.D1, D6.

Sachdev, P., N. Mondraty, W. Wen, and K. Gulliford. "Brains of Anorexia Nervosa Patients Process Self-Images Differently from Non-Self-Images: An fMRI Study." *Neuropsychologia*, 2008, *46*(8): 2161–2168.

Sacher, Ira, and Marc A. Simmer. *Dying to Be Thin: Understanding and Defeating Anorexia Nervosa and Bulimia — A Practical Lifesaving Guide*. New York: Grand Central, 1987. 288pp.

Sacher, Ira, and Sheila Buff. *Regaining Your Self: Breaking Free from the Eating Disorder Identity: A Bold New Approach*. New York: Hyperion, 2007. 208 pp.

Sansone, Randy A., and Lori A. Sansone. "Eating Disorders and Psychiatric Comorbidity: Prevalence and Treatment Modifications." In Yager, Joel, and Pauline Powers, eds., *Clinical Manual of*

Eating Disorders. Washington, D.C.: American Psychiatric Publishing, 2007, pp.79–111.

Schilder, Paul. *The Image and Appearance of the Human Body*. New York: International Universities Press, 1935.

Schnarch, David. *Constructing the Sexual Crucible: An Integration of Sexual and Marital Therapy*. New York: W.W. Norton, 1991. 636pp.

Schwartz, Donald M., and Michael G. Thompson. "Do Anorectics Get Well? Current Research and Future Needs." *American Journal of Psychiatry*, March 1981, *138*(3): 319–323.

Skrzypek, S., P.M. Wehmeier, and H. Remschmidt. "Body Image Assessment Using Body Size Estimation in Recent Studies on Anorexia Nervosa. A Brief Review." *European Child and Adolescent Psychiatry*, December 2001, *10*(4): 212–221.

Sodersten, P., R. Nergardh, C. Bergh, M. Zandian, and A. Scheurink. "Behavioral Neuroendocrinology and Treatment of Anorexia Nervosa." *Front Neuroendocrinology*, June 14, 2008 (Epub).

Stark, Arlynne, Simona Aronow, and Theresa McGeehan. "Dance/Movement Therapy with Bulimic Patients." In Hornyak, Lynne, and Ellen Baker, eds., *Experiential Therapies for Eating Disorders*. New York: Guilford, 1989, pp.121–143.

Stern, Steven. "Managing Opposing Currents: An Interpersonal Psychoanalytic Technique for the Treatment of Eating Disorder." In Johnson, Craig, ed., *Psychodynamic Treatment of Anorexia Nervosa*. New York: Guilford, 1991, pp. 86–105.

_____, Carl A. Whitaker, Nancy J. Hagemann, Richard B. Anderson, and Gerald J. Bargman. "Anorexia Nervosa: The Hospital's Role in Family Treatment." *Family Process*, December 1981, *20*(4): 395–408.

Stierlin, Helm, and Gunthard Weber. *Unlocking the Family Door: A Systemic Approach to the Understanding and Treatment of Anorexia Nervosa*. New York: Brunner/Mazel, 1989. 244pp.

Sugarman, Alan. "Bulimia: A Displacement from Psychological Self to Body Self." In Johnson, Craig, ed., *Psychodynamic Treatment of Anorexia Nervosa and Bulimia*. New York: Guilford, 1991, pp. 3–33.

_____, Donald Quinlan, and Luanna Devenis. "Anorexia Nervosa as a Defense against Anaclitic Depression." *The International Journal of Eating Disorders*, Autumn 1981, *1*(1): 44–61.

Swift, William James. "Bruch Revisited: The Role of Interpretation of Transference and Resistance in the Psychotherapy of Eating Disorders." In Johnson, Craig, ed., *Psychodynamic Treatment of Anorexia Nervosa and Bulimia*. New York: Guilford, 1991, pp.51–67.

Tamburrino, M.B., and R.A. McGinnis. "Anorexia Nervosa. A Review." *Panminerva Medica*, December 2002, *44*(4): 301–311.

Thomä, Helmut. *Anorexia Nervosa*. Trans. Gillian Brydone. New York: International Universities Press, 1967. 342pp.

Tiller, J., U. Schmidt, and J. Treasure. "Compulsory Treatment for Anorexia Nervosa: Compassion or Coercion?" *British Journal of Psychiatry*, 1993, *162*: 679–680.

Torem, Moshe. "The Use of Hypnosis with Eating Disorders." *Psychiatric Medicine*, 1992, *10*(4): 105–118.

Touyz, Stephen W., and Pierre J.V. Beaumont. "Behavioral Treatment to Promote Weight Gain." In Garner, David M., and Paul Garfinkel, eds., *Handbook of Treatment of Eating Disorders*. 2d ed. New York: Guilford, 1997, pp. 361–371.

Treasure, Janet, Ulrike Schmidt, and Eric van Furth, eds. *Handbook of Eating Disorders*. 2d ed. Chichester, West Sussex, England: John Wiley, 2003. 479 pp.

Tribole, Evelyn, and Elyse Resch. *Intuitive Eating: A Revolutionary Program That Works*. New York: St. Martin's Griffin, 2003. 284pp.

Tyre, Peg, Karen Springen, Ellise Pierce, Joan Raymond, and Dirk Johnson. "No One to Blame." *Newsweek*, December 5, 2005, *146*(23): 50–59.

University of South Carolina. http://www.state.sc.us/dmh/anorexia/statistics.htm. September 2008.

Vanderlinden, J., H. Buis, G. Pieters, and M. Probst. "Which Elements in the Treatment of Eating Disorders are the Necessary 'Ingredients' in the Recovery Process? A Comparison between the Patient and the Therapist's View." *European Eating Disorder Review*, September 2007, *15*(5): 357–65.

Wall, A. David, and Edward J. Cumella. "Anxiety and Eating Disorders: An Introduction." *The Remuda Review: The Christian Journal of Eating Disorders*, Fall 2005, *4*(4): 38–43.

Waller, Glenn, and Helen Kennerly. "Cognitive-Behavioural Treatments." In Treasure, Janet, et al., eds., *Handbook of Eating Disorders*. 2d ed. Chichester, West Sussex, England: John Wiley, 2003, pp.233–251.

Walsh, B.J. "Hypnotic Alteration of Body Image on the Eating Disordered." *American Journal of Clinical Hypnosis*, April 2008, *50*(4): 301–310.

Wang, Tzong-Shi, Yuan-Hwa Chou, and I-Shin Shiah. "Combined Treatment of Olanzapine and Mirtazapin in Anorexia Nervosa Associated with Major Depression." *Progress in Neuro-Psychopharmacology and Biological Psychiatry*. March 2006, *30*(2): 306–309.

Werne, Joellen, ed. *Treating Eating Disorders*. San Francisco, California: Jossey-Bass, 1996. 377 pp.

Wilson, G.T., S. Touyz, S.M. Dunn, and P. Beaumont. "The Eating Behavior Rating Scale (EBRS): A Measure of Eating Pathology in Anorexia Nervosa." *International Journal of Eating Disorders*, September 1989, *8*(5): 583–592.

Winnicott, David. *Playing and Reality*. London: Tavistock, 1971. 156pp.

Woodall, Camay, and Arnold E. Andersen. "The Use of Metaphor and Poetry Therapy in the Treatment of the Reticent Subgroup of Anorectic Patients." In Hornyak, Lynne, and Ellen Baker, eds., *Experiential Therapies for Eating Disorders*. New York: Guilford, 1989, pp.191–206.

Woodman, Marion. *Addiction to Perfection: The Still Unravished Bride*. Toronto, Canada: Inner City, 1982. 204pp.

_____. *The Owl Was a Baker's Daughter: Obesity, Anorexia Nervosa, and the Repressed Feminine*. Toronto, Canada: Inner City, 1980. 134pp.

Yager, Joel. "Management of Patients with Chronic, Intractable Eating Disorders." In Yager, Joel, and Pauline Powers, eds., *Clinical Manual of Eating Disorders*. Washington, D.C.: American Psychiatric Publishing, 2007, pp.407–439.

_____, and _____, eds. *Clinical Manual of Eating Disorders*. Washington, D.C.: American Psychiatric Publishing, 2007. 462pp.

Yapko, M. "Hypnotic and Strategic Interventions in the Treatment of Anorexia Nervosa." *American Journal of Clinical Hypnosis*, April 1986, *28*(4): 224–232.

Zandian, M., I. Ioakimidis, C. Bergh, and P. Sodersten. "Cause and Treatment of Anorexia Nervosa." *Physiological Behavior*, September 10, 2007, *92*(1–2): 283–290.

Zerbe, Kathryn. *Integrated Treatment of Eating Disorders: Beyond the Body Betrayed*. New York: W.W. Norton, 2008. 370pp.

_____. "Psychodynamic Management of Eating Disorders." In Yager, Joel, and Pauline Powers, eds., *Clinical Manual of Eating Disorders*. Washington, D.C.: American Psychiatric Publishing, 2007, pp.307–334.

Internet References

Alcoholics Anonymous and the Twelve Steps
http://www.aa.org/en_pdfs/smf-121_en.pdf
Serenity Prayer: http://www.aa.org/lang/en/sub
  page.cfm?page=287

Bodywork Certifications
http://www.feldenkrais.com/classes/become_a_prac
  titioner
http://www.ncbtmb.org
http://www.rolf.org/become/training.htm
http://www.rosenmethod.org/#bodywork
http://www.thealexandertechnique.net/advice
http://www.traumahealing.com
www.naturalhealers.com/qa/massage.html#NCE%2
  0Examination

Controversy About Eating Disorder Websites
BBC News/Health/Pro-Anorexia Site Clampdown
  Urged. February 24, 2008. http://news.bbc.co.uk/
  go/pr/fr/-/2/hi/health/7259143.stm

Bremner, Charles and Marie Tourres. "French
  Anorexia Law Targets Websites." *The Australian*,
  April 10, 2008. *http://www.theaustralian.news.*
  com.au/story/0,25197,235159-2703,00.html
Head, Jacqueline, "Seeking "thinspiration," BBC
  News/UK/Magazine. August 8, 2007. http://news
  vote.bbc.co.uk/mpapps/pagetools/print/news.
  bbc.co.uk/2hi/uk_news/magazine/6935768.stm
Reaves, Jessica. "Anorexia Goes High Tech." *Times.*
  com, July 31, 2001. http://www.time.com/health/
  article/0,8599,169660,00.html

Nutritionists
http://www.eatright.org/cps/rde/xchg/ada/hs.xsl/
  index.html http://www.eatright.org/cps/rde/x
  chg/ada/hs.xsl/CADE_748_ENU_HTML.html

Statistics on Prevalence of Eating Disorders
http://www.state.sc.us/dmh/anorexia/statistics.htm

Index